The Toxicity of Environmental Pollutants

Edited by Daniel Junqueira Dorta and Danielle Palma de Oliveira

Published in London, United Kingdom

The Toxicity of Environmental Pollutants
http://dx.doi.org/10.5772/intechopen.98127
Edited by Daniel Junqueira Dorta and Danielle Palma de Oliveira

Contributors
Benjamin Ampomah Asiedu, Ahmed Nasri, Mohamed Allouche, Amel Hannachi, Abdelwaheb Aydi, Patricia Aïssa, Hamouda Beyrem, Ezzeddine Mahmoudi, Bamba Massa Ismaë, Sorho Siaka, Saganuwan Alhaji Saganuwan, Çiğdem Sevim, Mehtap Kara, Selma Yazar, Peter Ostoich, Michaela Beltcheva, Roumiana Metcheva, Jose Antonio Heredia Rojas, Luciana Maria Saran, Ane Gabriele Vaz Souza, Tainá Carolini Maria, Lucia Maria Carareto Alves, Deepak S. Khobragade, Raymundo Erazo, Benito Buendía Quispe, Mahipal S. Sankhla, Pritam P. Pandit, Anubhav Singh, Anuj Sharma, Varad Nagar, Rushikesh L. Chopde, Kumud K. Awasthi, Garima Awasthi, Vinay Aseri, Rohit K. Verma, Sumit K. Choudhary, Daniel Junqueira Dorta, Raul Ghiraldelli Miranda, Carolina Ferreira Sampaio, Fernanda Gomes Leite, Flavia Duarte Maia

First published in London, United Kingdom, 2022 by IntechOpen
IntechOpen is the global imprint of INTECHOPEN LIMITED, registered in England and Wales, registration number: 11086078, 5 Princes Gate Court, London, SW7 2QJ, United Kingdom

British Library Cataloguing-in-Publication Data
A catalogue record for this book is available from the British Library

Additional hard and PDF copies can be obtained from orders@intechopen.com

The Toxicity of Environmental Pollutants
Edited by Daniel Junqueira Dorta and Danielle Palma de Oliveira
p. cm.
Print ISBN 978-1-80355-579-9
Online ISBN 978-1-80355-580-5
eBook (PDF) ISBN 978-1-80355-581-2

For EU product safety concerns:
IN TECH d.o.o., Prolaz Marije Krucifikse Kozulić 3, 51000 Rijeka, Croatia,
info@intechopen.com or visit our website at intechopen.com.

Meet the editors

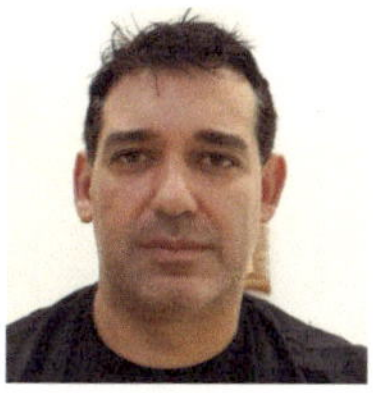

Daniel Dorta is a professor of toxicology and clinical chemistry at the University of São Paulo, Brazil. Dr. Dorta graduated in pharmacy and biochemistry, specializing in clinical pharmacology. He has a Ph.D. in toxicology, a Master's in pharmaceutical sciences, and a post-doctorate in pharmacology. He is a past president of the Brazilian Society of Toxicology and the Brazilian Society of Forensic Sciences. He was also a director of the Executive Committee of the International Union of Toxicology. He has written more than 50 articles and 17 book chapters. He is co-editor and author of *Forensic Toxicology* (in Portuguese) and *Toxicity Assessment – Methods and Protocols*. He has experience in the toxicological evaluation of ingredients applied to the pharmaceutical industry and in PDE/ADE determinations.

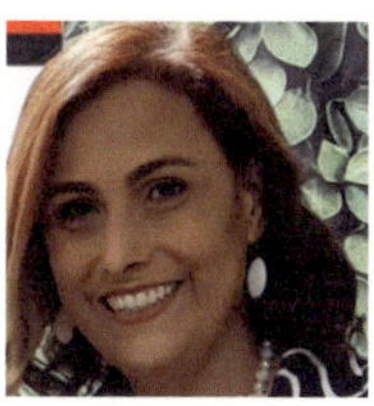

Danielle Palma de Oliveira graduated in pharmacy and biochemistry from the School of Pharmacy and Dentistry of Alfenas. She has a Master's and Ph.D. in toxicology and toxicological analysis. She is currently an associate professor at the Faculty of Pharmaceutical Sciences of Ribeirão Preto. She is a past president of the Brazilian Society of Toxicology and coordinator of the Environmental Toxicology Laboratory. She is the author of more than 60 articles and 15 book chapters. She is one of the editors and authors of *Toxicity Assessment – Methods and Protocols*. She has 20 years of experience in the field of toxicology, in the toxicological evaluation of ingredients applied to the pharmaceutical industry, and in PDE/ADE determinations according to ICH guidelines.

Contents

Preface

Until a few years ago, the major concern of environmental toxicology was compounds known to be toxic in the environment at high concentrations. Control and inspection by regulatory agencies around the world, in addition to concerted action between different countries, have reduced the release of various toxic substances. However, new or recurring problems have arisen, and much of this is due to technological advances of recent decades in various areas such as agriculture, medicine and the electronics industry.

While these advances have undeniably provided an improvement in people's quality of life, they are also responsible for the emergence of new problems that affect the environment and compromise the health of current and future generations. Our modern lifestyle is based on the production and widespread consumption of chemical compounds in the most diverse areas, and although there are already movements that recognize the need for sustainable development and "green" production practices, these are still insignificant in the face of the size and seriousness of the problem.

Thus, the current reality is the presence of a wide variety of chemical compounds found in different parts of the environment, such as soil, water, air and sediment, affecting not only human health but also several other non-target organisms for these compounds.

The Toxicity of Environmental Pollutants consists of 13 chapters that address topics ranging from the toxicity of environmentally relevant compounds such as organo-compounds, metals and radioisotopes, discuss the consequences of the interaction of these environmental contaminants with organisms, such as endocrine disruption, and introduce methodologies for assessing environmental contamination as well as forms of remediation.

We hope that the book has managed to achieve its initial objective of consolidating information that can be used to improve care for the environment and resolve the consequences of environmental contamination for the different organisms that inhabit the planet.

Daniel Junqueira Dorta
Faculty of Philosophy,
Sciences and Letters at Ribeirão Preto,
University of São Paulo (USP),
Ribeirão Preto, Brazil

Danielle Palma de Oliveira
School of Pharmaceutical Sciences of Ribeirão Preto,
University of São Paulo (USP),
Ribeirão Preto, Brazil

Section 1

Organocompounds

Chapter 1

Flame Retardants: New and Old Environmental Contaminants

Raul Ghiraldelli Miranda, Carolina Ferreira Sampaio, Fernanda Gomes Leite, Flavia Duarte Maia and Daniel Junqueira Dorta

Abstract

Flame retardants are a group of compounds used in a variety of consumer goods to inhibit or retard the spread of flames. Several classes of chemical compounds have such capabilities, however, the persistence of these compounds in the environment and their toxicity are crucial points for a risk assessment. Classes such as polybrominated diphenyl ethers (PBDEs) have already been banned in some parts of the world while they are still permitted and extensively used in other parts of the globe. In the need for substitutes for the toxic compounds used, new structures have been synthesized and suggested by the industry as an alternative and substitutives flame retardants. The objective of this review is to address the classes of compounds used as flame retardants in terms of their toxicity to human or non-human organisms and their persistence in the environment.

Keywords: brominated flame retardant, phosphorus-based flame retardants, ecotoxicity

1. Introduction

Materials with high carbon and hydrogen content are easily combustible, so most materials used nowadays, including plastics, are flammable. Over the last century, the furniture, electronics, upholstery, and textile industries have increasingly employed synthetic materials, which are also used in the transport sector (cars, airplanes, and trains) and at home. Using safety devices against fire, like flame retardants, is important to prevent these materials from burning and harming the society and the environment [1, 2].

But what are flame retardants? Flame retardants (FRs) are chemical compounds employed as safety devices to prevent fires from starting/spreading or to delay ignition, thereby reducing combustible material flammability, increasing escape time, and providing safety to humans and properties [3, 4]. The term "flame retardants" refers to the chemical compound action and not to the compound itself [5]. Various chemical compounds with different physicochemical properties and molecular structures can act as FRs. They can be added to (additive FRs) or incorporated into (reactive FRs) combustible materials, such as wood, plastics, kitchen utensils, appliances, computers, electrical cables, construction materials, textiles, and upholstery [6].

The global FR market is expected to reach about US$53 billion by 2024. In 2019, the world FR consumption amounted to over 2.4 million tons, corresponding to 4.9% growth in market size [1, 7, 8]. China is the largest FR consumer—it accounts for 26% of the global consumption, followed by Western Europe (23%), North America (22%), Asia (18%), and Japan (6%). Together, Central/Eastern Europe, Central/South America, and Middle East/Africa add up to 5% of the world's consumption. Over 175 chemicals are listed as FRs. They are classified on the basis of their chemical composition, but a single compound, aluminum trihydroxide ($Al(OH)_3$), tops the list as the most consumed FR in the world, corresponding to 38% of all the FRs consumed worldwide. Halogenated flame retardants (HFRs) come next (21%, being 17% brominated FRs and 4% chlorinated FRs), followed by organophosphorus (18%). Other classes like metal-based FRs amount to 14% of the global consumption, followed by FRs based on antimony oxides (9%) [7, 8]. **Figure 1** summarizes the consumption of flame retardants.

Despite the recent increase in FR use, the first reports on their application date back to 450 BC., when Egyptians employed aluminum to reduce wood flammability. Reports dating back to 200 BC. describe that the Roman civilization used aluminum with vinegar to decrease wood flammability [9]. In modern times, specifically in 1929, polychlorinated biphenyls (PCBs), the first class of FRs, were introduced in the United States of America to meet the need of the electrical industry for an insulator that could act as FR. Later, Europe and Japan also started to produce PCBs. After 37 years, PCB presence in the environment was reported for the first time: a Swedish biologist detected PCBs in fish. Two years later (1968) in Japan, about 1000 Japanese were intoxicated with rising oil contaminated with PCBs. PCBs were widely applied until the 1970s. Then, they were banned in Japan in 1972, and North America stopped producing them in 1976 [1, 10]. However, PCB presence in the environment is still relevant because they are Persistent Organic Pollutants (POPs) with the ability to bioaccumulate and biomagnify, consequently presenting high toxic potential [9, 11].

After PCBs were banned, brominated flame retardants (BFRs) emerged as an economically viable alternative to replace them. Although BFRs and PCBs differ because they belong to distinct chemical classes, the BRF mechanism of action resembles the PCB mechanism of action. In the gas phase, brominated and chlorinated FRs inhibit the combustion process of root chain reaction. HFRs neutralize the high-

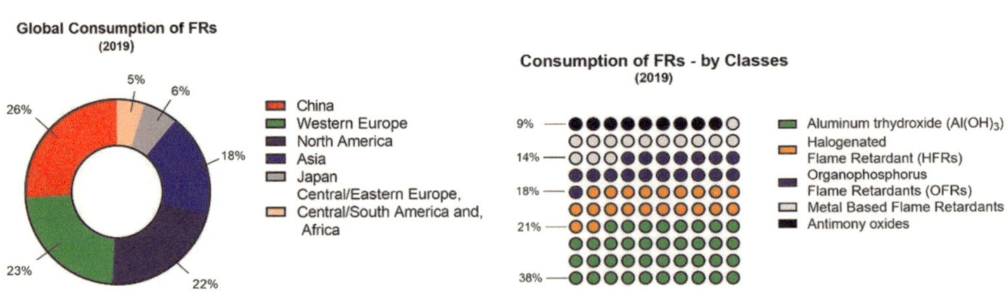

Figure 1.
Global consumption of flame retardants and their consumption by classes. (Designed using GraphPad prism 8.0.2. Adapted form FlameRetardant-online [7]).

energy $OH^{\cdot}$ and $H^{\cdot}$ radicals originating from a chain reaction in fire [12, 13]. However, concerns about HFR toxicity have been raised because they may leach into the environment, with high HFR concentrations being recorded in fish and marine mammals. Concerns about BFR toxic and ecotoxic effects, mainly their carcinogenic and endocrine-disrupting actions in humans, have pressed authorities to legislate about or even ban some BFRs. For example, commercial mixtures of polybrominated diphenyl ethers (PBDEs) and hexabromocyclododecane (HBCD) have been banned or phased out in North America and the European Union (E.U.) [14]. With the new legislation regarding BFRs, the global market has sought economically viable and environmentally friendly alternatives that act similarly to banned FRs. In this context, phosphorus flame retardants (PFRs) have emerged as suitable alternatives for BFRs although they have already been employed for over 150 years [4, 6].

Concerns about FRs being present in the environment grow every day. FRs may easily spread to environmental compartments (air, water, soil, sediments, and even house dust) through dissolution, volatilization, and attrition [4]. Improperly disposed electronic waste and furniture contribute to FR presence in the environment. Weak chemical interaction between manufactured products and FRs applied to them aggravates FR dispersion in the environment, not to mention that numerous compounds employed as FRs have serious effects on human health and the environment. Therefore, ensuring conscious use of these chemicals is crucial [14–16].

2. Brominated flame retardants

Despite laws discouraging or even banning BRF use, their global production continues to grow because new BFRs are being introduced to replace the banned or phased-out ones. About 75 different BFRs are marketed today, and most of them are found in the environment [12, 14]. The main classes of BFRs are polybrominated biphenyls (PBBs), tetrabromobisphenol A (TBBPA), HBCD, and PBDEs. PBDEs and HBCD are the most employed BFRs worldwide [12, 17]. **Table 1** shows the BFR chemical structures and physicochemical properties.

After some poisoning episodes and toxicity evidence involving BFRs, some countries started regulating their use in the same way they regulate the use of PBBs and the commercial PBDE mixture. In the early 1970s, accidental poisoning with PBBs occurred on Michigan Farms—animal feed contamination during production resulted in about 5 million eggs and 15.5 tons of milk products being contaminated and 1.5 million chicken, 30,000 cattle, 6000 hogs, and 1500 sheep dying. After this episode, PBBs were removed from the U.S. market, and this class was banned in the U.S. in 1973 [14, 17]. In the late 1980s, the development of analytical methods helped scientists to begin gathering data about FRs in Europe, North America, and Japan, and environmental and human health concerns started to increase when PBDE presence was reported in human milk [18] and marine animals [19] and rising PBDE levels were identified in environmental compartments including sediments, sewage sludge, the aquatic environment, and biological samples (fish, aquatic birds, and human tissues) [20].

Given the toxicological concern and the fact that POPs represent (some BFRs are included as POP) a growing threat to human health and the environment, in 1995, the council of the United Nations Environment Program (UNEP) requested an international process for evaluating an initial list of 12 POPs, and UNEP asked the Intergovernmental Forum on Chemical Safety (IFSC) to recommend international action on

Common name	Abbreviation	Structural formula	Molecular formula	Molecular weight	Log K_{ow}	Vapor pressure (kPa, 25°C)
Polybrominated biphenyls	PBBs	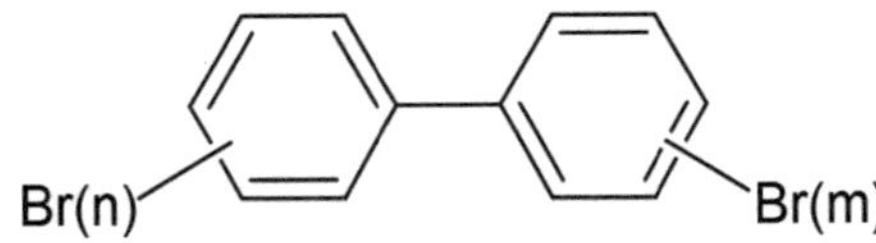	$C_{12}H_{10\text{-}x}Br_x$, where x = 1, 2, …, 10 = $m + n$	234.9–943.0	5.53–9.1	5.2×10^{-8}
Tetrabromobisphenol A	TBBPA	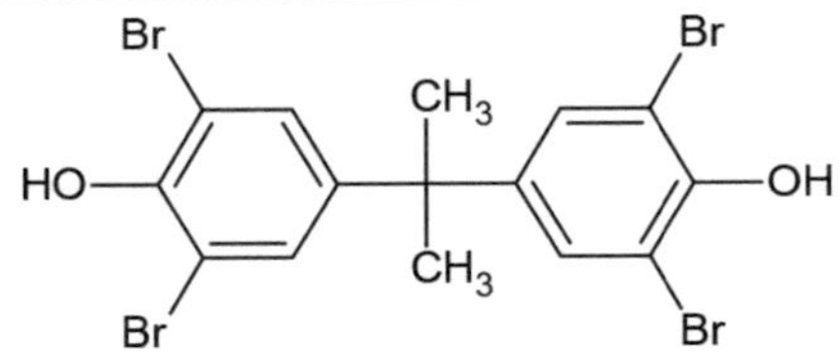	$C_{15}H_{12}Br_4O_2$	543.9	4.75	1.9×10^{-8}
Hexabromocyclododecane	HBCD	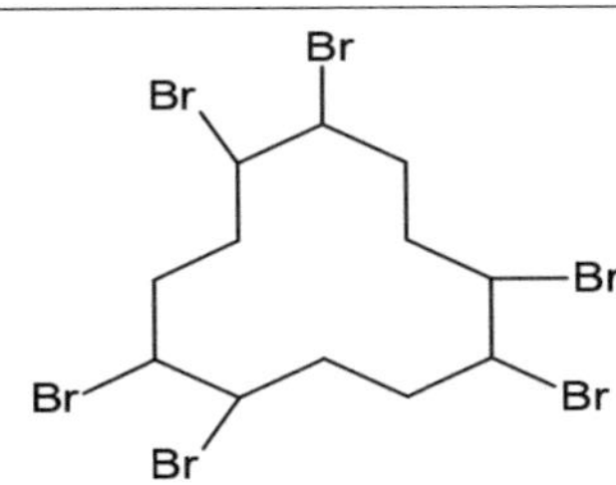	$C_{10}H_{14}Br_6$	613.6	6.6	10^{-10}
Polybrominated diphenyl ethers	PBDEs	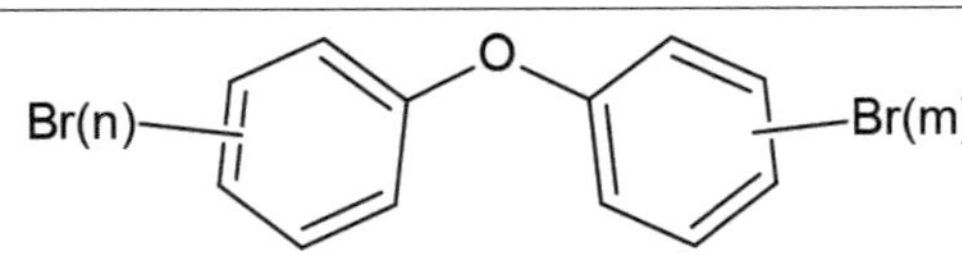	$C_{12}H_{10\text{-}x}Br_xO$, where x = 1, 2, …, 10 = $m + n$	248.9–959.0	6.26–6.97	2.2×10^{-7} – 3.47×10^{-8}

Source: Pubchem. Chemical structures were designed by the authors by using the software ACD/ChemSketch®.

Table 1.
Chemical structure of the main classes BFRs and their physicochemical properties [12, 17].

these pollutants. Thereafter, a negotiation process began; the Stockholm Convention on Persistent Organic Pollutants was created and adopted in 2001; and the Convention came into force three years later when 50 countries ratified it. Annex A lists PBDEs, PBBs, and HBCD as POPs to be eliminated [11]. In 2002, the European Union (E.U.) banned PBDEs and HBCD production, followed by the development of framework and directives such as the creation of the Registration, Evaluation, Authorization, and Restriction of Chemicals (REACH), the Restriction of Hazardous Substances, and the Waste Electrical and Electronic Equipment directives [14]. Other initiatives that aimed to reduce and eliminate the two main commercial PBDE mixtures (Penta- and Octa-diphenyl ether – Penta/OctaBDE) were also undertaken in North America (the U.S. and Canada). In 2004, several U.S. states prohibited the use of these two PBDE mixtures in some products. Canada also supported the virtual DecaBDE voluntary elimination by 2013. In 2017, the U.S. Consumer Product Safety Commission (CPSC) petitioned to restrict HFR use as additives and nonpolymeric constituents in electronics, furniture, and children's products [9, 14]. China added DecaBDE and HBCD to the priority list of substances, which implied restricted production or limited discharges. Taiwan and Japan follow similar examples: they have restrictions on PBDEs and HBCD. On the other hand, although Brazil and India are signatories of the Stockholm Convention on Persistent Organic Pollutants, no comprehensive legislation for FRs exists in these countries [14]. **Figure 2** shows a schematic timeline of the regulation of halogenated flame retardants.

BFRs are divided into three subgroups—additive, reactive, and polymeric—depending on how they are incorporated into manufactured materials. The incorporation mode directly influences BRF presence in the environment. Additive BFRs, such as PBDEs and HBCD, are just mixed at the time of manufacture, so they interact weakly with materials and easily leak into the environment. In contrast, reactive and polymeric BFRs establish a chemical interaction with materials, giving rise to a more stable interaction that results in less BRF bioavailability. Nevertheless, these BFRs

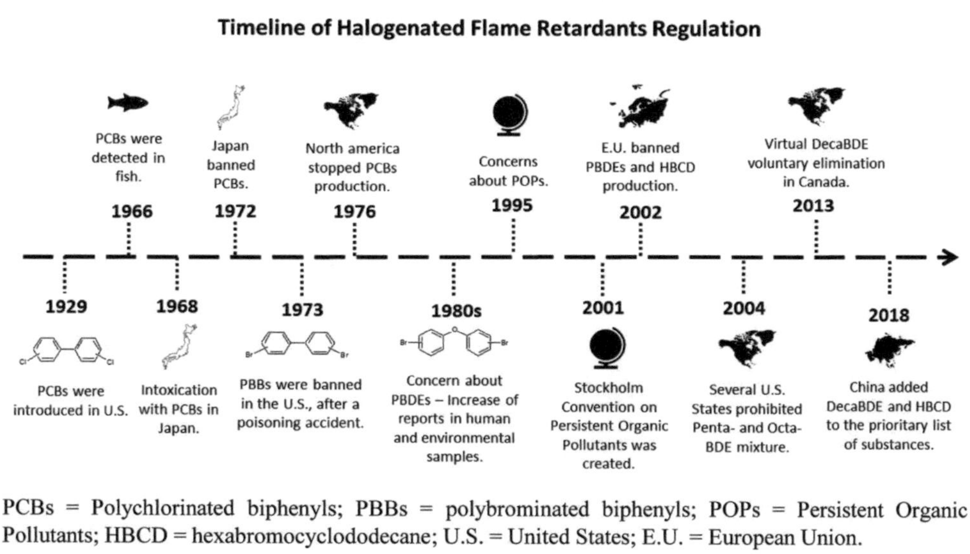

Figure 2.
Schematic timeline of regulation of halogenated flame retardant (HFRs). PCBs = polychlorinated biphenyls; PBBs = polybrominated biphenyls; POPs = persistent organic pollutants; HBCD = hexabromocyclododecane; U.S. = United States; E.U. = European Union.

should not be neglected because they may be lost to the environment during production or transport [21].

BFRs are ubiquitous in the environment. During the last decades, they have been detected in environmental samples even in places located far away from where they are produced or used (e.g., in the Artic) [22–24]. Once BFRs are released, they tend to persist, bioaccumulate, and biomagnify, and their physicochemical properties, mainly lipophilicity, may underlie potential toxic effects on the environment [24, 25].

2.1 Environmental occurrence and (eco)toxicological effects

2.1.1 Polybrominated diphenyl ethers (PBDEs)

PBDEs are sold as a mixture of congeners and have three commercial presentations: PentaBDE (pentabromodiphenyl ether), OctaBDE (octabromodiphenyl ether), and DecaBDE (decabromodiphenyl ether). The mixture name refers to the main congeners that compose it. Each PBDE congener varies in the number of bromine atoms and the arrangement of these substituted atoms in the aromatic ring. This gives 209 possible congeners, divided into ten groups: mono-, di-, tri-, tetra-, penta-, hexa-, hepta, octa-, nona-, and decabromo diphenyl ether. The number of isomers in these groups may be 3, 12, 24, 42, 46, 42, 24, 12, 3, and 1, respectively [26, 27]. Depending on the type of material, each mixture has a specific application. For example, DecaBDE is used in diverse polymeric materials, while Penta and OctaBDE are applied mainly in the textile and polyurethane foam industries [26].

PBDEs are released into the environment in different ways. First, they may be released during their industrial production. Second, materials containing PBDEs may release them. Third, goods with PBDEs in their composition may be inappropriately discharged. The latter situation is one of the main sources of environmental contamination with PBDEs. Other sources of exposure to PBDE congeners include use and recycling of products containing PBDEs, such as computers, household appliances in general, upholstery, and furniture [12, 27]. The PBDE physicochemical characteristics, including their high lipophilicity, hydrophobicity, low vapor pressure, and high affinity for particles, contribute to their presence in sediments in ambient compartments, particulate matter in the air, and foods. PBDEs are absorbed by inhalation of domestic and industrial dust, via the dermal route, and even by ingestion of contaminated food, which is aggravated by their ability to biomagnify in the food chain [17, 28].

Regarding the PBDE toxicological aspects, several studies have shown their high toxic potential. Their main effects include hepatotoxicity, neurotoxicity, immunological and endocrine alterations, and carcinogenicity. However, the mechanisms through which PBDEs exert their toxic action are not understood [17, 28]. PBDEs have been detected in human samples, especially blood and breast milk. The latter presentation is particularly alarming. Numerous studies involving human breast milk samples have reported different PBDE concentrations in all the analyzed samples, with the congeners BDE-47, -99, -100, and -153 being the most abundant and frequent [29–31].

PBDEs, mainly those with lower molecular weight, are structurally similar to thyroid hormones. Therefore, they may disrupt the endocrine system by interfering with hypothalamicpituitary-thyroid axis homeostasis [12, 32]. BDE-71 and -79 decrease thyroid hormone serum levels and induce liver enzyme biotransformation, as shown in studies carried out with mice and rats [33]. Moreover, many PBDE congeners damage mitochondria, increasing reactive oxygen species (ROS) production and oxidative stress, exerting genotoxicity, and inducing apoptotic cell death in isolated rat mitochondrial and hepatocarcinoma cells (HepG2) [34–36].

2.1.2 Hexabromocyclododecane (HBCD)

HBCD is a high-molecular-weight nonaromatic brominated cyclic alkane with six pairs of enantiomers. It is mainly used as an additive FR in thermoplastics for final application in styrene resins. Being an additive FR, HBCD is easily released into the environment. It has high lipophilicity (log K_{ow} = 5.6) and low solubility in water (0.0034 mg/l) [12, 37]. Due to these characteristics, HBCD is persistent, with a half-life of 3 days in the air and 2025 days in water. It bioaccumulates with a bioconcentration factor of approximately 18,100 in fathead minnows [38, 39]. Its commercial formulation consists of three isoforms: γ-HBCD (75–89%), α-HBCD (10–13%), and β-HBCD (1–12%) [37]. Enantiomers may behave differently in the environment; for example, γ-HBCD tends to be more toxic than α-HBCD, but α-HBCD is the enantiomer that occurs more often in environmental samples [40, 41].

HBCD has been measured in several environmental compartments, including air and dust, sediments, soil, and sewage sludge, and biological samples (aquatic organisms, marine mammals, birds, plants, and even human samples). In animals, HBCD tends to accumulate in lipid-rich organs, such as the liver, gonads, muscle, and adipose tissue [17, 37, 41].

HBCD presents high toxic potential. HBCD increases catalase transcription because this FR raises ROS concentration. Exposure to HBCD alters a protein involved in the mollusk immune system [42]. HBCD may lead to cellular apoptosis near the heart area, and zebrafish exposure to this compound induces cardiac hypertrophy and arrhythmia [43]. HBCD disrupts the endocrine system in Wistar rats and causes neuro- and hepatotoxicity in mice [44, 45]. HBCD induces cytotoxicity in human hepatocarcinoma cells (HepG2) and human neuroblastoma cells (SH-SY5Y), reducing cell viability. HBCD interferes with T4 metabolism in HepG2 cells and affects the estrogenic activity in breast cancer cells (MCF-7) [46–48], suggesting that it is hepatotoxic and neurotoxic and that it acts as an endocrine disruptor.

2.1.3 Tetrabromobisphenol A (TBBPA)

TBBPA is a reactive FR and one of the most prevalent FRs in the world. It is mainly applied in the epoxy resin used to produce printed circuit boards. It forms a covalent bond with the polymer structure, so it is less likely to be released into the environment. It is highly lipophilic (log K_{ow} = 4.75) and has low solubility in water (0.718 mg/l) [17, 37].

Although TBBPA release into the environment is more difficult, it may be released during production, processing, and final usage and disposal of the product it is incorporated into [49]. TBBPA is currently found in many kinds of abiotic and biotic matrixes, and it has been detected in air, water, soil, indoor dust sewage sludge, and sediments [37, 50, 51]. TBBPA may also accumulate in the food chain [52]. Indoor dust is the environmental matrix where TBBPA accumulates the most. This is a concern because human beings spend a considerable time indoors, which increases the risk of adverse effects [37].

Long exposure to TBBPA used to be considered harmless because it was believed to lie below levels that would produce a toxic effect [37, 53, 54]. However, several research studies have demonstrated that even low TBBPA doses disrupt the endocrine system, thyroid hormones, and neurobehavioral functions [37, 55]. Studies on animals have shown some toxic effects. Even at low doses, TBBPA induces toxicity in zebrafish, fathead minnow, and rainbow trout after exposure for 96 h (LC_{50} = 1.3 mg/l) [56]. In rodents, TBBPA induces nephrotoxicity, oxidative stress in the kidney, increased liver volume, hepatocyte necrosis, and endocrine disruption, but no neurological effects have been found in rats exposed to TBBA [37, 54].

The impacts of TBBPA on human health remain unclear. In vitro studies on human cells have suggested that TBBPA has the toxic potential [37, 55]. TBBPA increases caspase-3 activities and ROS generation; damages mitochondria; induces pathogenesis of several lung diseases in airway epithelial cells (A549) [57]; interferes with immune cell action [58]; induces liver cancer disorder promoting metastasis of liver cancer cells; promotes lysosome exocytosis; and decreases intracellular levels of hexosaminidase (HEXB), cathepsin B (CTSB), cathepsin D (CTSD), and lysosomal enzymes in HepG2 cells [59].

2.1.4 Novel brominated flame retardants (NBFRs)

The ban on some of the most widely used BFRs (PBDEs, HBCD, and TBBPA) has caused novel (or new) brominated flame retardants (NBFRs) to emerge. NBFR production and use have increased in the last decade [60]. Although NBFRs is applied as an alternative to replace traditional BFRs, they share a similar chemical structure with halogenic substitution in a cyclic hydrocarbon/aromatic hydrocarbon, so their physicochemical properties are generally analog. Some NBFRs are hydrophobic, semivolatile, relatively highly lipophilic, and little water-soluble [61, 62]. **Table 2** summarizes the NBFR chemical structure and physicochemical properties.

Information on NBFR toxicity and ecotoxicity is lacking, causing concern and increasing the number of studies about them. Like restricted and banned traditional BFRs, NBFRs are present in various environmental sources, including air, dust, sewage sludge, and sediments, and they also appear in biotic matrixes (human serum, fish, and birds) [62]. For example, BTBPE is usually measured in sediments associated with others BFRs, at a lower concentration than BDE-209, but higher concentrations than other PBDE congeners. Some studies have detected BTPE in household dust [60, 61, 63, 64].

Due to their physicochemical properties, NBFRs bioaccumulate and biomagnify. DBDPE has Bioaccumulation Factor (BAF) between 6.1 and 7.1 in three fish species (*Cirrhina molitorella*, *Tilapia nilotica*, and *Hypostomus Plecostomus*) from a Chinese river [65]. In southern China, the HBB trophic magnification in an aquatic food chain (invertebrates and fish) is about 2.1 [66], whereas PBT and PBEB biomagnify in waterbirds in the same region [67]. Metabolic rates in the organism influence NBFR bioaccumulation and biomagnification [62].

In vitro studies have reported that NBFRs are hepatotoxic. For instance, 0.1 and 0.2 μM DBDPE up-regulates CYP1A4/5 expression [68], modifying rainbow trout hepatocyte activity [69]. Additionally, it interferes in thyroid hormone deiodinase activity in human liver microsomes; its inhibitory concentration (IC_{50}) is 0.16 μM [70]. As for HBB, it activates the aryl hydrocarbon receptor (AhR), but to a lesser extent than 2,3,7,8-tetrachlorodibenzo-p-dioxin (TCDD). Furthermore, 100 μM HBB cannot activate the human androgen receptor (AR) in human hepatocarcinoma cells [71]. On the basis of the AMES test, PBEB and PBT have no mutagenic activity [72].

DOI: http://dx.doi.org/10.5772/intechopen.104886

Chemical name	Abbreviation	Structural formula	Molecular formula	Molecular weight	Log K_{ow}	Vapor pressure (kPa, 25°C)
1,2-bis-(2,3,4,5,6-pentabromophenyl) ethane	DBDPE	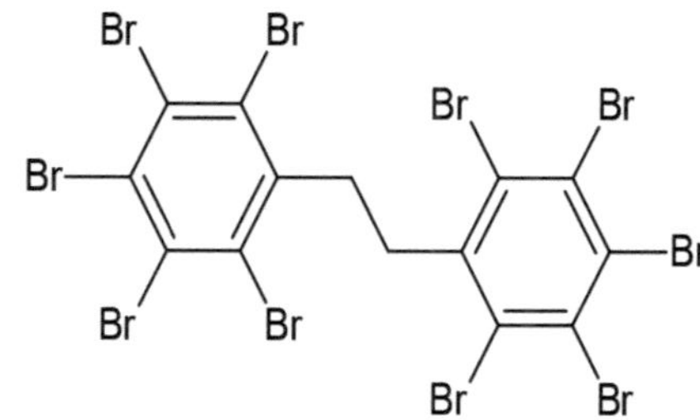	$C_{14}H_4Br_{10}$	971.22	13.64	1.90×10^{-13}
1,2-bis-(2,4,6 tribromophenoxy) ethane	BTBPE	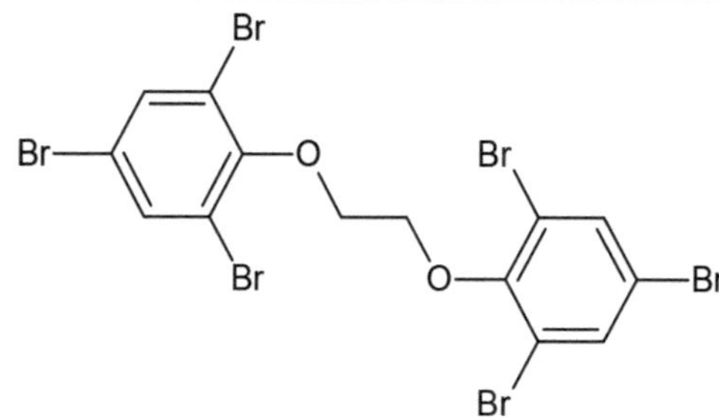	$C_{21}H_8Br_8O_2$	687.64	9.15	2.38×10^{-10}
tetrabromobisphenol A bis-(dibromopropyl ether)	TBBPA-DBPE	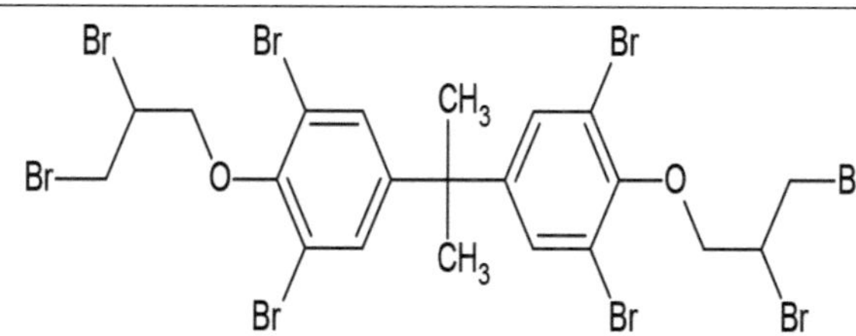	$C_{21}H_{20}Br_6O_2$	943.61	11.52	9.44×10^{-7}
2-ethylhexyl-2,3,4,5-tetrabromobenzoate	TBB	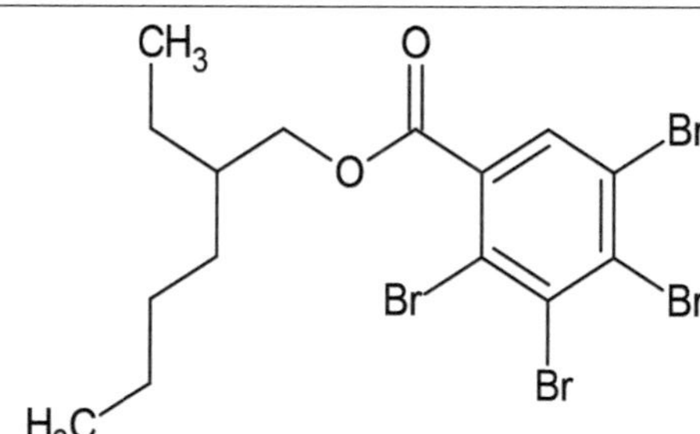	$C_{15}H_{18}Br_4O_2$	549.92	8.75	3.42×10^{-8}

Chemical name	Abbreviation	Structural formula	Molecular formula	Molecular weight	Log K_{ow}	Vapor pressure (kPa, 25°C)
bis-(2-ethylhexyl)-3,4,5,6-tetrabromo-phthalate	TBPH	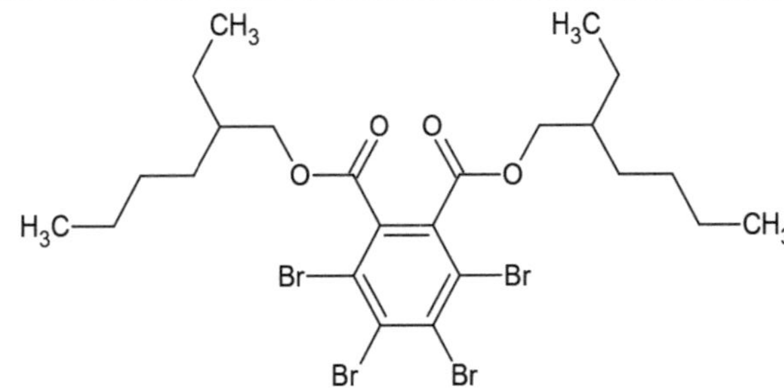	$C_{24}H_{32}Br_4O_4$	706.14	11.95	1.17×10^{-11}
2,3,4,5,6-pentabromotoluene	Penta-BT	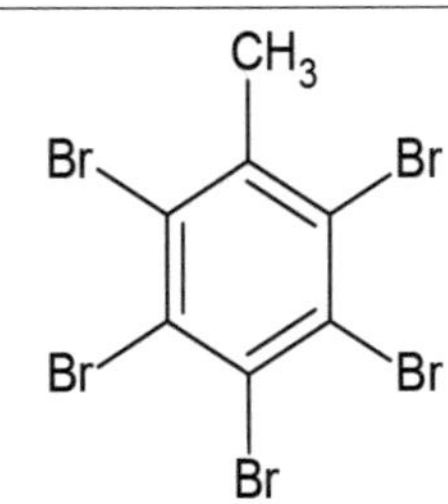	$C_7H_3Br_5$	486.62	6,99	1.46×10^{-7}
hexabromobenzene	HBB	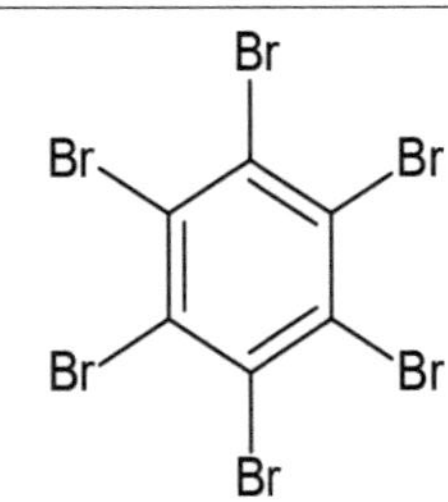	C_6Br_6	551.49	7,33	1.68×10^{-8}
2,3,4,5,6-pentabromoethylbenzene	PBEB	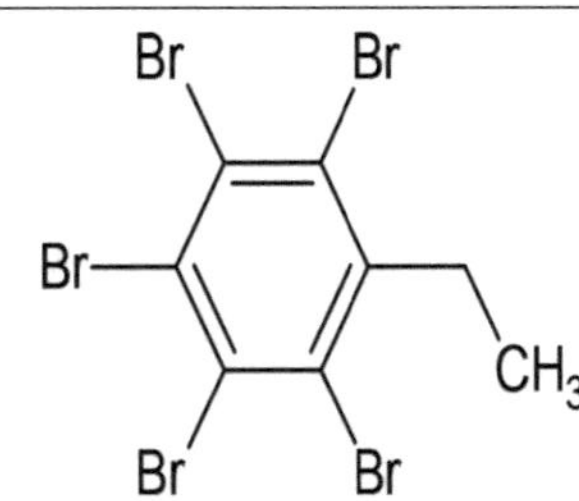	$C_8H_5Br_5$	500.65	7,48	6.65×10^{-6}

Chemical name	Abbreviation	Structural formula	Molecular formula	Molecular weight	Log K_{ow}	Vapor pressure (kPa, 25°C)
2,3-dibromopropyl-2,4,6-tribromophenyl ether	DPTE	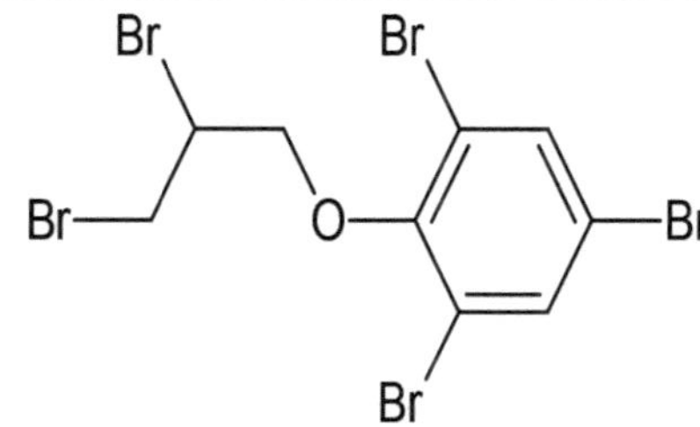	$C_9H_7Br_5O$	530.67	6,34	6.22×10^{-7}
2,4,6-tribromophenol	TBP	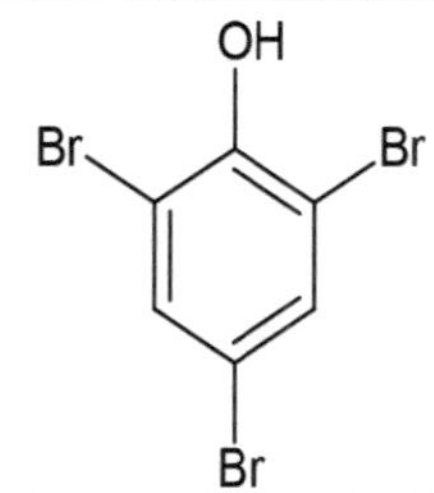	$C_6H_3Br_3O$	330.80	4,18	1.46×10^{-3}
1,2-dibromo-4-(1,2-dibromoethyl) cyclohexane	TBECH	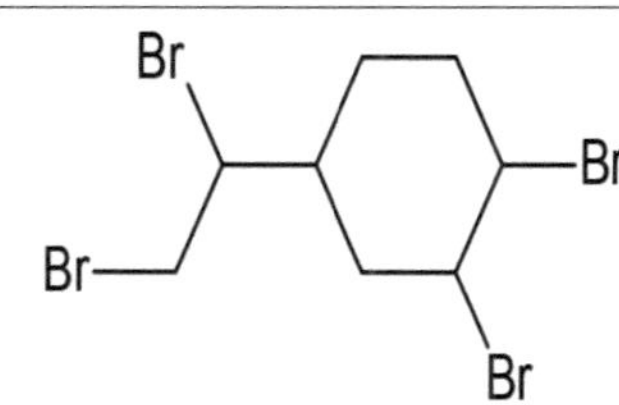	$C_8H_{12}Br_4$	427.82	5,24	1.05×10^{-4}

Adapted: [61]. Source: Pubchem—https://pubchem.ncbi.nlm.nih.gov/. Chemical structures were designed by the authors by using the software ACD/ChemSketch®.

Table 2.
Chemical structure and physicochemical properties of novel brominated flame retardants.

DBDPE does not show acute toxicity in rats or rabbits: the median lethal dose (LD_{50}) is greater than 5000 and 2000 mg/kg of bw, respectively [69]. However, subchronic and chronic exposure of mice and rats to DBDPE disrupt the endocrine system and alter thyroid hormone homeostasis, respectively [73, 74].

Ecotoxicological studies on aquatic organisms have shown acute DBDPE toxicity to water flea: 48 h EC_{50} is 19 μg/l. Besides that, zebrafish (*Danio rerio*) exposure to 12.5 and 25 μg/l DBDPE raises hatched larva mortality and reduces the zebrafish egg hatching rate [69]. Assessment of acute TBB and TBPH genotoxicity in fathead minnow revealed DNA damage in liver cells after oral exposure [75]. Exposure to TBB also increases zebrafish embryo mortality and malformation (LC_{50} = 7.0 mg/l). Zebrafish exposure to 20 mg/l TBPH (highest tested dose) has no adverse effects. **Table 3** summarizes the environmental occurrence and biological effects of the main classes of brominated flame retardants.

NBFRs used as an alternative to banned BFRs have frequently been detected in countless environmental compartments, with evidence of persistence under natural conditions—their physicochemical properties resemble the properties of banned BFRs. However, evidence of NBFR toxicity is lacking, and there is no legislation about them. Nevertheless, their in vitro and in vivo ecotoxicity to diverse organisms has been verified [22, 60, 62]. Therefore, finding new compounds that act as FRs and which are safer than older FRs like BFRs to human and environmental health is essential. Phosphorus-based flame retardants (PBFRs), which have already been used for over 150 years, could be suitable alternatives for BFRs [6].

3. Phosphorus-based flame retardants: organic compounds

Although several organophosphate FR categories exist, they are usually divided into three main groups, according to their chemical properties: organic, inorganic, and halogenated [6]. Organic organophosphates include phosphorus derivatives, such as phosphate esters, phosphonates, and phosphinate. Bisphenol-A diphenyl phosphate (BPA-DP), diethylphosphinic acid, diphenylcresylphosphate (DCP), melamine polyphosphate, resorcinol-bis-(diphenylphosphate) (RDP), tricresylphosphate (TCP), and triphenyl phosphate (TPhP) are examples of commonly employed organic organophosphates [6, 76].

Among organic organophosphates, Aluminum Diethylphosphinate (ALPi) is a new generation of halogen-free flame retardants. Despite having high performance in fire control, and gaining space in the manufacture of compounds, little is known about its long-term effects, both in the environmental scope and for human health [77].

Apart from being used as FRs, organic organophosphates have plasticizing and anti-foaming properties. Thus, they are present in various industrial and commercial products, such as eletronic equipment, paints, bedding, textiles, and building materials [78].

Smartphones deserve special attention because they represent a large portion of incorrectly discarded electronic waste, being an important contamination source. Zhang et al. [79] analyzed smartphone samples and found TPhP in all of them. This compound underlies environmental contamination.

Concern about the use of these compounds is related to the fact that they are used as additive FRs. Therefore, they are not chemically bound to the materials and products in which they are added, which facilitates their chronic release into the

	PBDEs	HBCD	TBBPA	NBFRs
Environmental occurrence	• Sediment; • Particulated matter air • Domestic and Industrial dust; • Food.	• Air and Dust; • Sediments, • Soil, • Sewage sludge • Biological Samples (aquatic organisms, marine mammals, birds, plants, and human samples).	• Air; • Water; • Soil; • Indoor dust; • Sewage sludge; • Sediments.	• Air; • Dust; • Sewage sludge; • Sediments; • Human serum; • Fish; • Birds.
Biological effects	• Hepatotoxicity; • Neurotoxicity; • Immunological alterations; • Endocrine Disruption; • Carcinogenicity.	• *In vivo:* o Increase oxidative stress (Raising ROS concentration ➔ Increase Catalase transcription); o Alters immune system of mollusk; o Cardiac toxicity in zebrafish; o Endocrine disruption in Wistar rats, o Neuro and hepaotoxicity in mice. • *In vitro:* o Neuro and hepatotoxicity in human cells lines (SH-SY5Y and HepG2 cells, respectively); o Affect estrogenic activity in breast cancer cells (MCF-7).	• Endocrine disruption; • Changes in neurobehavioral functions – even at low doses; • *In vivo:* o Induces toxicity in zebrafish, fathead minnow, and rainbow trout after 96 h of exposure; o Nephrotoxicity, hepatotoxicity, and endocrine disruption in rodents. • *In vitro:* o Increase apoptotic activity, oxidative stress, and mitochondria damage; o Induces pathogenesis of several lung diseases in airway epithelial cells (A549); o Interferes in immune cells action; o Induces carcinogenic effects in liver cells; o Alters intracellular levels of lysosomal enzymes.	• *In vitro:* o Hepatotoxicity o Up regulates CYP1A4/5 expression; o Interferes in thyroid hormone activity; o Activates the aryl hydrocarbon receptor (AhR) in HepG2 cell line; o Mutagenic activity in AMES test. • *In vivo:* o Hepatotoxicity in rainbow trout; o Endocrine disrupt in subchronic and chronic exposure in mice, and alter thyroid hormone homeostasis in rats; o Acute toxicity in zebrafish; o Hepatic genotoxicity in fathead minnow.
References	[17, 28]	[17, 37, 41, 44–48]	[37, 51, 55, 57, 59]	[62, 69, 71–75]

Table 3.
Summary of environmental occurrence and biological effect of brominated flame retardants classes.

environment [78]. Another issue is that their concentration in the product decreases over time, thereby reducing its FR properties [6].

To understand the chronic consequences related to the use, adverse effects on the environment, and toxicity of these FRs, their underlying mechanisms must be understood. Moreover, understanding the properties of these FRs and how they behave upon contact with living organisms and the ecosystem is crucial. Organic organophosphate FRs are considered emerging pollutants, and they have been widely studied in recent years.

3.1 Physicochemical characteristics

In general, organophosphates have different physicochemical characteristics. These organic compounds usually have reasonable solubility in water, but this varies according to molecular weight.

Organophosphates with low molecular weight are easily found in the aquatic environment, while compounds with high molecular weight are found in general nature. The octanol/water partition coefficient (log K_{ow}) of organophosphates ranges from −9.8 to 10.6, which means that they are more lipophilic than hydrophilic. However, they have better solubility in water than BFRs [6, 80].

Organophosphate distribution in the air and the environment varies. According to Henrys law, the vapor pressure also varies [6]. Variations in physicochemical characteristics are directly related to variations in biological effects. Thus, clarifying the mechanisms of these compounds is important [81].

BPA-DP is an organic additive FR with boiling point of 680°C and melting point ranging from 41 to 90°C, low solubility in water (∼ 0.4 mg/l), and log K_{ow} of 4.5. RDP is found in commercial blends with BPA-DP and is also an additive FR. It has a boiling point of 587°C, no melting point, and is even more insoluble in water (∼1.11×10^{-4} mg/l), with a log K_{ow} of 7.41. Both compounds are widely used together due to their advantageous characteristics, such as good thermal stability, high efficiency, and low volatility. They are primarily used as flat-screen protection for TVs and other electronics such as monitors and smartphones [6, 82].

Diethylphosphinic acid, on the other hand, has good solubility in water (4.52×10^4 mg/l), log K_{ow} of 0.68, melting point of −14°C, and lower boiling point (320°C). DCP also has a low boiling point (235°C), melting point of −38°C, but lower solubility in water (0.24 mg/l) and log K_{ow} of 4.51. Diethylphosphinic acid is an important compound because it is also a product of the thermal decomposition of aluminum diethyl phosphinate (AlPi), another FR that has been gaining visibility [6, 83].

Melamine polyphosphate is a nitrogen-containing FR. It is chemically linked to the polymer molecule, so it is not considered an additive FR [84]. This compound has the boiling point of 558°C, the melting point above 400°C, good solubility in water (around 1 g/l), and log K_{ow} of −2.3 [6].

TCP is an additive FR. It is an ester of cresols and phosphoric acid, with the boiling point of 439°C, melting point of 77°C, low solubility in water (∼0.36 mg/l), and log K_{ow} of 5.11. It is widely used in lubricants, hydraulic fluids, and engine oil. All its isomers (*ortho*-cresol, *para*-cresol, and *meta*-cresol) are active, but *o*-TCP has gained attention because it is related to cases of neuropathy induced by organophosphates [6, 85].

TPhP is one of the most commonly used additive organophosphates in the industry, and it is also the main contaminant in nature. Its boiling point is 370°C, its melting point is 49°C, it is sparingly soluble in water (∼1.9 mg/l), and its log K_{ow} is 4.59. Because TPhP has hydrophobic properties, it has a great affinity for sediments and soil, which is why it is frequently found in aquatic environments [6, 86]. Organophosphate distribution in air depends mainly on the values of the octanol-air coefficient (log K_{oa}). Compounds with log K_{oa} less than 10 are easily found in the gas phase, while higher values are necessary for compounds to be detected in the particulate form and associated with dust. Values for all the compounds are not yet clear. However, TPhP, for example, has a log K_{oa} of 10.5 and is easily found in many forms in the home environment [87, 88].

ALPi has excellent heat stability, producing less smoke during burning. The ALPi log K_{ow} is -0.44 and the water solubility is around 1 mg/l, suggesting low hydrophilic properties. Thus, soil and sediments can be the main target of the accumulation of this compound [89].

Organophosphates have relevant physicochemical characteristics for their applications. In general, they are interesting FRs because they decompose at a lower temperature than polymers used in the production of materials. Thus, heating compounds with phosphorus triggers phosphoric acid formation. This acid envelopes the material, protecting it from pyrolysis and preventing toxic gases from being formed [6, 90].

Table 4 summarizes the chemical structure and physicochemical properties of organic organophosphates.

3.2 Environmental occurrence and ecotoxicological effects

Although organic organophosphates have more interesting characteristics and offer more benefits than BFRs, they are often found in the environment (indoor dust, air, water, soil, and sediments) [91–93].

Because organophosphate particles are just additives and do not fully bind to the material they are incorporated into, they are easily dispersed. This causes them to be absorbed by suspended dust. Thus, indoor dust is an interesting indicator of indoor exposure to industrial chemicals [64].

Huang et al. [81] analyzed indoor dust from Australian homes, to find that TPhP is one of the most common compounds therein. This is expected if we consider the recurrent use of TPhP. The authors also found BPA-DP in abundance. In fact, this compound is used as a substitute for DecaBDE. The authors concluded that many organophosphates are present in the samples, presenting a high risk to human health [81].

Despite being mostly lipo-soluble, some organic organophosphates have good solubility in water. This has led to their detection in drinking water because treatment stations cannot eliminate these compounds effectively. Thus, the occurrence of organic organophosphates in the aquatic environment poses as much risk to human beings as to the aquatic ecosystem [94].

To identify the presence of organophosphates in water, Kim and Kannan [95] analyzed several samples, such as river water, rainwater, sea water, and tap water samples, collected from various locations in New York State. All the samples presented numerous organophosphates. Chlorinated compounds were identified as the most abundant due to their greater hydrophilicity. Among organic compounds, TPhP was found in over 90% of the river water samples.

On the other hand, compounds with greater lipophilicity are easily found in sediments and aquatic organisms, being the cause of bioaccumulation. In sediments, the composition is directly related to adsorption capacity. For example, clay-rich areas favor greater adsorption of these FRs [96].

Chemical name	Abbreviation	Structural formula	Molecular formula	Molecular weight	Log K_{ow}
Bisphenol A diphenyl phosphate	BPA-DP, BADP, BDP	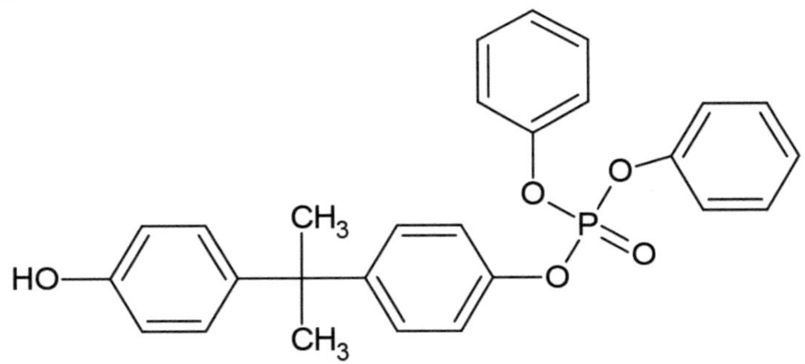	$C_{39}H_{34}O_8P_2$	692.6	4.5
Diethylphosphinic acid	—	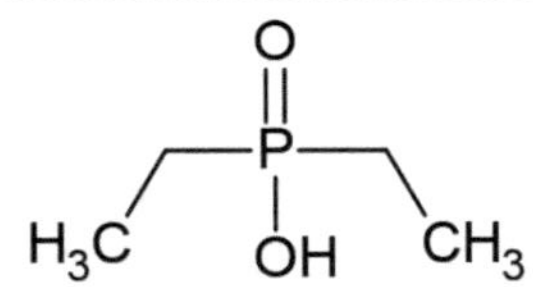	$C_4H_{11}O_2P$	122.10	0.68
Diphenylcresylphosphate	DCP, CDP, DPK	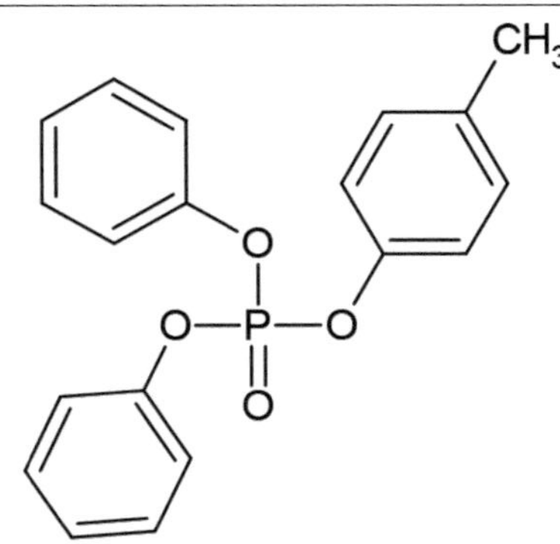	$C_{19}H_{17}O_4P$	340.31	4.51

DOI: http://dx.doi.org/10.5772/intechopen.104886

Chemical name	Abbreviation	Structural formula	Molecular formula	Molecular weight	Log K_{ow}
Melamine polyphosphate	—	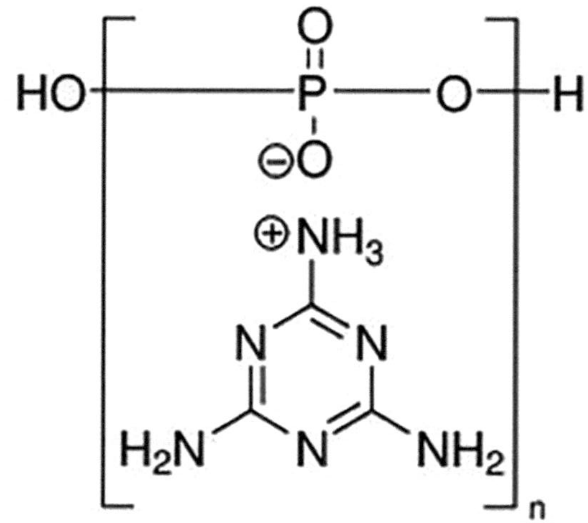	$C_3H_9N_6O_4P$	224.12	−2.3
Resorcinol-bis-(diphenyl) phosphate	RDP	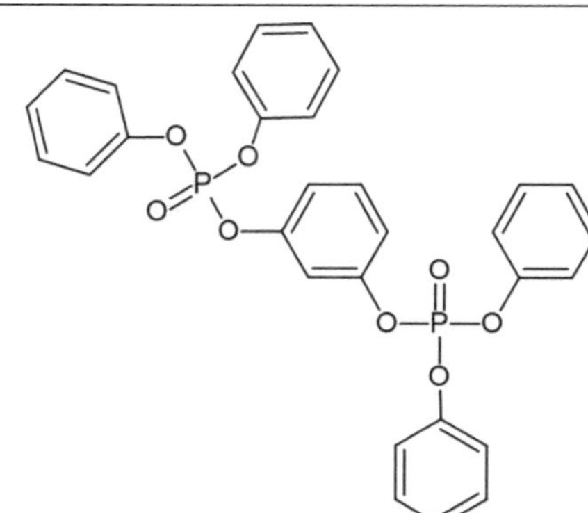	$C_{30}H_{24}O_8P_2$	574.5	7.41

Chemical name	Abbreviation	Structural formula	Molecular formula	Molecular weight	Log K_{ow}
Tricresyl phosphate	TCP	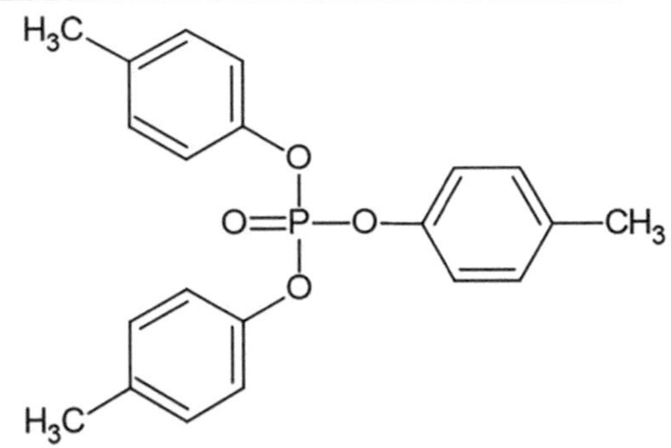	$C_{21}H_{21}O_4P$	368.4	5.11
Triphenyl phosphate	TPhP	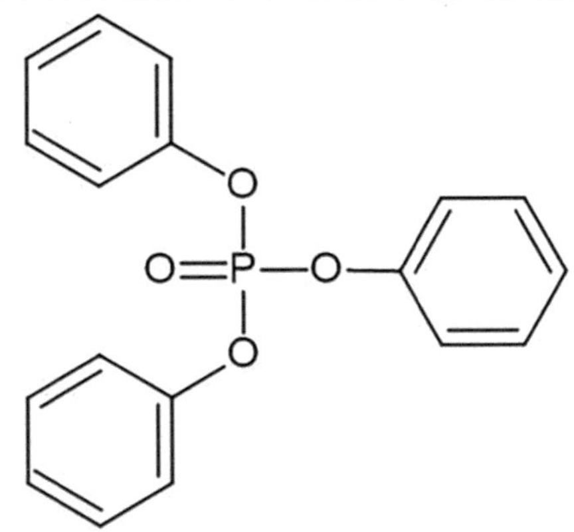	$C_{18}H_{15}O_4P$	326.3	4.59

Adapted: [6]. Source: Pubchem. Chemical structures were designed by the authors by using the software ACD/ChemSketch®.

Table 4.
Chemical structure and some physicochemical properties of novel organic organophosphate flame retardants.

Although organic compounds, such as TPhP, are found in sediments, halogenated compounds predominate. Lee et al. [97] and Chen et al. [98] analyzed the composition of water and sediments in lakes. In both studies, the halogenated ester tris-(chloroisopropyl) phosphate (TCPP) were found to predominate. Among non-halogenated compounds, tris-(2-butoxyethyl) phosphate (TBEP) was identified in most samples [97, 98].

Bioaccumulation and biomagnification affect biological characteristics negatively. In fish, for example, growth, sex, food, and maternal transfer are impacted, jeopardizing organism development and the ecosystem as a whole [99].

Organophosphate bioaccumulation has been studied since the 1970s. These compounds have been found in different tissues of rodents, fish, and birds, and they may accumulate in gills, kidneys, liver, and muscle tissue [100].

Wang et al. [101] evaluated the bioaccumulation and biomagnification potential of organophosphates in coral reef fish. These authors found several other types of organophosphates, including TCP. In addition to risking environmental health, this phenomenon may harm human health. Contamination of coral reef ecosystems is extremely relevant and further analysis will be needed in the future.

Indeed, water is an important factor in organophosphate distribution. Particles are dispersed in air through the mechanical friction of the materials. These particles may be included in rainwater and be the main cause of river water and soil contamination [102].

Recycling sites also impact soil contamination by organophosphates directly. In these sites, the soil is in direct contact with different types of materials, mainly electronic waste. Open-air storage of these residues determines local soil contamination and release of these compounds into the air [103].

According to Sánchez-Piñero et al. [104], several organic compounds, mainly BPA-DP and TPhP, are found in soil and dust in public places. Although these authors state that the values are within those authorized by legislation, investigating continuous exposure is necessary.

Thus, soil and water contamination are directly related to human health. Food and drinking water contamination and environmental contamination are directly related, as well.

As a reinforcement, the environmental effects caused by ALPi are still limited and not very specific, although the literature describes that bioaccumulation potential for free halogen compounds is low and that it is easily degraded in the environment [6].

3.3 Toxicokinetics

The prevalence of organic organophosphates in living organisms has become a research target. Toxicological research has suggested that chronic exposure may be directly related to damage to the endocrine system, with a high risk of reproduction being impaired. These compounds may also be related to systemic toxicity, affecting other important organs [101].

Unintentional dust ingestion and skin absorption are the routes with the highest organic organophosphate absorption rate. How these compounds are distributed in biological tissues has not been completely elucidated. However, the highest organophosphates levels have been found in the liver, muscle, and gonads [100].

Compounds are biotransformed through metabolization to diesters and hydroxylation by phase I reactions, followed by conjugation with glucuronide and sulfate in phase II reactions. These reactions happen both in humans and other living beings. Biotransformation products are important for monitoring and evaluating exposure to organophosphates: these products are eliminated fast because they are very hydrophilic [105].

Although organophosphate metabolism is relatively fast, even low concentrations of the metabolites may have physiological and endocrine effects. Considering that human exposure to these compounds is high and that multiple exposure pathways exist, the concern is enormous. For instance, children are generally less able to metabolize and to excrete xenobiotics, so these compounds are more toxic to them [106].

3.4 Toxicological effects

Among the potential adverse effects of organic organophosphates, reproductive and neurological effects are highlighted. Although the toxicity mechanisms of these compounds have not been fully elucidated, the consequences of being exposed to them involve cell apoptosis, ROS production, membrane disturbance, and mitochondrial alterations, among others [100].

Neurotoxic effects are concentration-dependent and inhibit DNA synthesis, decreasing the number of cells and altering neural differentiation. Acetylcholinesterase (AChE) inhibition is another reported mechanism. AChE is a widely used marker in neurotoxicity studies. Tris-(1,3-dichloro-2-propyl) phosphate (TDCPP) and TPhP have an affinity for the nervous system and are commonly associated with neurotrophic factor inhibition [107].

Aquatic organisms are often exposed to organophosphates, which tend to be neurotoxic to them. Sun et al. [108] analyzed the neurotoxicity of the halogenated tris-(2-chloroethyl) phosphate (TCEP) and the non-halogenated alkyl tri-*n*-butyl phosphate (TNBP) in zebrafish (*Dario rerio*). More specifically, these authors analyzed locomotor behavior, enzymatic activity, and AChE gene transcription. They found that zebrafish exposure to these compounds in early life stages affects locomotor behavior and gene transcription, suggesting that exposure to organophosphates may be relevant in humans, especially in children.

Exposure at developmental stages may also affect cardiac development. Cardiac development comprises several stages for increasing formation during embryogenesis. When the process occurs properly, chamber formation and maturation, septation, and valve formation take place correctly [109].

Using zebrafish as a model species for studies on developmental toxicity is advantageous and has been gaining ground in several areas of toxicology. Alzualde et al. [110] used zebrafish as a model in developmental toxicity assays to test not only the cardiotoxicity but also the neuro- and hepatotoxicity of organophosphates. These authors found that TPhP affects the heartbeat and reduces locomotor activity and hepatic edema. These data are extremely relevant when it comes to human biomonitoring.

Abe et al. [111] evaluated the toxicity of halogen-free flame retardants in zebrafish to trace a toxicity profile. At all concentrations used, ALPi did not show any sublethal or teratogenic effects, suggesting that ALPi may be a good alternative for brominated flame retardants. However, further studies are still needed to support this information [111].

The crustacean *Daphnia magna* is also a widely used model for toxicity testing. To test the chronic toxicity of ALPi, Waaijers et al. [112] exposed *D. magna* by 21 for toxicity tests. The toxicity of ALPi increased with the time of exposure, with low acute toxicity and moderate chronic toxicity [112].

DOI: http://dx.doi.org/10.5772/intechopen.104886

TDCPP and TPhP are also potential endocrine disruptors, altering hormone levels and decreasing semen quality in adult men. Furthermore, the concentration of these compounds in house dust has been correlated with decreased sperm concentration, increased prolactin level, and decreased free thyroxin (T4) level [113].

Given that reproductive system integrity also depends on the organism's redox state, An et al. [114] tested TPhP and TCPP cytotoxicity in HepG2, A549, and Caco-2 cells. In addition to inhibiting cell viability, these compounds increase ROS production, inducing DNA damage and mitochondrial dysfunction. These changes in redox balance may harm steroidogenesis and even estrogen metabolism, being directly related to reproductive changes.

Epidemiological studies on exposure to organophosphates are also gaining ground, especially when it comes to the early stages of development, when organophosphates may have greater consequences [115].

In a cohort study, Castorina et al. [116] evaluated how exposure to organophosphates, mainly TPhP, affected the cognitive or behavioral development of 310 school-age children. The authors monitored exposure by analyzing metabolites present in pregnant women's urine. They observed decreased intelligence quotient and working memory, associated with an increased level of the urinary metabolite diphenyl phosphate (DPhP).

Although some compounds have been widely used in research, and even though much information is available, the effects of other types of organophosphates remain to be elucidated. For example, toxicity data on BPA-DP and RDP are limited, so their consequences on human health are unknown [82].

Monitoring organic organophosphate metabolites is necessary to assess and control biological exposure, not to mention that these metabolites may play important biological roles in the toxicity of these compounds. In any case, many studies on organic organophosphates are still needed to understand their toxic effects and to reduce exposure to them [117].

4. Phosphorus-based flame retardants: halogenated compounds

Organophosphorus FRs can be divided into nonhalogenated and halogenated. Halogenated organophosphates have chlorinated forms, which are mainly used as FRs in furniture, building materials, textiles, and electronics [118]. According to the 2012 Chemical Data Reporting from the U.S. Environmental Protection Agency (EPA), about 22,700 tons/year of TDCPP, one of the most used organophosphorus FRs, were manufactured or imported by the U.S.A. in 2010 and 2011 [118, 119]. Tris-(chloropropyl)phosphate (TCPP), tris-(2-chloroethyl) phosphate (TCEP), tris-(1,3-dichloro-2-propyl) phosphate (TDCPP), and tetrakis-(2-chlorethyl) dichloroisopentyldiphosphate (V6) are the main halogenated organophosphates.

4.1 Physicochemical characteristics

4.1.1 Tris-(1,3-dichloro-2-propyl) phosphate (TDCPP)

Tris-(1,3-dichloro-2-propyl) phosphate is commonly abbreviated in the literature as TDCPP, TDCP, or TDCIPP. It a viscous colorless liquid with boiling of 457°C, water solubility of 1.5 mg/l, and log K_{ow} of 3.8 [6, 120, 121].

4.1.2 Tris-(chloropropyl)phosphate (TCPP)

TCPP is a clear, colorless liquid. Its commercial formulation consists of a mixture of tris-(chloroiso-propyl)phosphate (75%) and bis-(1-chloro-2-propyl)-2-chloropropyl-phosphate (15–30%). It has a boiling point of 342°C, the water solubility of 1.6 g/l, and log K_{ow} of 2.59 [6, 121].

4.1.3 Tris-(2-chloroethyl) phosphate (TCEP)

TCEP has boiling point of 351°C; however, above 220°C, it rapidly decomposes to carbon monoxide, hydrogen chloride, 2-chloroethane, and dichloroethane. It has a water solubility of 7.0 g/l and log K_{ow} of 1.44 [6, 121].

4.1.4 Tetrakis-(2-chlorethyl) dichloroisopentyldiphosphate (V6)

V6 has a boiling point of 620°C, the water solubility of 2.1 mg/l, and log K_{ow} of 1.9. In addition, V6 can be used in conjunction with TDCPP and TCPP, but with specific criteria [6, 121, 122].

Table 5 summarizes the chemical structure and physicochemical properties of Halogenated Organophosphates.

4.2 Environmental occurrence and ecotoxicological effects

Because organophosphate FRs are not chemically bound to the original material, they are slowly released into the environment by abrasion and volatilization [123, 124]. Consequently, they are widely distributed in indoor and outdoor environments [124]. In addition, dust and air are important means of human exposure to these compounds via skin and breathing [4]. Furthermore, dust may settle into water bodies, contaminate the water environment and affect aquatic organisms [4].

A study investigated organophosphate FR concentrations in air and dust in 63 homes in Canada, the Czech Republic, and the U.S [125]. The highest concentration of halogenated compounds was found in the U.S.—an average of 1440 ng/g TCEP to 4530 ng/g tris-(2,3-dibromopropyl) phosphate (TDBPP), followed by Canada, and the Czech Republic [11]. Regarding air, TCIPP was detected at the highest average concentration: 73.6 ng/m^3 in Canada, followed 26.3 ng/m^3 in the U.S. and 16.4 ng/m^3 in the Czech Republic [125].

A study carried out in Brazil investigated indoor dust concentrations in different places in Araraquara (Brazil) [22]. The authors observed that TDCIPP (up to 61,200 ng/g) was the second most abundant compound in homes and apartments, [12] and the most abundant compound in cars (from 1050 to 1,600,000 ng/g) [22].

Regarding halogenated compounds in outdoor dust, a study investigated FR concentrations in outdoor dust from urban and rural areas in Nanjing (China) [126]. The authors identified halogenated compounds as the most abundant in both the rural (median: 45.9%) and urban (median: 56.8%) areas [126] and TCPP as the most abundant FR in both studied areas [126].

Assessing sediments is important for monitoring aquatic ecosystems and the aquatic environments quality [127, 128]. Halogenated FRs may accumulate in sediments because they have low solubility in water and a relatively high octanolwater partition coefficient (K_{ow}) [129].

Chemical name	Abbreviation	Structural formula	Molecular Formula	Molecular weight	Log K_{ow}
Tris(1,3-dichloro-2-propyl) phosphate	TDCPP, TDCP, TDCIPP	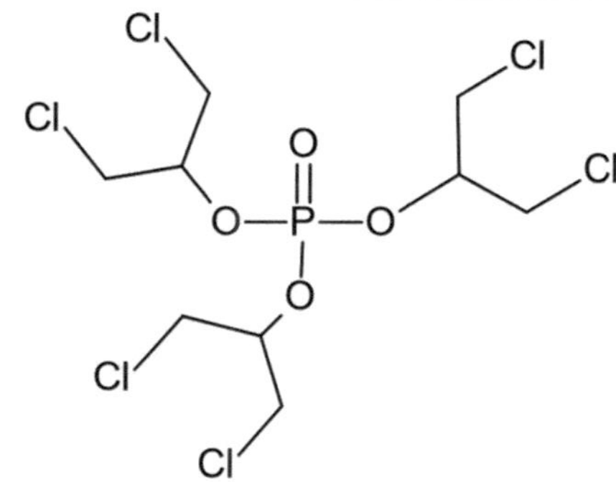	$C_9H_{15}C_{16}O_4P$	430.9	3.8
Tris(chloropropyl)phosphate	TCPP	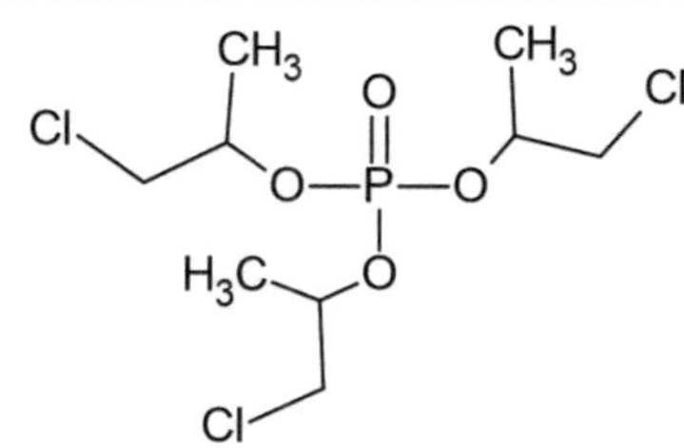	$C_9H_{18}Cl_3O_4P$	327.6	2.59
Tris(2-chloroethyl) phosphate	TCEP	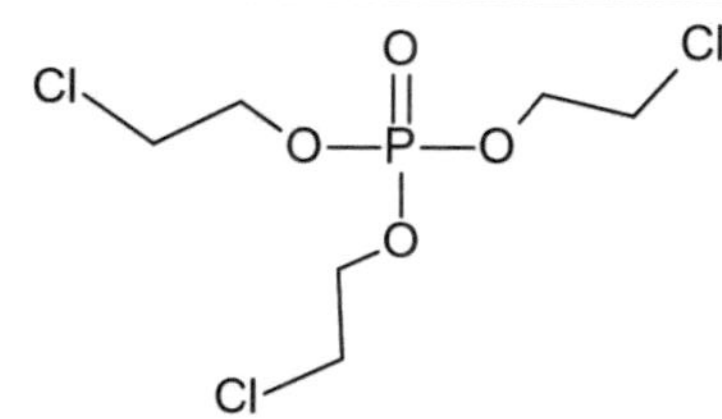	$C_6H_{12}Cl_3O_4P$	297.6	1.44

Chemical name	Abbreviation	Structural formula	Molecular Formula	Molecular weight	Log K_{ow}
Tetrekis(2-chlorethyl) dichloroisopentyldiphosphate	V6	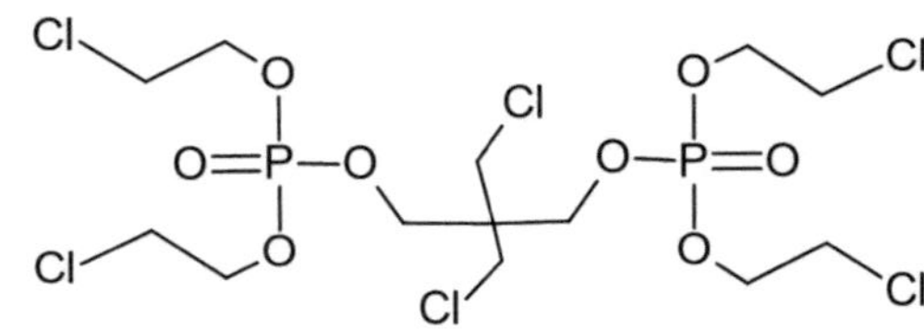	$C_{10}H_{20}C_{14}O_8P_2$	472.0	1.9

Adapted: [6, 143]. Source: Pubchem. Chemical structures were designed by the authors by using the software ACD/ChemSketch®.

Table 5.
Chemical structure and some physicochemical properties of novel halogenated organophosphate flame retardants.

A study analyzed sediment samples from the Bohai and Yellow Seas (China), to detect organophosphate FRs [130]. The authors identified halogenates as being more abundant than non-halogenated FRs [130]. In addition, TCEP was detected at the highest concentration (from 7 to 671 pg./g of dry weight) [130]. Another study evaluated sediments from rivers in Austria and found TCPP as the most abundant compound in the samples, with a maximum concentration of 1300 μg/kg [131].

Thus, evaluating FRs in sediments is important because, if they are present therein, they will be continuously ingested by aquatic organisms and will eventually accumulate in the food chain, thereby being a potential risk to aquatic organisms [4].

Organophosphate FRs are not completely removed during the wastewater treatment process. Besides that, chlorinated FRs (halogenated group) are more difficult to degrade than non-chlorinated ones [132]. Thus, halogenated FRs have the greatest potential to harm water quality and aquatic health [4, 133].

A study conducted in Germany evaluated the surface waters of the Elbe and Rhine rivers, to detect organophosphate FRs in the samples [134]. In the Elbe River, TCPP and TCEP were measured at concentrations between 40 and 250 ng/l and between 5 and 20 ng/l, respectively [134]. On the other hand, the Rhine river contained smaller concentrations of TCPP (75–160 ng/l) and TCEP (12–25 ng/l) [134].

A study evaluated samples from the Santa Clara River in Los Angeles (California, United States), to find halogenated organophosphate FRs as the main compounds, including TCPP (3.3 μg/l), TDCPP (1.4 μg/l), and TCEP (0.81 μg/l) [135].

Other works have evaluated the presence of halogenated compounds in seawater [136]. A study conducted in China analyzed samples from the Yellow Sea and the East China Sea and detected TCEP (134.44 ng/l), TCPP (84.12 ng/l), TDCPP (109.28 ng/l), and TDBPP (96.70 ng/l) [24]. The authors concluded that the source of these compounds is the municipal and industrial effluent of wastewater treatment plants [136].

Another study conducted in China evaluated types of drinking water samples including tap water, filtered drinking water, bottled water, barreled water, and well water in both urban and rural areas in Eastern China [137]. The authors identified TCPP as being more abundant in barreled water (8.04 ng/l) and well water (2.49 ng/l). The authors found TCEP in low amounts in all types of drinking water, making its carcinogenic risk unlikely [137]. The authors concluded that exposure to organophosphate FRs in drinking water in Eastern China poses no risk to human health [137].

Because halogenated FRs are not fully degraded during wastewater treatment, as already discussed above, they may occur in environmental compartments including air, sediments, and water [125, 130, 132, 137]. Therefore, investigating whether these compounds bioaccumulate in organisms is relevant, as it could damage the ecosystem and human health [138]. The appearance of halogenated FRs in mussels has already been reported in a study conducted in Maizuru Bay (Japan) [139], with TDCPP (18 ng/l), TCP (11 ng/l), and TCEP (11 ng/l) being detected. According to the study authors, these concentrations would not be able to promote adverse effects in the organisms [139]. Another study analyzed fish samples collected from the Pearl River in southern China and domestic birds (chicken and ducks) purchased from farmers living in Qingyuan County [28]. TCEP (82.7–4692 ng/g lipid weight in fish and 33.7–162 ng/g lipid weight in the bird) and TCPP (62.7–883 ng/g lipid weight in fish and 3.89–21.4 ng/g lipid weight in the bird) were detected in all the samples [140].

Studying human exposure to aquatic animals that bioaccumulate halogenated compounds is important. A study has evaluated fish, mussels, and breast milk samples [141]. Aquatic organisms were collected from Swedish lakes, and breast milk samples were collected from women in Swedish cities [141]. The authors found that all the samples contained TCPP at concentrations between 170 and 770 ng/g lipid weight (l.w), and they detected TDCPP only in fish, at a concentration between 49 and 140 ng/g l.w [141]. In addition, they identified TCPP (22–82 ng/g l.w) and TDCPP (1.6–5.3 ng/g l.w) in the breast milk samples [141]. The authors concluded that human exposure to organophosphate FRs via fish and human milk ingestion seems to have minor significance compared to the calculated exposure to these compounds in dust and air [141].

4.3 Toxicokinetics

Humans may be exposed to halogenated organophosphates through inhalation or oral or dermal contact; the general population is exposed to these compounds through food and drinking water [142]. Moreover, occupational exposure to these compounds occurs through vapor inhalation and dermal contact [143]. Consumer exposure includes exposure through vapor inhalation, direct skin contact with halogenated organophosphates on the surface of objects, incidental ingestion of air-suspended particulates or resuspended dust, and ingestion via object-to-mouth behavior by children [144–146].

TCDCPP, TCEP, and TCPP are rapidly absorbed by the oral route of exposure. Furthermore, TDCPP dermal absorption is significant in rats, and TCPP dermal absorption is significant in humans as revealed by in vitro studies [147]. In addition, TCEP is extensively absorbed during nebulized exposure [148]. After halogenated compounds are absorbed, they are distributed throughout the body without specific accumulation in tissue or organs, but TCEP has been reported to be present in breast milk [149].

These compounds are rapidly metabolized during Phase I and Phase II metabolism. TDCPP is metabolized by a combination of hydrolase, MFO (mixed function oxidase), and GST reactions synthesizing glutathione conjugates, so the main metabolite is BDCPP (bis-(1,3-dichloro-2-propyl)phosphate) [147, 150]. TCEP and TCPP are metabolized by hydroxylation possibly by MFO and CYP 450 enzymes conjugated with glucuronic acid [147]. After that, the metabolic products of halogenated organophosphate FRs are rapidly excreted, primarily in the urine [147].

4.4 Toxicological effects

Exposure to halogenated organophosphate compounds may cause some toxic effects in humans. According to Freudenthal and Henrich, chronic exposure to TDCPP causes benign tumors to appear in Sprague–Dawley rats [151]. A study conducted with patients at a Duke Cancer Institute suggested that increased incidence of thyroid cancer may be associated with exposure to TCEP in the home environment [152]. Additionally, under regulation EC 1272/2008, TDCPP is classified as a category 2 carcinogen with hazard statement H351 “suspected of causing cancer” and TCEP is classified as a “potential human carcinogen” by the E.U [145, 153].

In recent years, endocrine disruption effects of halogenated compounds have been observed. Stapleton and Meeker associated TDCPP concentrations in house dust with hormone levels [64]. They analyzed TDCPP in-house dust collected from 50 men recruited through a U.S. infertility clinic, to observe that increased TDCPP was associated with 3% lower free thyroxine concentration and 17% higher prolactin level [64]. Increased prolactin is a positive effect because it serves a number of important functions involving reproduction, metabolism, and angiogenesis [64, 154]. Studies have also shown that exposure to TDCPP causes thyroid endocrine disruption—exposure of female zebrafish to TDCPP decreases T3 and T4 hormone levels, whereas exposure of Sprague–Dawley rats to TDCPP decreases serum thyroid stimulating hormone [155, 156].

Halogenated FRs and organophosphorus pesticides, such as chlorpyrifos, have similar chemical structures, so these FRs might also exert neurotoxic effects like organophosphate pesticides do [157]. Stapleton performed studies on PC12 cells and observed that TDCPP inhibits DNA synthesis and causes high oxidative stress, without adverse effects on cell viability or growth [157]. Moreover, TDCPP promotes differentiation into dopaminergic and cholinergic neurophenotypes, while TCEP and TCPP only promote the cholinergic phenotype [157].

Finally, there are very limited human health and toxicity data available for organophosphate halogenated FRs, so further studies are needed to understand how they affect humans.

5. Phosphorus-based flame retardants: inorganic compounds

Inorganic FRs act mainly in the solid phase, with thermal decomposition through the release of phosphoric acid. This leads to substrate carbonization, resembling phosphorus-containing FRs [158].

The German report “Substituting Environmentally Relevant Flame Retardants: Assessment Fundamentals” analyzed some FRs on the basis of several evaluation criteria, including potential to accumulate in environmental media (occurrences in humans and the environment), chronic and acute toxicity, emission trend (production, use, and waste disposal), fire by-products (smoke density, gas toxicity, and corrosivity, and fire extinguishing water charges, etc.), and concluded that red phosphorus and ammonium polyphosphate are the least problematic FRs [158].

5.1 Red phosphorus (RP)

RP is a very effective FR in many polymer applications is. It is a stable form of the element phosphorus, which has an amorphous structure [158].

RP acts as an FR via a solid-phase mechanism. It forms a rigid layer that prevents flammable material replenishment in the gas phase, reducing fire and decreasing fire gas toxicity [159]. For polyphosphoric acid (the main component of the aforementioned rigid layer) to be formed, oxygen must be supplied by the polymer or another material used as matrix. Therefore, RP is a more efficient FR in materials with high oxygen content (such as cellulose or plastics containing oxygen) [158]. The RP concentration varies from 2 to 10% of the total weight. RP reduces the toxic smoke formation and heat release, preventing large fires from occurring [160]. Its use restrictions are based on color—because it is red, it cannot be used in white or light products given that it is difficult to mask even with dyes, [158].

RP is mainly used in condensation polymers (polyamide, polyester, polyurethane, polyisocyanurate, and epoxy resins), but it can also be used in dispersions for textile finishing, polyamide components for electrical and electronic devices, fiberglass reinforced plastics for electrical applications, synthetic glues, and automotive textiles [158].

According to some studies, the use of RP as FR is not problematic because it does not dissolve in water easily, making the risk of environmental contamination with phosphorus unlikely. Organ intoxication effects are also unlikely, and RP may only cause skin irritation. Therefore, the use of this FR has a low ecological and human health impact, as long as it is not mixed with white or yellow phosphorus [158].

The risks of contaminating the environment with phosphorus as a result of using RP as FR are unlikely. There are no data on RP concentrations in air, soil, or water. Like microencapsulated phosphorus, inert RP does not pose a threat to the environment [158].

The occurrence of phosphorus compounds in environmental samples cannot be analyzed separately from the natural occurrences of phosphorus compounds and cannot be seen as a consequence of the use of RP as FR [158]. Accumulation is hardly a consequence of RP used in plastics because this FR degrades fast, with phosphine and phosphoric acid formation. The effects on aquatic systems are not alarming because phosphorus concentrations are low compared to natural occurrences [158].

RP oral ingestion is unlikely because it is degraded in the environment when it is eliminated in sewage plants through adsorption to sewage sludge. Whether resorption occurs when RP is microencapsulated and ingested orally has not been examined, but resorption is more likely negligible and organ effects are improbable [158].

If inhaled, RP LD50 in rats is 4.3 mg/l, which indicates moderate acute toxicity because metabolism is rapid. Eyes and mucous membranes may become irritated probably due to acid formation. Therefore, affected individuals should not be taken for toxicological evaluation because phosphoric acid may be formed due to the high reactivity of phosphine. Nevertheless, oxides released during a fire should not be ignored because they may irritate the affected persons skin [158].

The RP physicochemical properties prevent it from evaporating at room temperature and from solubilizing in water. Because oxygen is present in the environment, RP forms some phosphates that generate phosphine (PH) through a complex chain of chemical reactions. As toxic as phosphine is (with prescribed exposure limits for humans being TLV/TWA—0.3 ppm or 0.4 mg/m^3; TLV/STEL—0.75–1 ppm), it is also very reactive and produces non-toxic phosphates [159].

Some techniques for RP production have been developed and improved, so phosphine is no longer a problem. Phosphine arises if RP is treated at high temperatures or if it is exposed to humidity. If during compounding the RP levels are kept below the TLV/TWA limit, phosphine formation may be drastically reduced, and they can be removed in a well-ventilated area [159]. RP should not be stored in closed containers because phosphine may be formed [158].

RP in the powder form is flammable and has therefore been regulated as a potentially hazardous material. The safest and most ecological way to transport RP is to microencapsulate it. But the newly developed RP grade is highly stable, safer to use, and easier to handle in terms of cleaning and service life [159].

During a fire, RP is easily oxidized to phosphorus oxides that do not form phosphine: in fact, phosphorus oxides remain as polymeric phosphoric acid or phosphates that can be removed in the incinerators' flue gas treatment system [159].

5.2 Ammonium polyphosphates (APP)

APP is a crystalline inorganic salt with the chemical formula NH_4PO_3. This FR retardant is found in the crystalline or liquor form and contains nitrogen and phosphorus (**Figure 3**). Like most FRs containing phosphorus, APP begins to decompose at temperatures above 225°C and acts by releasing phosphoric acid and carbonizing [158].

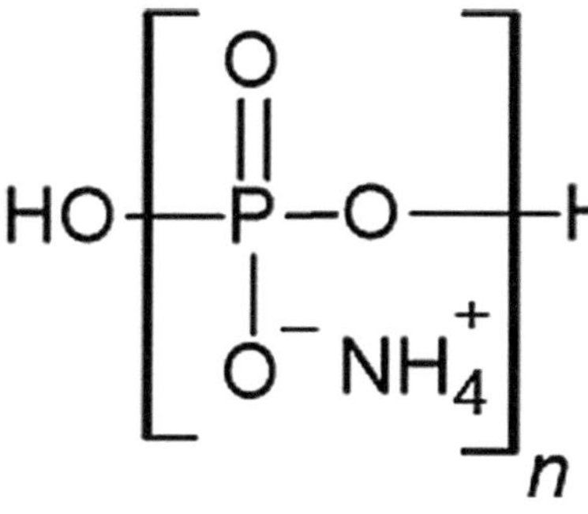

Figure 3.
APP chemical structure.

The composition of ingredients varies depending on the manufacturer. For example, APP 422 from Clariant GmbH, contains 31.5% phosphorus and 14.5% nitrogen [158]. APP is often used in conjunction with other compounds such as polyalcohol as a carbon dioxide dispenser, melamine as a blowing agent, and aluminum trihydrate (ATH) in resins [158].

In intumescent systems, APP is combined with carbonic compound distributors and blowing agents. This mechanism releases non-flammable gases, preventing oxygen from being supplied to the flammable substrate. APP is used in polyurethane foams (hard and flexible), polypropylene, epoxy and polyester resins, cellulose-containing systems, and wash-resistant textile backings [158].

Some studies have reported that, from a toxicological viewpoint, APP is not problematic, or that it has a very low ecological and human health impact. Air contamination caused by APP is unlikely due to its physicochemical properties [158].

There are no data available on APP reabsorption by oral ingestion, but a high rate can be predicted from experiments with similar compounds. APP is metabolized to ammonia and phosphate, which integrate with the nitrogen and phosphate cycle. However, there are no considerable concentrations in the body or toxic effects that need to be feared. If APP comes into contact with skin, it causes some irritating or sensitizing effect because hydrolysis occurs in the presence of acid and ammonia salts in an aqueous medium. The LD50 data (>2000 mg/kg) allows no conclusions about chronic toxicity [158].

Rapid APP decomposition into ammonia and phosphate occurs in soil and sewage sludge, so water eutrophication must be taken into account. However, there are no exact data on the relevance of the volume. During a fire from plastics containing APP, nitrogen oxide and ammonia are formed, as well as phosphorus oxide. These gases are aggressive, and the health effects cannot be ignored [158].

Table 6 summarizes the biological effects caused by organic, halogenated, and inorganic phosphorus-based flame retardants.

6. Conclusion

Fire has always been an enemy of humanity and can cause a lot of destruction. Over time, more and more people live with materials with high flammability, creating the need to control the flammability of these materials. Thus, flame retardants are widely used to reduce the risk of fire, as a safety device. However, other risks can arise

Abbreviation	Type	Toxic effect	Reference
TPhP	Organic	• Neurotoxic—AChE inhibition; • Cardiotoxicity, affecting heartbeat and reduces locomotor activity and hepatic edema; • Decreased sperm concentration, increased prolactin level, and decreased free thyroxin (T4) level; • Cytotoxicity in HepG2, A549, and Caco-2 cells, increasing ROS production, inducing DNA damage and mitochondrial dysfunction; • Affect the cognitive or behavioral development.	[107, 110, 113, 114, 116]
TNBP	Organic	• Affect locomotor behavior and gene transcription.	[73]
ALPi	Organic	• Any sublethal or teratogenic effects, suggesting that ALPi may be a good alternative for brominated flame retardants; • Increase with the time of exposure, with low acute toxicity and moderate chronic toxicity (*Daphnia magna)*.	[111, 113]
BPA-DP	Organic	• Toxicity data are limited.	[6]
RDP	Organic	• Toxicity data are limited.	[6]
TDCPP	Halogenated	• Affinity for the nervous system and are commonly associated with neurotrophic factor inhibition; • Altering hormone levels and decreasing semen quality in adult men;	[107, 113]
TCPP	Halogenated	• Cytotoxicity in HepG2, A549, and Caco-2 cells. • Increasing ROS production, inducing DNA damage and mitochondrial dysfunction.	[114]
TCEP	Halogenated	• Inducing thyroid cancer	[152]
RP	Inorganic	• Low human health impact as long as it is not mixed with white • and yellow phosphorus	[158]
APP	Inorganic	• Low human health impact	[158]

Table 6.
Summary of biological effects caused by organic, halogenated, and inorganic inorganic phosphorus-based flame retardants.

with the wide use of this class of compounds, including the risks to environmental and human health.

As flame retardants are being used, research and new knowledge are being generated to understand the behavior of these substances in the environment and the consequences for the ecosystem and human health. Classes of flame retardants begin to be legislated and controlled due to their highly toxic potentials, such as PCBs, PBDEs, and HBCD. On the other hand, new compounds have been introduced to

DOI: http://dx.doi.org/10.5772/intechopen.104886

replace the legislated flame retardants, here, phosphorus-based flame retardants emerge as an effective and possibly ecofriendly alternative to the old flame retardants.

As the need arises for alternatives to the old flame retardants, new substances are being introduced into the market with the purpose of reducing the damage that could be caused. However, this insertion occurs without full knowledge of the toxic effects of these new products. Furthermore, over the last decades, we can observe a pattern of substitution of harmful or legislated flame retardants to another that initially was human and ecofriendly but, after few years it turns out and it was harmful. In this way, the environmental consequences can be exacerbated, as can the exposure of ecosystems. In this chapter, we provide a review of the main classes of flame retardants and its possible substitutes, trying to understand the behavior of these substances in the environment and their toxicological consequences for the ecosystem and human health.

Author details

Raul Ghiraldelli Miranda[1], Carolina Ferreira Sampaio[1], Fernanda Gomes Leite[1], Flavia Duarte Maia[2] and Daniel Junqueira Dorta[2]*

1 Department of Clinical, Toxicological and Food Sciences, School of Pharmaceutical Sciences of Ribeirão Preto, University of São Paulo, Ribeirão Preto, Brazil

2 Faculdade de Filosofia, Departamento de Química, Ciências e Letras de Ribeirão Preto, Universidade de São Paulo, Ribeirão Preto, Brazil

*Address all correspondence to: djdorta@ffclrp.usp.br

References

[1] Wypych G. Introduction. In: Handbook of Flame Retardants. Toronto, Canada: ChemTec Publishing; 2021. pp. 1-2

[2] de Boer J. Fire. Chemosphere. Toronto, Canada: ChemTec Publishing. 2019;**217**:A1-A2

[3] Innes A, Innes J. Flame retardants. In: Handbook of Environmental Degradation of Materials. 2nd ed. Waltham, USA: William Andrew Publishing; 2012. pp. 306-335

[4] Yao C, Yang H, Li Y. A Review on Organophosphate Flame Retardants in the Environment: Occurrence, Accumulation, Metabolism and Toxicity. Science of the Total Environment. Vol. 795. Amsterdam, Netherland: Elsevier B. V.; 2021

[5] NIEHS NI of EHS. Flame Retardants Fact Sheet. National Institute of Environmental Health Sciences, 2016 [Internet]. Available from: https://www.niehs.nih.gov/health/materials/flame_retardants_508.pdf [Accessed: Nov 22, 2021]

[6] van der Veen I, de Boer J. Phosphorus flame retardants: Properties, production, environmental occurrence, toxicity and analysis. Chemosphere. 2012;**88**(10): 1119-1153

[7] FlameRetardant-Online. The flame retardants market [Internet]. 2020. Available from: https://www.flameretardants-online.com/flame-retardants/market [Accessed: Nov 21, 2021]

[8] Ekpe OD, Choo G, Barceló D, Oh JE. Introduction of emerging halogenated flame retardants in the environment. Comprehensive Analytical Chemistry. 2020;**88**:1-39

[9] Sauvé S, Desrosiers M. A review of what is an emerging contaminant. Chemistry Central Journal. 2014;**8**(15): 1-7

[10] Aznar-Alemany Ò, Eljarrat E. Food contamination on flame retardants. Comprehensive Analytical Chemistry. 2020;**88**:141-189

[11] UNEP. Stockholm Convention on Persistent Organic Pollutants (POPS)—Texts and Annexes. United Nations Environment programme (UNEP). Switzerland: Châtelaine; 2017

[12] Kodavanti PRS, Stoker TE, Fenton SE. Brominated flame retardants. In: Reproductive and Developmental Toxicology. 2nd ed, Cambridge, USA: Academic Press; 2017. pp.681-710

[13] Wypych G. Mechanisms of action of flame retardants. Handbook of Flame Retardants. Toronto, Canada: ChemTec Publishing. 2021:53-88

[14] De Boer J, Stapleton HM. Toward fire safety without chemical risk. Science. 2019;**364**(6437):231-232

[15] Ferrari RS, de Souza AO, Annunciação DLR, Sodré FF, Dorta DJ. Assessing surface sediment contamination by PBDE in a recharge point of Guarani aquifer in Ribeirão Preto, Brazil. Water (Switzerland). 2019; **11**(8):1-13

[16] Osimitz TG, Kacew S, Hayes AW. Assess flame retardants with care. Science (Letters). 2019;**365**(6457):6-9

[17] Kodavanti PRS, Loganathan BG. Polychlorinated biphenyls, polybrominated biphenyls, and brominated flame retardants. In:

Biomarkers in Toxicology. 2nd ed. Cambridge, USA: Academic Press;. 2019: 501-518

[18] Norén K, Meironyté D. Certain organochlorine and organobromine contaminants in Swedish human milk in perspective of past 20–30 years. Chemosphere. 2000;**40**(9–11):1111-1123

[19] De Boer J, Wester PG, Klamer HJC, Lewis WE, Boon JP. Do flame retardants threaten ocean life? Nature. 1998; **394**(6688):28-29

[20] De Wit CA. An overview of brominated flame retardants in the environment. Chemosphere. 2002; **46**(5):583-624

[21] Guerra P, Alaee M, Eljarrat E, Barceló D. Introduction to brominated flame retardants: Commercially products. Applications, and Physicochemical Properties. Brominated Flame Retardants. The Handbook of Environmental Chemistry, vol. 16. Berlin Heidelberg: Springer; 2010. pp. 1-17

[22] Cristale J, Aragão Belé TG, Lacorte S, Rodrigues de Marchi MR. Occurrence and human exposure to brominated and organophosphorus flame retardants via indoor dust in a Brazilian city. Environmental Pollution. 2018;(237): 695-703

[23] de Wit CA, Herzke D, Vorkamp K. Brominated flame retardants in the Arctic environment—Trends and new candidates. Science of The Total Environment. 2010;**408**(15): 2885-2918

[24] Yu G, Bu Q, Cao Z, Du X, Xia J, Wu M, et al. Brominated flame retardants (BFRs): A review on environmental contamination in China. Chemosphere. 2016;**150**:479-490

[25] Waaijers SL, Parsons JR. Biodegradation of brominated and organophosphorus flame retardants. Current Opinion in Biotechnology. 2016; **38**:14-23

[26] La Guardia MJ, Hale RC, Harvey E. Detailed polybrominated diphenyl ether (PBDE) congener composition of the widely used penta-, octa-, and deca-PBDE technical flame-retardant mixtures. Environmental science & technology. 2006;**40**(20):6247-6254

[27] Rahman F, Langford KH, Scrimshaw MD, Lester JN. Polybrominated diphenyl ether (PBDE) flame retardants. The Science of the Total Environment. 2001;**275**(1–3):1-17

[28] Costa LG, de Laat R, Tagliaferri S, Pellacani C. A mechanistic view of polybrominated diphenyl ether (PBDE) developmental neurotoxicity. Toxicology letters. 2014;**230**(2):282-294

[29] Chen MW, Castillo BAA, Lin DY, Chao HR, Tayo LL, Gou YY, et al. Levels of PCDD/Fs, PBDEs, and PBDD/Fs in breast milk from southern Taiwan. Bulletin of Environmental Contamination and Toxicology. 2018; **100**(3):369-375

[30] Toms LML, Harden FA, Symons RK, Burniston D, Fürst P, Müller JF. Polybrominated diphenyl ethers (PBDEs) in human milk from Australia. Chemosphere. 2007;**68**(5):797-803

[31] Zhang J, Chen L, Xiao L, Ouyang F, Zhang QY, Luo ZC. Polybrominated diphenyl ether concentrations in human breast milk specimens worldwide. Epidemiology. 2017;**28**(October):S89-S97

[32] Zota AR, Park JS, Wang Y, Petreas M, Zoeller RT, Woodruff TJ. Polybrominated diphenyl ethers,

hydroxylated polybrominated diphenyl ethers, and measures of thyroid function in second trimester pregnant women in California. Environmental Science & Technology. 2011;**45**(18): 7896-7905

[33] Zhou T, Ross DG, Devito MJ, Crofton KM. Effects of short-term in vivo exposure to polybrominated diphenyl ethers on thyroid hormones and hepatic enzyme activities in weanling rats. Toxicological Sciences. 2001;**61**(1):76-82

[34] Pazin M, Pereira LC, Dorta DJ. Toxicity of brominated flame retardants, BDE-47 and BDE-99 stems from impaired mitochondrial bioenergetics. Toxicology Mechanisms and Methods. 2015;**25**(1):34-41

[35] Pereira LC, Souza AO, Tasso MJ, Oliveira AMC, Duarte FV, Palmeira CM, et al. Exposure to decabromodiphenyl ether (BDE-209) produces mitochondrial dysfunction in rat liver and cell death. Journal of Toxicology and Environmental Health, Part A, 80. 2017; **80**(19-21):1129-1144. DOI: 10.1080/15287394.2017.1357370

[36] Pereira LC, de Souza AO, Meireles G, Franco-Bernardes MF, Tasso MJ, Bruno V, et al. Comparative study of genotoxicity induced by six different PBDEs. Basic & Clinical Pharmacology & Toxicology. 2016; **119**(4):396-404

[37] Feiteiro J, Mariana M, Cairrão E. Health toxicity effects of brominated flame retardants: From environmental to human exposure. Environmental Pollution. 2021;**285** (May):117475

[38] Lyman WJ, Reehl WF, Rosenblatt DH. Handbook of Chemical Property Estimation Methods. Washington, DC (USA): American Chemical Society; 1990

[39] Veith GD, DeFoe DL, Bergstedt BV. Measuring and estimating the bioconcentration factor of chemicals in fish. 1979;**36**(9):1040-1048. DOI: 101139/f79-146

[40] Ruan Y, Zhang X, Qiu JW, Leung KMY, Lam JCW, Lam PKS. Stereoisomer-specific trophodynamics of the chiral brominated flame retardants HBCD and TBECH in a marine food web, with implications for human exposure. Environmental Science and Technology. 2018;**52**(15): 8183-8193

[41] Zhang Q, Yao Y, Wang Y, Zhang Q, Cheng Z, Li Y, et al. Plant accumulation and transformation of brominated and organophosphate flame retardants: A review. Environmental Pollution. 2021; **288**:117742

[42] Zhang H, Pan L, Tao Y, Tian S, Hu Y. Identification and expression of differentially expressed genes in clam Venerupis philippinarum in response to environmental pollutant hexabromocyclododecane (HBCD). Journal of Experimental Marine Biology and Ecology. 2013;**445**:166-173

[43] Du M, Zhang D, Yan C, Zhang X. Developmental toxicity evaluation of three hexabromocyclododecane diastereoisomers on zebrafish embryos. Aquatic Toxicology. 2012;**112–113**:1-10

[44] Germer S, Piersma AH, Van Der Ven L, Kamyschnikow A, Fery Y, Schmitz HJ, et al. Subacute effects of the brominated flame retardants hexabromocyclododecane and tetrabromobisphenol a on hepatic cytochrome P450 levels in rats. Toxicology. 2006;**218**(2–3):229-236

[45] van der Ven LTM, van de Kuil T, Leonards PEG, Slob W, Lilienthal H, Litens S, et al. Endocrine effects of hexabromocyclododecane (HBCD) in a one-generation reproduction study in Wistar rats. Toxicology Letters. 2009; **185**(1):51-62

[46] Al-Mousa F, Michelangeli F. The sarcoplasmic–endoplasmic reticulum Ca^{2+}-ATPase (SERCA) is the likely molecular target for the acute toxicity of the brominated flame retardant hexabromocyclododecane (HBCD). Chemico-Biological Interactions. 2014; **207**(1):1-6

[47] Al-Mousa F, Michelangeli F. Some commonly used brominated flame retardants cause Ca^{2+}-ATPase inhibition, beta-amyloid peptide release and apoptosis in SH-SY5Y neuronal cells. PLoS One. 2012;7(4): e33059

[48] Zhang X, Yang F, Xu C, Liu W, Wen S, Xu Y. Cytotoxicity evaluation of three pairs of hexabromocyclododecane (HBCD) enantiomers on hep G2 cell. Toxicology in Vitro. 2008;**22**(6): 1520-1527

[49] European Chemical Agengy (ECHA). Risk assessment of 2,2′,6,6′-tetrabromo-4,4′-isopropylidene diphenol (tetrabromobisphenol A). 2008; [Internet] Available from: https://echa.europa.eu/documents/10162/17c7379e-f47b-4a76-aa43-060da5830c07 [Accessed: Nov 22, 2021]

[50] Zhou H, Yin N, Faiola F. Tetrabromobisphenol A (TBBPA): A controversial environmental pollutant. Journal of Environmental Sciences. 2020;**97**:54-66

[51] Covaci A, Voorspoels S, Abdallah MAE, Geens T, Harrad S, Law RJ. Analytical and environmental aspects of the flame retardant tetrabromobisphenol-a and its derivatives. Journal of Chromatography A. 2009; **1216**(3):346-363

[52] Shi Z, Zhang L, Zhao Y, Sun Z, Zhou X, Li J, et al. Dietary exposure assessment of Chinese population to tetrabromobisphenol-A, hexabromocyclododecane and decabrominated diphenyl ether: Results of the 5th Chinese Total Diet Study. Environmental Pollution. 2017;**229**: 539-547

[53] World Health Organization (WHO). Tetrabromobisphenol A and Derivatives. 1995, Environmental Health Criteria 172. International Programme on Chemical Safety [Internet] Available from: https://inchem.org/documents/ehc/ehc/ehc172.htm [Accessed: Nov 22, 2021]

[54] Yu Y, Yu Z, Chen H, Han Y, Xiang M, Chen X, et al. Tetrabromobisphenol a: Disposition, kinetics and toxicity in animals and humans. Environmental Pollution. 2019; **253**:909-917

[55] Lyche JL, Rosseland C, Berge G, Polder A. Human health risk associated with brominated flame-retardants (BFRs). Environment International. 2015;**74**:170-180

[56] Godfrey A, Abdel-moneim A, Sepúlveda MS. Acute mixture toxicity of halogenated chemicals and their next generation counterparts on zebrafish embryos. Chemosphere. 2017;**181**: 710-712

[57] Wu S, Wu M, Qi M, Zhong L, Qiu L. Effects of novel brominated flame retardant TBBPA on human airway epithelial cell (A549) in vitro and proteome profiling. Environmental Toxicology. 2018;**33**(12):1245-1253

[58] Yasmin S, Whalen M. Flame retardants, hexabromocyclododecane (HCBD) and tetrabromobisphenol a (TBBPA), alter secretion of tumor necrosis factor alpha (TNFα) from human immune cells. Archives of Toxicology. 2018;**92**(4):1483-1494

[59] Lyu L, Jin X, Li Z, Liu S, Li Y, Su R, et al. TBBPA regulates calcium-mediated lysosomal exocytosis and thereby promotes invasion and migration in hepatocellular carcinoma. Ecotoxicology and Environmental Safety. 2020;**192**: 110255

[60] Ezechiáš M, Covino S, Cajthaml T. Ecotoxicity and biodegradability of new brominated flame retardants: A review. Ecotoxicology and Environmental Safety. 2014;**110**:153-167

[61] Hou R, Lin L, Li H, Liu S, Xu X, Xu Y, et al. Occurrence, bioaccumulation, fate, and risk assessment of novel brominated flame retardants (NBFRs) in aquatic environments—A critical review. Water Research. 2021;**198**:117168

[62] Xiong P, Yan X, Zhu Q, Qu G, Shi J, Liao C, et al. A review of environmental occurrence, fate, and toxicity of novel brominated flame retardants. Environmental Science and Technology. 2019;**53**(23):13551-13569

[63] Klinčić D, Dvoršćak M, Jagić K, Mendaš G, Herceg RS. Levels and distribution of polybrominated diphenyl ethers in humans and environmental compartments: A comprehensive review of the last five years of research. Environmental Science and Pollution Research. 2020;**27**(6):5744-5758

[64] Meeker JD, Stapleton HM. House dust concentrations of organophosphate flame retardants in relation to hormone levels and semen quality parameters. Environmental Health Perspectives. 2010;**118**(3):318-323

[65] He MJ, Luo XJ, Chen MY, Sun YX, Chen SJ, Mai BX. Bioaccumulation of polybrominated diphenyl ethers and decabromodiphenyl ethane in fish from a river system in a highly industrialized area, South China. Science of The Total Environment. 2012;**419**: 109-115

[66] Zhang Y, Luo XJ, Wu JP, Liu J, Wang J, Chen SJ, et al. Contaminant pattern and bioaccumulation of legacy and emerging organhalogen pollutants in the aquatic biota from an e-waste recycling region in South China. Environmental Toxicology and Chemistry. 2010;**29**(4):852-859

[67] Zhang XL, Luo XJ, Liu HY, Yu LH, Chen SJ, Mai BX. Bioaccumulation of several brominated flame retardants and dechlorane plus in waterbirds from an e-waste recycling region in South China: Associated with trophic level and diet sources. Environmental Science and Technology. 2011;**45**(2):400-405

[68] Egloff C, Crump D, Chiu S, Manning G, McLaren KK, Cassone CG, et al. In vitro and in ovo effects of four brominated flame retardants on toxicity and hepatic mRNA expression in chicken embryos. Toxicology Letters. 2011; **207**(1):25-33

[69] Nakari T, Huhtala S. In vivo and in vitro toxicity of decabromodiphenyl ethane, a flame retardant. Environmental Toxicology. 2010;**25**(4): 333-338

[70] Smythe TA, Butt CM, Stapleton HM, Pleskach K, Ratnayake G, Song CY, et al. Impacts of unregulated novel brominated flame retardants on human liver thyroid deiodination and Sulfotransferation. Environmental

Science and Technology. 2017;**51**(12): 7245-7253

[71] Larsson A, Eriksson LA, Andersson PL, Ivarson P, Olsson PE. Identification of the brominated flame retardant 1,2-Dibromo-4-(1,2-dibromoethyl)cyclohexane as an androgen agonist. Journal of Medicinal Chemistry. 2006;**49**(25): 7366-7372

[72] Harju M, Heimstad ES, Herzke D, Sandanger T, Posner S, Wania F. Emerging "new" brominated flame retardants in flame retarded products and the environment. Oslo, Norway: Statens Forurensningstilsyn, Norwegian Pollution Control Authority. 2009;1–114

[73] Wang F, Wang J, Dai J, Hu G, Wang J, Luo X, et al. Comparative tissue distribution, biotransformation and associated biological effects by decabromodiphenyl ethane and decabrominated diphenyl ether in male rats after a 90-day oral exposure study. Environmental Science & Technology. 2010;**44**(14):5655-5660

[74] Sun RB, Shang S, Zhang W, Lin BC, Wang Q, Shi Y, et al. Endocrine disruption activity of 30-day dietary exposure to decabromodiphenyl ethane in Balb/C mouse. Biomedical and Environmental Sciences: BES. 2018; **31**(1):12-22

[75] Bearr JS, Stapleton HM, Mitchelmore CL. Accumulation and DNA damage in fathead minnows (Pimephales promelas) exposed to 2 brominated flame-retardant mixtures, Firemaster 550 and Firemaster BZ-54. Environmental Toxicology and Chemistry. 2010;**29**(3):722-729

[76] Laoutid F, Bonnaud L, Alexandre M, Lopez-Cuesta JM, Dubois P. New prospects in flame retardant polymer materials: From fundamentals to nanocomposites. Materials Science and Engineering R: Reports. 2009;**63**(3): 100-125

[77] Tang G, Zhou L, Zhang P, Han Z, Chen D, Liu X, et al. Effect of aluminum diethylphosphinate on flame retardant and thermal properties of rigid polyurethane foam composites. Journal of Thermal Analysis and Calorimetry. 2020;**140**(2):625-636

[78] Chen Y, Liu Q, Ma J, Yang S, Wu Y, An Y. A review on organophosphate flame retardants in indoor dust from China: Implications for human exposure. Chemosphere. 2020;**260**:127633

[79] Zhang Y, Su H, Ya M, Li J, Ho SH, Zhao L, et al. Distribution of flame retardants in smartphones and identification of current-use organic chemicals including three novel aryl organophosphate esters. Science of The Total Environment. 2019;**693**:133654

[80] Wang Q, Zhao H, Xu L, Wang Y. Uptake and translocation of organophosphate flame retardants (OPFRs) by hydroponically grown wheat (*Triticum aestivum* L.). Ecotoxicology and Environmental Safety. 2019;**174**:683-689

[81] Huang Y, Tan H, Li L, Yang L, Sun F, Li J, et al. A broad range of organophosphate tri- and di-esters in house dust from Adelaide, South Australia: Concentrations, compositions, and human exposure risks. Environment International. 2020;**142**:105872

[82] Kubwabo C, Fan X, Katuri GP, Habibagahi A, Rasmussen PE. Occurrence of aryl and alkyl-aryl phosphates in Canadian house dust. Emerging Contaminants. 2021;7: 149-159

[83] Ma C, Wang J, Yuan Y, Mu X, Pan Y, Song L, et al. An insight into gas phase flame retardant mechanisms of AHP versus AlPi in PBT: Online pyrolysis vacuum ultraviolet photoionization time-of-flight mass spectrometry. Combustion and Flame. 2019;**209**:467-477

[84] Jiang H, Bi M, Ma D, Li B, Cong H, Gao W. Flame suppression mechanism of aluminum dust cloud by melamine cyanurate and melamine polyphosphate. Journal of Hazardous Materials. 2019;(368):797-810

[85] Al-Salem AM, Saquib Q, Siddiqui MA, Ahmad J, Wahab R, Al-Khedhairy AA. Organophosphorus flame retardant (tricresyl phosphate) trigger apoptosis in HepG2 cells: Transcriptomic evidence on activation of human cancer pathways. Chemosphere. 2019;**237**: 124519

[86] Wang D, Zhu W, Chen L, Yan J, Teng M, Zhou Z. Neonatal triphenyl phosphate and its metabolite diphenyl phosphate exposure induce sex- and dose-dependent metabolic disruptions in adult mice. Environmental Pollution. 2018;**237**:10-17

[87] Persson J, Wang T, Hagberg J. Organophosphate flame retardants and plasticizers in indoor dust, air and window wipes in newly built low-energy preschools. Science of The Total Environment. 2018;**628–629**:159-168

[88] Zhang X, Sühring R, Serodio D, Bonnell M, Sundin N, Diamond ML. Novel flame retardants: Estimating the physical–chemical properties and environmental fate of 94 halogenated and organophosphate PBDE replacements. Chemosphere. 2016;**144**: 2401-2407

[89] Niu Y, Liu J, Liang Y, Hao Z, Liu J, Liu Y, et al. Aluminum dialkyl phosphinate flame retardants and their hydrolysates: Analytical method and occurrence in soil and sediment samples from a manufacturing site. Environmental Science and Technology. 2014;**48**(6):3336-3343

[90] Chen X, Hu Y, Song L. Thermal behaviors of a novel UV cured flame retardant coatings containing phosphorus, nitrogen and silicon. Polymer Engineering & Science. 2008; **48**(1):116-123

[91] Tao F, Abdallah MA-E, Harrad S. Emerging and legacy flame retardants in UK indoor air and dust: Evidence for replacement of PBDEs by emerging flame retardants? Environmental Science & Technology. 2016;**50**(23):13052-13061

[92] Björnsdotter MK, Romera-García E, Borrull J, de Boer J, Rubio S, Ballesteros-Gómez A. Presence of diphenyl phosphate and aryl-phosphate flame retardants in indoor dust from different microenvironments in Spain and the Netherlands and estimation of human exposure. Environment International. 2018;**112**:59-67

[93] Giulivo M, Capri E, Eljarrat E, Barceló D. Analysis of organophosphorus flame retardants in environmental and biotic matrices using on-line turbulent flow chromatography-liquid chromatography-tandem mass spectrometry. Journal of Chromatography A. 2016;**1474**:71-78

[94] Li J, Yu N, Zhang B, Jin L, Li M, Hu M, et al. Occurrence of organophosphate flame retardants in drinking water from China. Water Research. 2014;**54**:53-61

[95] Kim U-J, Kannan K. Occurrence and distribution of organophosphate flame retardants/plasticizers in surface waters, tap water, and rainwater: Implications

for human exposure. Environmental Science & Technology. 2018;**52**(10): 5625-5633

[96] Zha D, Li Y, Yang C, Yao C. Assessment of organophosphate flame retardants in surface water and sediment from a freshwater environment (Yangtze River, China). Environmental Monitoring and Assessment. 2018;**190**(4):222

[97] Lee S, Cho HJ, Choi W, Moon HB. Organophosphate flame retardants (OPFRs) in water and sediment: Occurrence, distribution, and hotspots of contamination of Lake Shihwa, Korea. Marine Pollution Bulletin. 2018;**130**: 105-112

[98] Chen P, Ma S, Yang Y, Qi Z, Wang Y, Li G, et al. Organophosphate flame retardants, tetrabromobisphenol a, and their transformation products in sediment of e-waste dismantling areas and the flame-retardant production base. Ecotoxicology and Environmental Safety. 2021;**225**:112717

[99] Choo G, Lee IS, Oh JE. Species and habitat-dependent accumulation and biomagnification of brominated flame retardants and PBDE metabolites. Journal of Hazardous Materials. 2019; **371**:175-182

[100] Du J, Li H, Xu S, Zhou Q, Jin M, Tang J. A review of organophosphorus flame retardants (OPFRs): Occurrence, bioaccumulation, toxicity, and organism exposure. Environmental Science and Pollution Research. 2019;**26**(22): 22126-22136

[101] Wang W, Qing X, Wang J, He T, Fan R, Huang Y. Bioaccumulation and potential risk of organophosphate flame retardants in coral reef fish from the Nansha Islands, South China Sea. Chemosphere. 2022;**287**(P1): 132125

[102] Fang Y, Kim E, Strathmann TJ. Mineral- and base-catalyzed hydrolysis of organophosphate flame retardants: Potential major fate-controlling sink in soil and aquatic environments. Environmental Science & Technology. 2018;**52**(4):1997-2006

[103] Wang Y, Sun H, Zhu H, Yao Y, Chen H, Ren C, et al. Occurrence and distribution of organophosphate flame retardants (OPFRs) in soil and outdoor settled dust from a multi-waste recycling area in China. Science of The Total Environment. 2018;**625**: 1056-1064

[104] Sánchez-Piñero J, Bowerbank SL, Moreda-Piñeiro J, López-Mahía P, Dean JR. The occurrence and distribution of polycyclic aromatic hydrocarbons, bisphenol A and organophosphate flame retardants in indoor dust and soils from public open spaces: Implications for human exposure. Environmental Pollution. 2020;**266**:115372

[105] Tang B, Poma G, Bastiaensen M, Yin SS, Luo XJ, Mai BX, et al. Bioconcentration and biotransformation of organophosphorus flame retardants (PFRs) in common carp (*Cyprinus carpio*). Environment International. 2019;**126**:512-522

[106] Li N, Ho W, Sun Wu RS, Ying GG, Wang Z, Jones K, et al. Organophosphate flame retardants and bisphenol a in children's urine in Hong Kong: Has the burden been underestimated? Ecotoxicology and Environmental Safety. 2019;**183**:109502

[107] Gu Y, Yang Y, Wan B, Li M, Guo LH. Inhibition of O-linked N-acetylglucosamine transferase activity in PC12 cells—A molecular mechanism of organophosphate flame retardants developmental neurotoxicity.

Biochemical Pharmacology. 2018;**152**: 21-33

[108] Sun L, Xu W, Peng T, Chen H, Ren L, Tan H, et al. Developmental exposure of zebrafish larvae to organophosphate flame retardants causes neurotoxicity. Neurotoxicology and Teratology. 2016;**55**:16-22

[109] Du Z, Wang G, Gao S, Wang Z. Aryl organophosphate flame retardants induced cardiotoxicity during zebrafish embryogenesis: By disturbing expression of the transcriptional regulators. Aquatic Toxicology. 2015; **161**:25-32

[110] Alzualde A, Behl M, Sipes NS, Hsieh JH, Alday A, Tice RR, et al. Toxicity profiling of flame retardants in zebrafish embryos using a battery of assays for developmental toxicity, neurotoxicity, cardiotoxicity and hepatotoxicity toward human relevance. Neurotoxicology and Teratology. 2018; **70**:40-50

[111] Abe FR, de Oliveira AÁS, Marino RV, Rialto TCR, Oliveira DP, Dorta DJ. A comparison of developmental toxicity of brominated and halogen-free flame retardant on zebrafish. Ecotoxicology and Environmental Safety. 2021;**208**:111745

[112] Waaijers SL, Bleyenberg TE, Dits A, Schoorl M, Schütt J, Kools SAE, et al. Daphnid life cycle responses to new generation flame retardants. Environmental Science and Technology. 2013;**47**(23):13798-13803

[113] Liu X, Ji K, Choi K. Endocrine disruption potentials of organophosphate flame retardants and related mechanisms in H295R and MVLN cell lines and in zebrafish. Aquatic Toxicology. 2012;**114–115**: 173-181

[114] An J, Hu J, Shang Y, Zhong Y, Zhang X, Yu Z. The cytotoxicity of organophosphate flame retardants on HepG2, A549 and Caco-2 cells. Journal of Environmental Science and Health, Part A. 2016;**51**(11):980–988

[115] Patisaul HB, Mamta B, Birnbaum LS, Blum A, Diamond ML, Fernández SR, et al. Beyond cholinesterase inhibition: Developmental neurotoxicity of organophosphate Ester flame retardants and plasticizers. Environmental Health Perspectives. 2021;**129**(10):105001

[116] Castorina R, Bradman A, Stapleton HM, Butt C, Avery D, Harley KG, et al. Current-use flame retardants: Maternal exposure and neurodevelopment in children of the CHAMACOS cohort. Chemosphere. 2017;**189**:574-580

[117] Lee JS, Morita Y, Kawai YK, Covaci A, Kubota A. Developmental circulatory failure caused by metabolites of organophosphorus flame retardants in zebrafish, Danio rerio. Chemosphere. 2020;**246**:125738

[118] Chupeau Z, Bonvallot N, Mercier F, Le BB, Chevrier C, Glorennec P. Organophosphorus flame retardants: A global review of indoor contamination and human exposure in Europe and epidemiological evidence. International Journal of Environmental Research and Public Health. MDPI AG. 2020;**17**:1-24

[119] Rhyu DY, Lee H, Tanguay RL, Kim KT. Tris(1,3-dichloro-2-propyl) phosphate (TDCIPP) disrupts zebrafish tail fin development. Ecotoxicology and Environmental Safety. 2019;**182**:109449

[120] Wang C, Chen H, Li H, Yu J, Wang X, Liu Y. Review of Emerging Contaminant Tris(1,3-Dichloro-2-Propyl)Phosphate: Environmental

Occurrence, Exposure, and Risks to Organisms and Human Health, Environment International. Vol. 143. Amsterdam, Netherland: Elsevier Ltd; 2020:105946

[121] World Health Organization (WHO). Flame Retardants: Tris (chloropropyl) Phosphate and Tris(2-Chloroethyl) Phosphate. 1998. World health Organization [Internet] Available from: https://apps.who.int/iris/handle/10665/42148. [Accessed: Nov 18, 2021]

[122] Scientific Committee on Health and Environmental Risks (SCHER). Risk Assessment Report on 2,2-Bis (chloromethyl)trimethylene bis[bis(2-chloroethyl)phosphate] (V6) Environmental Part. 2007. European Commission [Internet] Available from: https://ec.europa.eu/health/ph_risk/committees/04_scher/docs/scher_o_067.pdf. [Accessed: Nov 18, 2021]

[123] Marklund A, Andersson B, Haglund P. Screening of organophosphorus compounds and their distribution in various indoor environments. Chemosphere. 2003; **53**(9):1137-1146

[124] Van den Eede N, Dirtu AC, Neels H, Covaci A. Analytical developments and preliminary assessment of human exposure to organophosphate flame retardants from indoor dust. Environment International. 2011;**37**(2):454-461

[125] Vykoukalová M, Venier M, Vojta Š, Melymuk L, Bečanová J, Romanak K, et al. Organophosphate esters flame retardants in the indoor environment. Environment International. 2017;**106**: 97-104

[126] Chen Y, Zhang Q, Luo T, Xing L, Xu H. Occurrence, distribution and health risk assessment of organophosphate esters in outdoor dust in Nanjing, China: Urban vs. rural areas. Chemosphere. 2019;**231**:41-50

[127] Li-zhing Z, Xue-fen C, Jing W. PAHs in aquatic sediment in Hangzhou, China: Analytical methods, pollution pattern, risk assessment and sources. Jounal of Environmental Sciences. 2005; **17**(5):748-755

[128] Luo Q, Gu L, Wu Z, Shan Y, Wang H, Sun L. Distribution, source apportionment and ecological risks of organophosphate esters in surface sediments from the Liao River, Northeast China. Chemosphere. 2020;250:126297

[129] Mihajlović I, Miloradov MV, Fries E. Application of twisselmann extraction, SPME, and GC-MS to assess input sources for organophosphate esters into soil. Environmental Science and Technology. 2011;**45**(6):2264-2269

[130] Zhong M, Wu H, Mi W, Li F, Ji C, Ebinghaus R, et al. Occurrences and distribution characteristics of organophosphate ester flame retardants and plasticizers in the sediments of the Bohai and yellow seas. China. Science of the Total Environment. 2018;**615**: 1305-1311

[131] Martínez-Carballo E, González-Barreiro C, Sitka A, Scharf S, Gans O. Determination of selected organophosphate esters in the aquatic environment of Austria. Science of the Total Environment. 2007;**388**(1–3): 290-299

[132] Meyer J, Bester K. Organophosphate flame retardants and plasticisers in wastewater treatment plants. Journal of Environmental Monitoring. 2004;**6**(7):599-605

[133] Greaves AK, Letcher RJ, Chen D, McGoldrick DJ, Gauthier LT,

Backus SM. Retrospective analysis of organophosphate flame retardants in herring gull eggs and relation to the aquatic food web in the Laurentian Great Lakes of North America. Environmental Research. 2016;**150**:255-263

[134] Bollmann UE, Möller A, Xie Z, Ebinghaus R, Einax JW. Occurrence and fate of organophosphorus flame retardants and plasticizers in coastal and marine surface waters. Water Research. 2012;**46**(2):531-538

[135] Maruya KA, Dodder NG, Sengupta A, Smith DJ, Lyons JM, Heil AT, et al. Multimedia screening of contaminants of emerging concern (CECS) in coastal urban watersheds in southern California (USA). Environmental Toxicology and Chemistry. 2016;**35**(8):1986-1994

[136] Hu M, Li J, Zhang B, Cui Q, Wei S, Yu H. Regional distribution of halogenated organophosphate flame retardants in seawater samples from three coastal cities in China. Marine Pollution Bulletin. 2014;**86**(1–2): 569-574

[137] Ding J, Shen X, Liu W, Covaci A, Yang F. Occurrence and risk assessment of organophosphate esters in drinking water from eastern China. Science of the Total Environment. 2015;**538**:959-965

[138] Campone L, Piccinelli AL, Östman C, Rastrelli L. Determination of organophosphorous flame retardants in fish tissues by matrix solid-phase dispersion and gas chromatography. In: Analytical and Bioanalytical Chemistry, vol. 397, 2010. pp. 799-806

[139] Harino H, Yatsuzuka E, Yamao C, Ueno M, Ohji M. Current status of organophosphorus compounds contamination in Maizuru Bay, Japan. Journal of the Marine Biological Association of the United Kingdom. 2014;**94**(1):43-49

[140] Ma Y, Cui K, Zeng F, Wen J, Liu H, Zhu F, et al. Microwave-assisted extraction combined with gel permeation chromatography and silica gel cleanup followed by gas chromatography-mass spectrometry for the determination of organophosphorus flame retardants and plasticizers in biological samples. Analytica Chimica Acta. 2013;**786**:47-53

[141] Sundkvist AM, Olofsson U, Haglund P. Organophosphorus flame retardants and plasticizers in marine and fresh water biota and in human milk. Journal of Environmental Monitoring: JEM. 2010;**12**(4):943-951

[142] Poma G, Sales C, Bruyland B, Christia C, Goscinny S, Van Loco J, et al. Occurrence of organophosphorus flame retardants and plasticizers (PFRs) in Belgian foodstuffs and estimation of the dietary exposure of the adult population. Environmental Science and Technology. 2018;**52**(4):2331-2338

[143] Kim UJ, Wang Y, Li W, Kannan K. Occurrence of and human exposure to organophosphate flame retardants/ plasticizers in indoor air and dust from various microenvironments in the United States. Environment International. 2019;(125):342-349

[144] Abdallah MAE, Covaci A. Organophosphate flame retardants in indoor dust from Egypt: Implications for human exposure. Environmental Science and Technology. 2014;**48**(9): 4782-4789

[145] Abou-Elwafa Abdallah M, Pawar G, Harrad S. Human dermal absorption of chlorinated organophosphate flame retardants; implications for human

exposure. Toxicology and Applied Pharmacology. 2016;**291**:28-37

[146] Sugeng EJ, de Cock M, Leonards PEG, van de Bor M. Toddler behavior, the home environment, and flame retardant exposure. Chemosphere. 2020;**252**:126588

[147] United States Environmental Protection Agency (EPA). TSCA Workplan Chemical Problem Formulation and Initial Assessment Chlorinated Phosphate Ester Cluster Flame Retardants. 2015 [Internet] Available from: https://www.epa.gov/assessing-and-managing-chemicals-under-tsca/tsca-work-plan-chemical-problem-formulation-and-0. [Accessed: Nov 18, 2021]

[148] Yoshida K, Ninomiya S, Esumi Y, Kurebayashi H, Ohno Y, Takahashi A. Pharmacocinetic study of tris(2-chloroethyl)phosphate (TCEP) after inhalation exposure. Toxicology and Environmental Health. 1997;**43**:9

[149] Kim JW, Isobe T, Muto M, Tue NM, Katsura K, Malarvannan G, et al. Organophosphorus flame retardants (PFRs) in human breast milk from several Asian countries. Chemosphere. 2014;**116**:91-97

[150] Nomeir' AA, Kato S, Matthews HB, Nomeir AA, Kato S. The metabolism and disposition of tris(l,3-dichloro-2-propyl) phosphate (Fyrol FR-2) in the rat the metabolism and disposition of tris(1,3-dichloro-2-propyl) phosphate (Fyrol FR-2) in the rat. Oxicology and Applied Pharmacology. 1981;**57**:401-413

[151] Freudenthal RI, Henrich RT. Chronic toxicity and carcinogenic potential of tris-(1,3-dichloro-2-propyl) phosphate in Sprague-Dawley rat. International Journal of Toxicology. 2000;**19**:119-125

[152] Hoffman K, Lorenzo A, Butt CM, Hammel SC, Henderson BB, Roman SA, et al. Exposure to flame retardant chemicals and occurrence and severity of papillary thyroid cancer: A case-control study. Environment International. 2017;**107**:235-242

[153] ECHA. European Chemicals Agency: Annex1-Document to RAC Opinion on TDCP. 2010. [Internet] Available from: https://www.echa.europa.eu/documents/10162/26d19254-81a6-f16a-8182-e7824d66bfec. [Accessed: Nov 18, 2021]

[154] Ben-Jonathan N, LaPensee CR, LaPensee EW. What can we learn from rodents about prolactin in humans? Endocrine Reviews. 2008;**29**:1-41

[155] Xu T, Wang Q, Shi Q, Fang Q, Guo Y, Zhou B. Bioconcentration, metabolism and alterations of thyroid hormones of tris(1,3-dichloro-2-propyl) phosphate (TDCPP) in zebrafish. Environmental Toxicology and Pharmacology. 2015;**40**(2):581-586

[156] Zhao F, Wang J, Fang Y, Ding J, Yang H, Li L, et al. Effects of tris(1,3-dichloro-2-propyl)phosphate on pathomorphology and gene/protein expression related to thyroid disruption in rats. Toxicology Research. 2016;**5**(3):921-930

[157] Dishaw LV, Powers CM, Ryde IT, Roberts SC, Seidler FJ, Slotkin TA, et al. Is the PentaBDE replacement, tris (1,3-dichloro-2-propyl) phosphate (TDCPP), a developmental neurotoxicant? Studies in PC12 cells. Toxicology and Applied Pharmacology. 2011;**256**(3):281-289

[158] Leisewitz A, Kruse H, Schramm E. Substituting environmentally relevant flame retardants: Assessment

fundamentals. In: Results and Summary Overview. Federal Environmental Agency, Berlin, Germany. Vol. 1. 2001. p. 1-204

[159] Gatti N. New red phosphorus masterbatches find new application areas in thermoplastics. Plastics, Additives and Compounding. 2002;**4**(4): 34-37

[160] Levchik SV, Weil ED. A review of recent progress in phosphorus-based flame retardants. Journal of Fire Science. 2016;**24**(5):345-364. DOI: 101177/ 0734904106068426

Section 2

Metals and Metalloids

Chapter 2

Heavy Metal Contamination of Water and Their Toxic Effect on Living Organisms

Anubhav Singh, Anuj Sharma, Rohit K. Verma, Rushikesh L. Chopade, Pritam P. Pandit, Varad Nagar, Vinay Aseri, Sumit K. Choudhary, Garima Awasthi, Kumud K. Awasthi and Mahipal S. Sankhla

Abstract

Water has become a major threat in today's world. Collection of heavy metals, a few of them, is potentially toxic and these get distributed to different areas through different pathways. With an increase in the earth's population, development and industrialization are taking place rapidly and these get the major source of water contamination. With heavy metals in lakes, rivers, groundwater, and various water sources, water gets polluted by the increased concentration of heavy metals and metalloids through release from the suddenly mine tailings, disposal of high metal wastes, growing industrial areas, leaded gasoline and paints, usage of fertilizers inland, animal manures, E-waste, sewage sludge, pesticides, wastewater irrigation, coal, etc. Exposure to heavy metals has been linked to chronic and acute toxicity, which develops retardation; neurotoxicity can damage the kidneys, lead to the development of different cancers, damage the liver and lungs; bones can become fragile; and there are even chances of death in case of huge amount of exposure. This chapter mainly focuses on heavy metal pollution in water and its toxic effect on living organisms.

Keywords: heavy metal, water, toxicity, pollution, living organisms

1. Introduction

Expeditious expansion and industrial development near the rivers have led to more stress on the river, and with increased stress, the water becomes polluted, and worsening environmental health is observed [1]. The water-soil interface and the water-atmosphere interface are the medium through which the heavy metals travel [2, 3]. Both anthropogenic activities and geochemical processes are responsible for heavy metal contamination in ecosystems [4]. Elements that have high density and are less noxious are known as heavy metals. Examples of heavy metals are lead, iron, mercury, cadmium, zinc, arsenic, copper, and chromium and the actual volume of these heavy metals is more than 6 g/m^3 [5]. Heavy metals have the property of

IntechOpen

environmental persistence and bioaccumulation, and these heavy metals enter the aquatic system through various routes. These heavy metals not only impair the quality of the aquatic ecosystem but also human health [6, 7]. These heavy metals can be found on the layer of earth in their regular form. These heavy metals are so dangerous that they cannot be degraded or decomposed and they have the arability to bioaccumulate [8]. These heavy metals once get into the ecosystem through the air, via drinkable water, or multiple chemicals and products that are manmade. The route of administration of these heavy metals is via inhalation, ingestion, and skin absorption. These heavy metals get into the biosphere via human activities, which include industrial production, mining, agriculture, and transportation [9]. Some methods are fossil fuel burning, smelting of different, waste from the municipality, fertilizers, pesticides, and sewage these all are considered to be the primary sources of metal pollution [10–13]. The toxicity of these heavy metals in the human body reduces energy levels; disrupts brain functioning; disturbs the functioning of various other organs such as the brain, lungs, liver, and kidney; and also hinders blood composition. If the contact with heavy metals continues, then it can hinder the physical, neurological, and muscular functioning. And due to these diseases like multiple sclerosis, Parkinson's disease and muscular dystrophy, and Alzheimer's disease. Chronic exposure to some of the heavy metals and their compounds may even cause cancer [14]. Pollution of these heavy metals into the river may cause distressing effects on the ecological balance of the aquatic environment, and with the extent of contamination, the diversity of aquatic organisms becomes limited [15]. The fish in the aquatic ecosystem can be used for examining the well-being of biota. Due to pollutants in the food chain of organisms, harmful effects can be seen and the aquaculture can become dead [16]. These heavy metals are neurotoxins for the fish living in the aquatic environment. When these heavy metals enter the fish body, they interact with them to generate biochemical reaction inside the fish, which makes it difficult for fish to communicate with their surroundings [17]. The presence of these heavy metals leads to diseases like Minamata, which is organic mercury poisoning. When these heavy metals get bioaccumulated, they become a threat to both the human population and animals who uses that water [18]. Modeling of risk assessment is divided into four stages, i.e.,

Heavy metal ions	WHO's permissible limit (mg L^{-1})
Se	0.02
Hg	0.001
Mn	0.02
Ag	0.1
Cd	0.05
Cr	0.003
Pb	0.01
Zn	3.00
Fe	0.30
Cu	0.02
As	0.01

Table 1.
Permissible limit of heavy metal ions in water [21].

exposure assessment, toxicity (dose-response) assessment, hazard identification, and risk characterization. There are three pathways through which humans get exposed to traced metals, which include directly ingesting, inhaling through the mouth or nose, and via skin absorption when it gets exposed. From the water, the heavy metals usually enter through ingestion and dermal absorption. To assess exposure, the average daily dose is measured for pollutants through different identified paths. In a dose-response assessment for no carcinogens, reference doses (RfD) are calculated, and for carcinogens, slope factors (SF) are obtained by the United States Environment Protection Agency (USEPA) Integrated Risk Information System (IRIS) database. With the help of the facts which are discussed above, there was a study done with an aim to evaluate the water quality of the Subarnarekha River relating to metals, their temporal classification, source of identification, and assessment of human health risk when that water was ingested or the contaminate when absorbed through the skin. Through this, it is possible to know the contamination level and accordingly, the strategies were planned (**Table 1**) [19, 20].

2. Source of contamination in water

The presence of these heavy metals on the surface of the water can be due to natural or anthropogenic activities. In natural activities, weathering of rocks that contain metals, an eruption from volcanos, fires in the forest, and naturally occurring processes of weathering can be included. From these activities, metal enters the different sections of the environment. Heavy metals can be found in the forms of sulfates, hydroxides, oxides, sulfides, phosphates, and silicates [12, 22]. A huge amount of accumulation of heavy metals into the water is mainly due to anthropogenic and natural activities. Some more examples of natural source through which heavy metals contaminates water are, wet and dry deposition of atmospheric salts, water-rock interaction, or water interaction with the soil. While the sudden increase in urbanization and industrialization are an example of anthropogenic sources through which water get contaminated (**Table 2**; **Figure 1**) [23].

2.1 Natural sources

Trace metals are found in excess levels in the environment, they are formed by geographical processes such as volcanic eruptions, weathering of rocks, and leaching into rivers, lakes, and oceans due to the action of water [25]. The presence of heavy metals in water depends on the local geology, hydrogeology, and geochemical characteristics of the aquifer [26]. One of the main sources of pollution is weathering. The weathering of the sedimentary rocks such as limestone or dolomite or shale makes the water contaminated or polluted. When there is an interaction of water with rock element, it also leads addition of these elements into the water; thus, contamination occurs. Examples of such elements are granite, syenite, basalt, gabbro, nepheline, and andesite. Due to the particular ore or the minerals, the element level increases. Elements examples are magnetite, hematite, goethite, siderite, calcite, cuprite, malachite, azurite, chromite, kaolinite, montmorillonite, arsenic trioxide, orpiment, arsenopyrite, calamine, smithsonite, pyrolusite, and rhodochrosite [27–30]. The sulfide deposition also increases as it is associated with the mineralization of the gold and hydrous iron oxide ores [31].

Heavy metal ion	Common sources
Copper (Cu)	Fertilizers, tanning, and photovoltaic cells
Zinc (Zn)	Soldering, cosmetics, and pigments
Silver (Ag)	Refining of copper, gold, nickel, zinc, jewelry, and electroplating industries
Chromium (Cr)	Leather industry, tanning, and chrome plating industries
Arsenic (As)	Wooden electricity poles that are treated with arsenic-based preservatives, pesticides, fertilizers, the release of untreated effluents, oxidation of pyrite (FeS) and arsenopyrite (FeAsS)
Mercury (Hg)	Combustion of coal, municipal solid waste incineration, and volcanic emissions
Cadmium (Cd)	Paints, pigments, electroplated parts, batteries, plastics, synthetic rubber, photographic and engraving process, photoconductors, and photovoltaic cells
Lead (Pb)	PVC pipes in sanitation, agriculture, recycled PVC lead paints, jewelry, lead batteries, lunch boxes, etc.

Table 2.
Major sources of some heavy metal ions in water [24].

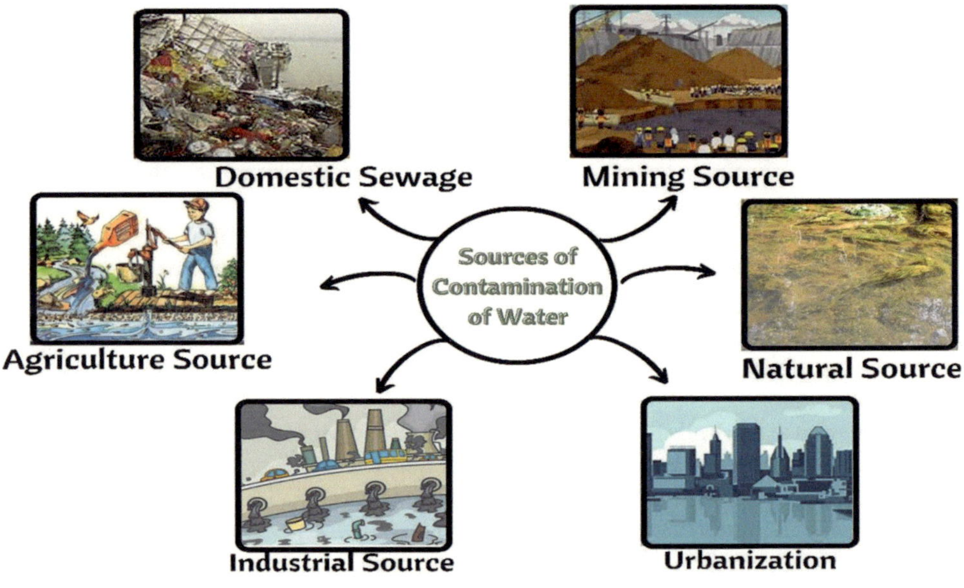

Figure 1.
Contamination of water through different sources.

2.2 Anthropogenic sources

Anthropogenic events, in which human settlement replaced the natural forest and agricultural activities have increased the environmental impacts. Such activities have contaminated the aquatic ecosystems, which include spring waters from the river like the Amala and Nyangores, tributaries of Mara River, Indonesia in Mau Complex. The maximum of forest land is converted into human settlement and agriculture. People who live near the Mara River Basin use that spring water for the purpose of animal and agricultural purposes [21]. The water carrying capacity has decreased with the rapid increase in industrialization and urbanization. Hg concentration in water has increased with agriculture activities and human activities. Activities like domestic sewage into the water, solid waste burning, coal and oil combustions, and pyrometallurgical processes and mining are the main reason for this. Water, by either snow or rain, brings the contaminated soil with Hg into the adjacent water areas [32, 33]. The source of Ni is the corroded metal pipes and containers [34]. The major source of lead in water majorly comes from additives of paints and petrol and aerosol precipitation, which is formed due to the high temperature used in industrial processes for the purpose of coal combustion, smelting, and cement production [35], and chloralkali, batteries, fluorescent lamps, thermometers, and electronic switches production. Chemical industries are some industrial activities through which Hg pollutes the water system and these activities are the largest contributor to Hg contamination in the environment [36].

2.3 Domestic sewage

Huge amount of untreated sewage from domestic is thrown into the river. This untreated waste from domestic has the presence of toxins. These toxins are due to the presence of solid waste or from the litter of plastic, or the contamination of bacteria due to the presence of these the water can get polluted. Domestic untreated water is thrown directly into the water resource and this majorly causes pollution inside the water and harms the ecosystem [37]. These pollutants majorly depend upon what kind of industry has thrown those pollutants. When these toxic metals get inside the water, they decrease the quality of the water [38]. Around 25% of pollution inside the water is caused only by these industries [39]. When the water gets contaminated, the water gets enriched by the nitrogen and phosphorous elements. With the presence of these nutrients, the growth rate of algae gets multiplied, and then it competed with the surrounding aquatic biota for the dissolved oxygen in water [40]. The presence of nitrite and nitrate anions leads to a major threat to the exposed organisms; examples of such threats are methemoglobinemia. It is more common in small children, and the symptoms caused by this are cyanotic color in the skin due to blood alterations [41]. Water sources that get deposited by this sewage also become anions rich, due to the presence of chlorine in urine, and NaCl is used in the human diet. On the side of the sea, there is the presence of chloride in high concentrations due to the leakage of salt into the sewerage system. It also may be increased by industrial processes [42].

2.4 Industrial source

Contamination of heavy metals in the aquatic environment is very harmful since these elements cannot be degraded and they get accumulated inside the living organisms [43]. Residue from the industry is the major source through which these heavy metals get into the aquatic ecosystems, and their accumulation in water varies with the type of wastewater treatment used [44]. Effects known as deleterious can be observed when the metal particles are introduced into the water system [45, 46]. Different metals from the Amazon River (Brazil) and the Yukon River (Alaska) were analyzed in the solid-state only. Plants have the presence of these metals in water. In tissue, the concentration of several metals is slow, and their concentration should be kept in less range only as more concentration can be harmful to the biological development of the pant [47]. Through the food chain, fish contaminants can reach man [48]. Effluent from industries, water tank leakages, dumping beside marines, and due to radioactive waste and atmospheric deposition, are some sources of water contamination. Disposed of heavy metals and waste from industries they get accumulated in rivers and lakes thus causing harmful impacts on animals and humans. For suppression of the immune, reproductive failure and acute poisoning toxins are responsible [49]. Then there is direct damage to plant or animal nutrition at that time human health is affected. The pollutants that are polluting the water are killing marine organisms such as mollusks, marine birds, fishes, and other organisms that live in the sea [50].

2.5 Urbanization

With an increase in the population has created many issues and one of the issues is the pollution of water [38]. An increase in the population leads automatically leads to more generations of solid waste [51]. Both solid waste and liquid waste are deposited into the water without any treatment. Human excreta also contaminate the water. Thus, contaminated water leads to a generation of a large number of bacteria, which is a threat to human well-being [39]. Government is unable to supply vital requirements to the People because of the increase in the number of people. Facility for sanitization is more in urban areas as compared to rural areas. Plastic bag and waste are a major contribution to pollution. People throw the waste in plastic bags into water sources [24]. From the research, it was found that around three crore people of the population defecate in the open, while 77% population use flush and around 8% use the pit latrines. Urbanization can cause many infectious diseases. Overpopulation, unhealthy conditions, and dangerous drinkable water are these major health problems in urban areas. One-third of urban people are vulnerable to disease [37].

2.6 Agriculture source

The population in rural areas is less but the use of fertilizers, pesticides, and eroded soil contaminates the water. When it rains the water from the surface runoff and that rainwater enters the nearby water resource and thus pollutes the existing water [52]. Agricultural runoff cases freshwater bodies' eutrophication. Half of the lakes in the US are eutrophic. Phosphate has one of the major contributions to eutrophication. And the high concentration of phosphates promotes cyanobacteria and algae growth, which leads to the excessive use of the biologically dissolved oxygen inside the water [53]. Fertilizers that are too enriched with nitrogen decrease the dissolved oxygen in rivers and coastal zones thus bringing hazardous effects to the biota. Since 2006, the nitrogen in fertilizers is being controlled in America and Northwest Europe [54]. Like pesticides, which are used as pest control, these pesticides leach into groundwater, thus polluting groundwater. The pesticides that are water-soluble leach more and the sandy soil favors the process of leaching [55].

2.7 Atmospheric source

Small pollutants particles which are present in the air, get into the water stream through the rain, when it rains these particles come down and then with the flow of water enters into the sea, thus polluting the water there. These pollutants that are present in the air usually get from the burning of fossil fuels e.g. is CO_2, which combines with water and produces sulfuric acid. Sulfur dioxide, which is formed via volcanic eruption and from industries, also gets attached to a water molecule to form the sulfuric acid. When coal is combusted then also sulfuric dioxide is produced and it is also produced from petroleum products. Just like this nitrogen dioxide also combines with the water and forms the nitric acid. And with the help of rainwater, they enter the water resources (**Figure 2**) [52, 56–59].

2.8 Mining source

Heavy metals are present on the earth and thus they can enter the water system through various pathways and one of them is through mining sources. When it rains or through flowing water, it leaches heavy metals out from their geological formation. These processes get disturbed when manmade economic activities such as mining are done. Through these processes, the area that is already mined out gets exposed to water and air and this leads to the acid mine drainage (AMD). The low pH conditions associated with AMD mobilize heavy metals, including radionuclides where these are present [60].

2.9 Heavy metal intake through water

Soil gets polluted with the presence of heavy metal on surface and underground water and the pollution rises when mined ores are discarded on the ground surface for manual dressing [61]. Due to the dumping over the surface, the metals get exposed to air and rain thereby generating huge AMD. If soil is polluted at that time, it gets into the plant tissue and gets accumulated there. And when those plants are grazed

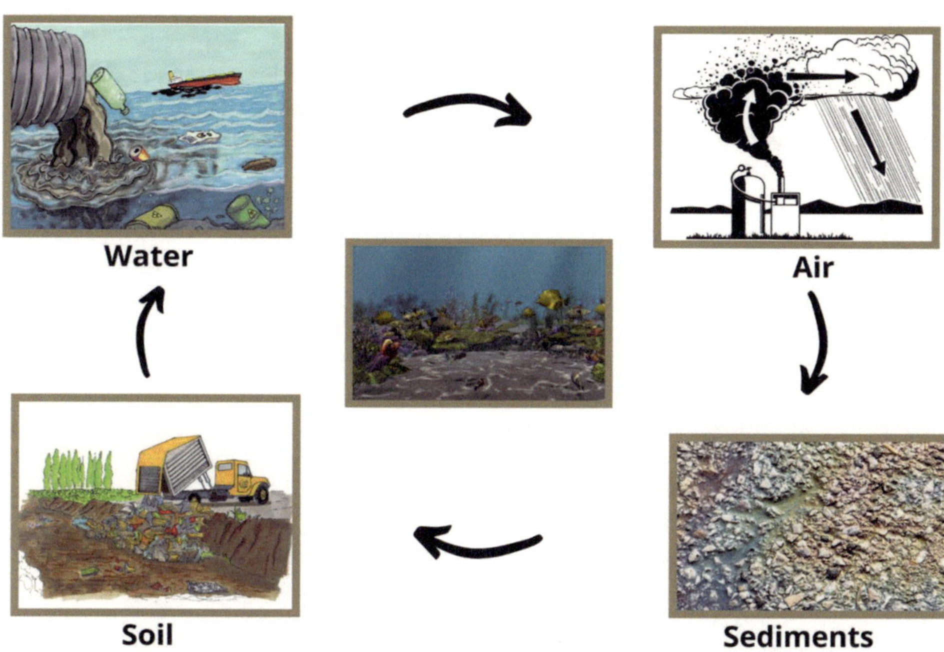

Figure 2.
Circulation of contaminants between environmental sources under the effect of atmospheric sources.

by animals and water is used for the drink from polluted waters, through there these heavy metals enter the body. Also, marine lives, which reproduce in contaminated water, also have the presence of heavy metals inside their body tissues, if they are lactating then inside their milk. As an overview, all organisms within a given ecosystem are contaminated via these pollutants through their food chains [62]. When nutrition from these contaminated vegetables is taken, the presence of heavy metals in those vegetables can lead to different chronic diseases. Toxic effects due to these heavy metals usually depend on the amount of concentration and the oxidative state of the particular heavy metals [63]. Heavy metals have a very dangerous impact as they are non-biodegradable in nature, have long biological half-lives, and have the potential to accumulate inside the body. Also, there are some heavy metals that are extremely toxic only because of their solubility. Fewer concentrations of heavy metals inside the food chain also show severe effects as there is no particular procedure through which these heavy metals pollutants can be extracted from the body of an organism. Nowadays presence of these toxic heavy metals is everywhere because of their extreme use in industries. In case of the wastewater, it contains a huge concentration of heavy metals, which create various health-related problems [64, 65].

3. Effect on living organism

3.1 Effect on aquatic environment

Water from estuaries and freshwater is not polluted till now to some extent, but that water is also at threat of being polluted in the long term due to metal deposition because of human past activities [66]. The water in the river and lakes can be highly polluted depending on the volume of flow and proximity to the point sources. Due to the human civilization, the element content in water is raised. Such elements are cadmium, lead, mercury, zinc, and chromium. Unlike organic chemicals, there are some metals that cannot be converted into compounds with lesser toxicity, and one of its characteristics is the loss of biodegradability. Once the heavy metals enter the water system it gets redistributed throughout the column and gets accumulated in the sediments [67]. The sediments constitute a partial contribution to polluting the natural phenomena due to their activity and metal remobilization processes. Metal residues that are present in the contaminated surroundings have the flexibility to get bioaccumulated into the aquatic environment [68]. Growth in fish larvae and juveniles is rapid. But when these heavy metals enter they might inhibit the growth rate. The fish grows in length and bulk when given the right conditions, such as a specific temperature and an acceptable amount of food. Fish growth, on the other hand, may be impeded in water contaminated with toxicants, such as heavy metals. One of the most noticeable signs of metal toxicity in fish larvae is growth inhibition. As a result, the length and bulk of fish are indications of environmental conditions [69]. Heavy metals are introduced in liquid form and surface water constituents (carbonate, sulfate, organic substances humic, fulvic, and amino acids) cause the formation of non-soluble salts or complexes. Aquatic species are not expected to be harmed by these salts and compounds. Some of them sink and collect in the sediments at the bottom. A decrease in pH of water either due to acid rain or any other acidic incidents, due to the heavy metal's deposition into the water column, causes aquatic biota to become poisonous. Low levels of heavy metals can also make chronic stress, through fish might not get dead but can cause them to lose weight and become smaller, reducing their capacity to compete for food and habitat [70]. Pollution poses a hazard to both freshwater and marine habitats. Heavy metal poisoning of water is a significant environmental hazard that has detrimental consequences for organisms who are exposed to it be that plant-animal or humans. Fish from freshwater are majorly exposed to various heavy metals, which are added into the water bodies through the different-different sources. Contamination of these heavy metals into aquaculture has intensified global issues because it shows a risk to fish and has harmful impacts on fish buyers [71]. There are three different modes through which heavy metals enter the fish. These methods are either through the gills of fish, by the body of the fish, or by the digestive tract of the fish. Heavy metals immediately enter the fish body through the gills, while the body surface takes time for uptaking of these heavy metals through this mode [72]. Mostly the metals get accumulated in the liver, kidney, and gills. In fishes, the muscles have most of the metals present there as compared to the other body parts of the fish. Too much accumulation of these heavy metals inside the fish organ can cause lesions and operative disturbances [73]. These heavy metals also interfered with the embryo's shape and the metabolic processes of the fishes. Structural and functional defects throughout the development of the embryo resulted in fewer larvae hatching. Several freshly born larvae die shortly after hatching owing to lead and copper absorption [74, 75]. Heavy metals get into the fish through three routes: the first is via the fish gills, the second is through the digestive tract of the fish and the last one is through the body of the fish. The gills of fish are the area that is known for the primary metal intake from the contaminated water. On the fish gills, zinc accumulates. It suggests a depressing influence on tissue respiration, which leads to hypoxia and mortality. Zinc pollution also causes alterations in the structure of the lungs and heart [76]. Humans and fish are both affected by mercury. Brain damage, with postnatal and fetal problems, leads to abortions, congenital deformity, and development differences in young fry due to Monomethyl. Minamata illness and Hg poisoning (via methyl Hg) both showed considerable neurotoxicity [77]. Nickel is necessary for tiny amounts for the formation of RBC, but when its concentration gets increased, at that time, it becomes harmful or poisonous. Cd has been linked to an increase in blood pressure and cardiac illness in fish. Blood vessels damage, hemorrhages, and depletion of blood cell count of a fish are induced by Hg, from previous research. Anemia, eosinophilia, lymphocytosis, bronchial, and renal injuries can affect chromium levels in the blood [18]. Malformations in fish are caused by cadmium, nickel, mercury, chromium, lead, and arsenic. The accumulation of these heavy metals in excessive amounts causes a variety of physiological effects. Fin loss, gill underdevelopment, liver dysfunction, and fin function in fingerlings were all prevalent findings in the studies [78]. The harmful effects of heavy metals have the greatest impact on the death rate, reproduction, individual development rates, and physiological capacity of fish. There have been effects on physical functioning and chemical parameters in the tissues and blood of fish living in water that is polluted via metals. It has been reported that fish exposed to metals developed immune system defects, making them more susceptible to infectious infections and increasing their chances of dying (**Figure 3**) [79].

3.2 Effects on aquatic plants

For the growth of plants, few HMs like As, Cd, Hg, Pb, and Se are not important as they do not perform any known physiological function in them. Others, such as Co, Cu, Fe, Mn, Mo, Ni, and Zn, are key elements that are required for regular plant

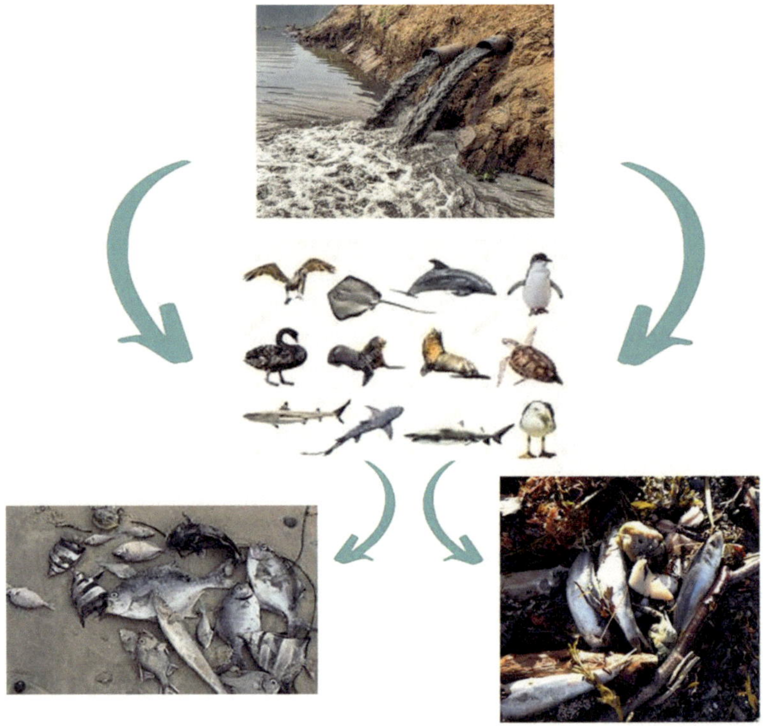

Figure 3.
Harmful effects on the aquatic environment.

development and metabolism, but their amounts can quickly exceed the appropriate levels, resulting in poisoning [80, 81]. Heavy metal concentrations in plants vary by plant species, and the efficiency with which various plants absorb metals is measured by plant absorption or metal transfer factors from soil to plant. An increased amount of Pb in agricultural soil decreases the productivity rate of the soil, and a less lead amount may hinder some important processes of plant, dark green leaves, withering of older leaves, stunted foliage, and brown short roots are poisonous indicators of photosynthesis, mitosis, and water absorption [82]. Heavy metals are poisonous and phytotoxic to plants, resulting in diseases such as chlorosis, poor plant development, and yield depression, as well as decreased nutrient absorption, plant metabolic problems, and a reduced capacity to fix molecular nitrogen in leguminous plants. Seed germination was gradually reduced in the presence of increasing levels of lead, it may be due to exposure to lead for a longer duration, some methods, such as leaching, chelation, metal binding, or microbe accumulation, have resulted in the neutralization of lead's harmful effects [83]. Heavy metals such as Cd, Pb, and Ni even their small concentration in plants can be hazardous to them. Poisoning due to this heavy metal will result in the complex interplay between the primary unpleasant ions and additional necessary or non-essential ions. Metals affect the activity of enzymes by swapping metal ions from metal enzymes, as well as preventing plant growth [84]. Some exceptional metals are vital for plants, as they reveal their roles in the catabolism of plants and biosynthesis, together as cofactors for enzymes and as metabolic yields. For example, Zn, Fe, Cu, Cr, and Co are the important nutrients but when their amounts are increased, they become toxic. Comparatively, Pb and Cd have no effect, which is favorable to the plant and is solely lethal [85]. The most abundant hazardous elements in the soil are lead. Pb poisoning in the soil is caused by municipal sewage sludge discharge, mining and smelting operations, Pb-containing paints, paper and pulp, gasoline, and explosives. They do not have any role in the shape of the plant or their growth and photosynthetic process of the plant. Pb poisoning also inhibits enzyme action, creates an imbalance of the water, alters membrane permeability, and disrupts mineral feeding [86].

3.3 Effects on fish

One of the main sources of contamination of the water is heavy metals, as it overwhelms the important species indirectly through biological chains or directly via chemical modifications in water. Three potential ways are there, through which heavy metals get into the fish body: though fish gills, through the body of the fish, and through the fish digestive tract. Gills are responsible for the immediate absorption of metals from the water, whereas the body surface is thought to have a smaller role in the intake of these elements in fish [87]. By altering the normal activities of numerous enzymes and metabolites, the accumulation of these heavy metals in the tissues causes significant biochemical, physiological, and histological changes in fish and other freshwater fauna. Fish are one of the most widely dispersed creatures in the aquatic ecosystem, and their susceptibility to metal poisoning may indicate the extent of metal pollution's biological impact [88]. Heavy metals, such as As, Cd, Cu, Cr, Fe, Pb, Mn, Hg, Ni, Zn, and tin (Sn), are major contaminants that cause serious toxicity in fish. Due to the heavy metals, the physiological and biochemical functions both in tissues and in blood Carpi can be altered. The compounds of As and inorganic As, Cd, Ni, silica in its crystal form, beryllium, and its compounds are considered to be chemical carcinogens, which results in the development of cancer inside the fishes. The drop in hematological parameters indicated that the exposed fishes had become anemic as a result of Cr exposure. This dangerous heavy metal was released into the aquatic ecosystem via trash, causing severe anemia and changes in hematological parameters in the *Labeo rohita* fish [89]. There are various studies on different fish such as *Noemacheilus barbatulus*, *Perca fluviatilis*, *Catostomus commersonii*, *Oreochromis mossambicus*, and *Oreochromis aureus*, and increased quantities of zinc, lead, cadmium, copper, mercury, and cadmium were found in the gonads of fish, according to the study. This causes contamination of eggs and sperm, as well as a reduction in fish fertility and embryonic development [90]. The number of hatched larvae was reduced due to anatomical and functional abnormalities during embryonic development. A percentage of freshly born larvae died shortly after hatching as a result of lead and copper absorption [75]. The sensitivity of heavy metals inhibits estrogenic and androgenic secretion and produces pathological differentiation in fish. The reproductive tissues of fish gonads are affected by effluents such as industrial and agricultural waste, pesticides, and heavy metals [91, 92]. Zinc gets accumulated over the gills of fish. It entails a depressing influence on tissue respiration, which leads to hypoxia and death. Zinc contamination also causes abnormalities in the structure of the ventilator and heart. Zinc is a toxicant that destroys gill tissue, disrupts acid–base and ion balance, and causes hypoxia in fish [93]. More importantly, heavy metal for neurotoxicity is Hg. While other factors play a role in neurotoxicity, mercury has a major impact on both fish and humans. Japan's rivers have been contaminated with mercury. Minamata illness and Hg poisoning (via methyl Hg) both showed considerable neurotoxicity [77]. Arsenic coagulates proteins, binds to coenzymes, and reduces the production of adenosine triphosphate (ATP) during respiration. It can induce cancer in all of its oxidation states in combination, and high-level articulation can result in mortality. Carcinogenic metals such as cadmium, arsenic, nickel, and chromium [94] can damage DNA by deleting base pairs, mutating it, or attacking it with radical oxygen. Malformations in fish are caused by cadmium, nickel, mercury, chromium, lead, and arsenic. When the accumulation of these heavy metals gets excessive inside the water through this, many physical effects on fish can be seen. Fins get shortened; gills are underdeveloped; and liver and fin functions of fingerlings were commonly observed. The harmful effects of heavy metals have the greatest impact on the death rate, individual growth rates, reproduction, and physiological capacity of fish. The effects of metal pollution on physiological processes and biochemical parameters in the blood and tissue of fish have been studied. Fish that are exposed to heavy metals reveal faults in the immune system and thus are more exposed to diseases and chances of death increase [79].

4. Conclusion

Water pollution is a global problem, and the world's population is suffering the consequences of tainted water. Living organisms are also affected by the polluted water very much and it is very harmful to the environment. Acute and choric illnesses are caused by heavy metal concentrations in drinking water that exceed the permissible limits set by several national and international organizations. These can range from nonfatal, such as muscle and physical weakness, to fatal, such as brain, nervous system, and even cancer. Water quality testing is necessary for the protection of human health and the environment.

Author details

Anubhav Singh[1], Anuj Sharma[2], Rohit K. Verma[3], Rushikesh L. Chopade[2], Pritam P. Pandit[2], Varad Nagar[2], Vinay Aseri[2], Sumit K. Choudhary[1], Garima Awasthi[4], Kumud K. Awasthi[4] and Mahipal S. Sankhla[2]*

1 School of Forensic Science and Risk Management, Rashtriya Raksha University, Gujarat, India

2 Department of Forensic Science, Vivekananda Global University, Jaipur, Rajasthan, India

3 Dr. APJ Abdul Kalam Institute of Forensic Science and Criminology, Bundelkhand University, U.P., India

4 Department of Life Sciences, Vivekananda Global University, Jaipur, Rajasthan, India

*Address all correspondence to: mahipal.sankhla@vgu.ac.in

References

[1] Giri S, Singh AK. Risk assessment, statistical source identification and seasonal fluctuation of dissolved metals in the Subarnarekha River, India. Journal of Hazardous Materials. 2014;**265**:305-314

[2] Ali MM et al. Assessment of toxic metals in water and sediment of Pasur River in Bangladesh. Water Science and Technology. 2018;**77**(5):1418-1430

[3] Varol M. Assessment of heavy metal contamination in sediments of the Tigris River (Turkey) using pollution indices and multivariate statistical techniques. Journal of Hazardous Materials. 2011;**195**:355-364

[4] Li GH, Cao ZM, Lan DZ, Xu J, Wang SS, Yin W. Spatial variations in grain size distribution and selected metal contents in the Xiamen Bay China. Environmental Geology. 2007;**52**(8):1559-1567

[5] Tavakoli-Hosseinabady B et al. Detoxification of heavy metals from leafy edible vegetables by agricultural waste: Apricot pit shell. Journal of Environmental & Analytical Toxicology. 2018;**8**(1):548

[6] Meng T et al. Determinants of urban consumer expenditure on aquatic products in Shanghai, China. Aquaculture Economics & Management. 2021:1-24

[7] Sharma M et al. Kinetics of sorption of lead on bed sediments of River Hindon, India. Environmental Monitoring and Assessment. 2009;**157**(1):11-21

[8] Baby J et al. Toxic effect of heavy metals on aquatic environment. International Journal of Biological and Chemical Science. 2010;**4**(4):1-39

[9] Sardar K et al. Heavy metals contamination and what are the impacts on living organisms. Greener Journal of Environmental Management and Public Safety. 2013;**2**(4):172-179

[10] Nriagu JOJN. A global assessment of natural sources of atmospheric trace metals. Nature. 1989;**338**(6210):47-49

[11] Nriagu JOJN. Global inventory of natural and anthropogenic emissions of trace metals to the atmosphere. Nature. 1979;**279**(5712):409-411

[12] Kabata-Pendias A, Pendias H. Trace Elements in Soil and Plants. London: CRC Press; 1984

[13] Rai PK. Technology, Heavy metal phytoremediation from aquatic ecosystems with special reference to macrophytes. Critical Reviews in Environmental Science and Technology. 2009;**39**(9):697-753

[14] Ghosh L, Adhikari S, Ayyappan SJRJET. Assessment of toxic interactions of heavy metals and their effects on accumulation in tissues of fresh water fish. Research Journal of Environmental Toxicology. 2007;**1**:37-44

[15] Ay T et al. Bioconcentration of metals in the body muscle and gut of Clarias gariepinus exposed to sublethal concentrations of soap and detergent effluent. Journal of Cell and Animal Biology. 2009;**3**(8):113-118

[16] Sankhla MS, Kumar R. New and advanced technologies in aquaculture to support environmentally sustainable development. In: Microbial

Biotechnology: Basic Research and Applications. Germany: Springer; 2020. pp. 249-263

[17] Baatrup EJCB, Pharmacology PPCC. Structural and functional effects of heavy metals on the nervous system, including sense organs, Fisheries. Comparative Biochemistry and Physiology Part C: Comparative Pharmacology. 1991;**100**(1-2):253-257

[18] Sonone SS et al. Water contamination by heavy metals and their toxic effect on aquaculture and human health through food Chain. Letters in Applied NanoBioScience. 2020;**10**(2):2148-2166

[19] Means B. Risk-Assessment Guidance for Superfund. Volume 1. Human Health Evaluation Manual. Part A. Interim report (Final). Washington, DC (USA): Environmental Protection Agency; 1989 Office of Solid Waste

[20] Wu B et al. Preliminary risk assessment of trace metal pollution in surface water from Yangtze River in Nanjing Section, China. Bulletin of Environmental Contamination and Toxicology. 2009;**82**(4):405-409

[21] Sankhla et al. Seasonal Variations of Lead and chromium concentration in the water samples from Yamuna River in Delhi, India. Iranian Journal of Toxicology. 2021;**15**(2):109-114

[22] Salgarello M, Visconti G, Barone-Adesi L. Interlocking circumareolar suture with undyed polyamide thread: A personal experience. Aesthetic Plastic Surgery. 2013;**37**(5):1061-1062

[23] Priti P, Paul B. Assessment of heavy metal pollution in water resources and their impacts: A review. Journal of Basic and Applied Engineering Research. 2016;**3**(8):671-675

[24] Gumpu MB et al. A review on detection of heavy metal ions in water–An electrochemical approach. Sensors and Actuators B: Chemical. 2015;**213**:515-533

[25] Bagul V et al. New perspective on heavy metal pollution of water. Journal of Chemical and Pharmaceutical Research. 2015;**7**(12):700-705

[26] Wang S, Mulligan CN. Occurrence of arsenic contamination in Canada: Sources, behavior and distribution. Science of the Total Environment. 2006;**366**(2-3):701-721

[27] Wedepohl KH. The composition of the continental crust. Geochimica et cosmochimica Acta. 1995;**59**(7):1217-1232

[28] Ball JW, Izbicki JJAG. Occurrence of hexavalent chromium in ground water in the western Mojave Desert, California. Applied Geochemistry. 2004;**19**(7):1123-1135

[29] Viers J et al. Evidence of Zn isotopic fractionation in a soil–plant system of a pristine tropical watershed (Nsimi, Cameroon). Chemical Geology. 2007;**239**(1-2):124-137

[30] Hüffmeyer N, Klasmeier J, Matthies M. Geo-referenced modeling of zinc concentrations in the Ruhr river basin (Germany) using the model GREAT-ER. Science of the Total Environment. 2009;**407**(7):2296-2305

[31] Nordstrom DKJS. Worldwide Occurrences of Arsenic in Ground Water. Washington D.C.: American Association for the Advancement of Science; 2002. pp. 2143-2145

[32] Kowalski A, Siepak M, Boszke L. Mercury Contamination of Surface and Ground Waters of Poznań, Poland.

Polish Journal of Environmental Studies. 2007;**16**(1)

[33] Wang Q et al. Sources and remediation for mercury contamination in aquatic systems—A literature review. Environmental Pollution. 2004;**131**(2):323-336

[34] Cempel M, Nikel GJPJS. Nickel: A review of its sources and environmental toxicology. Polish Journal of Environmental Studies. 2006;**15**(3):375-382

[35] Li Y et al. The distribution of dissolved lead in the coastal waters of the East China Sea. Marine Pollution Bulletin. 2014;**85**(2):700-709

[36] Li P et al. Mercury pollution in Asia: A review of the contaminated sites. Journal of Hazardous Materials. 2009;**168**(2-3):591-601

[37] Kamble SM. Water pollution and public health issues in Kolhapur city in Maharashtra. International Journal of Scientific and Research Publications. 2014;**4**(1):1-6

[38] Ho Y et al. Industrial discharge and their effect to the environment. Industrial Waste, Intech. 2012:1-39

[39] Desai N. SmtVanitaben. A study on the water pollution based on the environmental problem. Indian Journal of Research. 2014;**3**(12):95-96

[40] Moore JW, Moore EA. Resources in environmental chemistry. I. An annotated bibliography of the chemistry of pollution and resources. Journal of Chemical Education. 1976;**53**(3):167

[41] Sankhla et al. Impact of variation in climatic changes in concentration of Lead & Nickel in Yamuna River Water, Delhi, India. Materials Today: Proceedings. Elsevier; 2022

[42] Baird RB et al. Standard Methods for the Examination of Water and Wastewater. Vol. 23. Washington, DC: American Public Health Association; 2017

[43] Jardim WDF. Metais pesados: Um dano irreparável. Rev. Bras. Tecno. 1983;**14**(2):41-42

[44] Magossi L, P.J.S.P.E.M. Bonacella, Poluição das águas–coleção desafios. 9ª. 1992

[45] Tavares TM, Carvalho FMJQN. Avaliação de exposição de populações humanas a metais pesados no ambiente: Exemplos do recôncavo baiano. Química nova. 1992;**15**(2):147-154

[46] Gibbs RJ. Transport phases of transition metals in the Amazon and Yukon Rivers. Geological Society of America Bulletin. 1977;**88**(6):829-843

[47] Allaway W. Agronomic controls over the environmental cycling of trace elements. In: Advances in Agronomy. Netherlands: Elsevier; 1968. pp. 235-274

[48] Pfeiffer W et al. Metais pesados no pescado da Baía de Sepetiba, Estado do Rio de Janeiro. Ciência e Cultura. 1985;**37**(2):297-302

[49] Juneja T, Chaudhary A. Assessment of water quality and its effects on the health of residents of Jhunjhunu district, Rajasthan: A cross sectional study. Journal of Public Health and Epidemiology. 2013;**5**(4):186-191

[50] Khan MA, Ghouri AM. Environmental pollution: Its effects on life and its remedies. Researcher World: Journal of Arts, Science & Commerce. 2011;**2**(2):276-285

[51] Jabeen S et al. Health impact caused by poor water and sanitation in district

Abbottabad. Journal of Ayub Medical College Abbottabad. 2011;**23**(1):47-50

[52] Letchinger M. Pollution and water quality, neighbourhood water quality assessment. Project Oceanography. 2000

[53] Werner W. Fertilizers, 6. Environmental aspects. Ullmann's Encyclopedia of Industrial Chemistry. 2000

[54] Van Grinsven H et al. Management, regulation and environmental impacts of nitrogen fertilization in northwestern Europe under the Nitrates Directive; A benchmark study. Biogeosciences. 2012;**9**(12):5143-5160

[55] Ramdwar MN, Maharaj R, Siew NJSFP. Sustaining the environment: Farm and beyond the farm. 2 Sustainable Food Production: 209

[56] Larry W. World Water Day. A Billion people Worldwide Lack Safe Drinking. 2006

[57] Florescu D et al. The influence of pollution monitoring parameters in characterizing the surface water quality from Romania southern area. Romanian Journal of Physics. 2011;**56**(7-8):1001-1010

[58] Tietenberg T. Economics of pollution control, Chapter 15: Environmental and natural resource economics. 7th ed. New York, Boston: Pearson; 2006

[59] Moss B. Water pollution by agriculture. Philosophical Transactions of the Royal Society B: Biological Sciences. 2008;**363**(1491):659-666

[60] Sankhla MS et al. Heavy metals contamination in water and their hazardous effect on human health—A review. International Journal of Current Microbiology and Applied Sciences. 2016;**5**(10):759-766

[61] Garbarino J. et al. Contaminants in the Mississippi River US Geological Survey Circular 1133. 1995

[62] Truby, P., Impact of Heavy Metals on Forest Trees from Mining Areas. 2003

[63] Duruibe JO, Ogwuegbu M, Egwurugwu JN. Heavy metal pollution and human biotoxic effects. International Journal of physical sciences. 2007;**2**(5):112-118

[64] Chen Y, Wang C, Wang Z. Residues and source identification of persistent organic pollutants in farmland soils irrigated by effluents from biological treatment plants. Environment International. 2005;**31**(6):778-783

[65] Singh KP et al. Impact assessment of treated/untreated wastewater toxicants discharged by sewage treatment plants on health, agricultural, and environmental quality in the wastewater disposal area. Chemosphere. 2004;**55**(2):227-255

[66] Forstner U, Wittmann GT. Metal Pollution in the Aquatic Environment. Germany: Springer-Verlag; 1979

[67] Meybeck M, Chapman DV, Helmer R. Global freshwater quality: A first assessment. Global Freshwater Quality: A First Assessment. 1990:306-306

[68] Joshi R, Ahmed SJCES. Status and challenges of municipal solid waste management in India: A review. Cogent Environmental Science. 2016;**2**(1):1139434

[69] Sarnowski P, Jezierska B. A new coefficient for evaluation of condition of fish Electronics. Journal of Ichthyology. 2007;**2**:69-76

[70] Jadhav J. et al, Evaluation of the efficacy of a bacterial consortium for the removal of color, reduction of heavy metals, and toxicity from textile dye effluent. Bioresource Technology. 2010;**101**(1):165-173

[71] Atici T et al. The accumulation of heavy metals (Cd, Pb, Hg, Cr) and their state in phytoplanktonic algae and zooplanktonic organisms in Beysehir Lake and Mogan Lake, Turkey. African Journal of Biotechnology. 2010;**9**(4):475-487

[72] Roméo M et al. Heavy metal distribution in different fish species from the Mauritania coast. Science of the Total Environment. 1999;**232**(3):169-175

[73] Jezierska B, Witeska M. The metal uptake and accumulation in fish living in polluted waters. In: Soil and Water Pollution Monitoring, Protection and Remediation. Germany: Springer; 2006. pp. 107-114

[74] Perry DM et al. Cytogenetic effects of methylmercury in embryos of the killifish, Fundulus heteroclitus. Archives of Environmental Contamination and Toxicology. 1988;**17**(5):569-574

[75] Jezierska B et al. The effects of heavy metals on embryonic development of fish (a review). Fish Physiology and Biochemistry. 2009;**35**(4):625-640

[76] Beijer K. Sources, transport and transformation of metals in the environment. Handbook of the Toxicology of Metals. 1986;**1**:68

[77] Pandey G, Madhuri S. Heavy metals causing toxicity in animals and fishes. Research Journal of Animal, Veterinary and Fishery Sciences. 2014;**2**(2):17-23

[78] Nwabunike MO. The effects of bioaccumulation of heavy metals on fish fin over two years. Global Journal of Fisheries and Aquaculture. 2016;**4**(1):281-289

[79] Amundsen P-A et al. Heavy metal contamination in freshwater fish from the border region between Norway and Russia. Science of the Total Environment. 1997;**201**(3):211-224

[80] Garrido S et al. Heavy metals in soil treated with sewage sludge composting, their effect on yield and uptake of broad bean seeds (Vicia faba L.). Water, Air, and Soil Pollution. 2005;**166**(1):303-319

[81] Rascio N, Navari-Izzo F. Heavy metal hyperaccumulating plants: How and why do they do it? And what makes them so interesting? Plant Science. 2011;**180**(2):169-181

[82] Bhattacharyya P et al. Fractionation and bioavailability of Pb in municipal solid waste compost and Pb uptake by rice straw and grain under submerged condition in amended soil. Geosciences Journal. 2008;**12**(1):41-45

[83] Ashraf R, Ali TA. Effect of heavy metals on soil microbial community and mung beans seed germination. Pakistan Journal of Botany. 2007;**39**(2):629

[84] Agarwal SJA. Studies on the Effect of the Auto Exhaust Emission on the Mitragyna Patriflora. India: MDS University; 1999

[85] Radojevic M, Bashkin VJ.U.K. The Royal Society of Chemistry Cambridge. 1999

[86] Sharma P, Dubey RS. Lead toxicity in plants. Brazilian Journal of Plant Physiology. 2005;**17**:35-52

[87] Tekin Özan S, Aktan NJJZ. Relationship of heavy metals in water, sediment and tissues with total length,

weight and seasons of cyprinus carpio L, 1758 From Işikli Lake (Turkey). Journal of Zoology. 2012;**44**(5):1405-1416

[88] Vanisree et al. Heavy metal contamination of food crops: Transportation via food chain, human consumption, toxicity and management strategies. Environmental Impact and Remediation of Heavy Metals. Intech Open; 2022

[89] Praveena M et al. Impact of tannery effluent, chromium on hematological parameters in a fresh water fish, Labeo Rohita (Hamilton). Research Journal of Animal, Veterinary and Fishery Sciences. 2013;**1**(6):1-5

[90] Allen P. Accumulation profiles of lead and cadmium in the edible tissues of Oreochromis aureus during acute exposure. Journal of Fish Biology. 1995;**47**(4):559-568

[91] Johnson LL et al. Patterns of oocyte development and related changes in plasma 17-β estradiol, vitellogenin, and plasma chemistry in English sole Parophrys vetulus Girard. Journal of Experimental Marine Biology and Ecology. 1991;**152**(2):161-185

[92] Lye C, Frid C, Gill MJMEPS. Seasonal reproductive health of flounder Platichthys flesus exposed to sewage effluent. Marine Ecology Progress Series. 1998;**170**:249-260

[93] Vosylienė MZ, Mikalajūnė AJE. Effect of heavy metal model mixture on rainbow trout biological parameters. Ekologija. 2006;**4**:12-17

[94] Landolph JR. Molecular mechanisms of transformation of C3H/10T1/2 C1 8 mouse embryo cells and diploid human fibroblasts by carcinogenic metal compounds. Environmental Health Perspectives. 1994;**102**(suppl. 3):119-125

Chapter 3

The Toxicity of Environmental Pollutants

Bamba Massa Ismaël and Sorho Siaka

Abstract

In view of the growing threat of trace metals to human health, this work set itself the objective of documenting the toxicity of the trace metals most in contact with humans on human health through food. Thus, this study revealed that organic matter, pH and CEC are the main soil parameters that influence the passage of trace metals from soil to plants. The study also revealed that agriculture, industry and road traffic contribute greatly to the input of trace metals into the environment. Regarding the mechanisms of toxicity, the study showed that chromium VI and copper manifested their toxicity by the formation of free radicals after reduction, those of zinc, nickel, manganese and nickel resulting from the disfunctioning of homeostasis. The study showed that lead caused toxic effects by replacing certain cations such as Ca^{2+}, Mg^{2+}, Fe^{2+}, Na^{+} which have important functions in the cell. Cadmium expresses its toxicity by binding to albumin, thus altering the homeostasis of metals such as calcium. All these mechanisms have revealed both acute and chronic toxic effects.

Keywords: trace metal element, toxicological profile, toxicity

1. Introduction

The term metallic trace elements or heavy metals denote the elements of the periodic table having densities greater than 5.0 $g.cm^{-3}$. They contain metals and metalloids [1]. They are naturally present in the environment, but the various industrial revolutions and the exponential progress of heavy industries have led to an increasingly massive release of these pollutants into the environment.

The environment is made up of several compartments, which are the final recipients of these heavy metal discharges. One of these compartments is the soil. Soils are the precursors of food for the majority of the world's inhabitants; their pollution by these metals therefore presents a threat to human health. Indeed, metallic trace elements can, under certain conditions, pass from soils to crops grown on them.

Among the metallic trace elements most in contact with human food, we can cite lead, cadmium, manganese, chromium, copper, nickel and zinc. Manganese, copper, zinc and nickel are considered as trace elements. However, depending on their concentrations, studies have shown that these trace elements can have different toxicities on human health. Lead, chromium and cadmium are considered strict pollutants because of the harmful effects they can have on human health. Faced with this increasingly growing threat, several questions may arise: What are the soil parameters that influence the penetration of metals into the plants we or animals eat? Once contaminated food is consumed, what health problems are we exposed to?

To provide some answers to these concerns, the main objective of this work is to document the toxicity of the metallic trace elements mentioned above on human health through food. Specifically, it will be a question of recalling the main sources of contamination of these metallic trace elements, showing their behaviour in soils and drawing up their toxicological profiles.

2. Sources of metallic trace elements

2.1 Natural sources

Soil naturally contains metallic trace elements. They are generally in the natural pedogeochemical background (FPGN) resulting solely from the geological and pedological evolution of the soil. This natural pedogeochemical background varies greatly depending on the nature of the rock and the type of soil that has developed there [2, 3]. Other natural phenomena such as wind erosion and volcanic activities can transport metallic trace elements from one soil to another [4]. Indeed, according to Ilyinskaya and al [5], in 2018, emissions from a volcano in Hawaii had concentrations of cadmium, lead, and zinc respectively of 4.10^{-3} $\mu g.m^{-3}$, 2.10^{-3} $\mu g .m^{-3}$, 0.04 $\mu g.m^{-3}$. In addition, Ma and al in 2019 [6] showed in volcanic ash, the presence of chromium, copper, lead, zinc and manganese respectively at concentrations of 0.824 $mg.kg^{-1}$, 0.95 $mg. kg^{-1}$, 16.16 $mg.kg^{-1}$, 367 $mg.kg^{-1}$, 518.6 $mg.kg^{-1}$.

2.2 Anthropogenic origins of trace metals in soils

The main anthropogenic sources of increased fluxes of heavy metals in soils are urban and industrial discharges as well as agricultural activities [7, 8].

With regard to pollution linked to agricultural activities, inputs of trace metals come mainly from the spreading of NPK and phosphate fertilizers [9]. These types of fertilizers generally provide agricultural soils with cadmium, arsenic, chromium and lead. In addition, the application of certain pesticides, and the use of sewage sludge, untreated industrial wastewater, and landfill compost to amend agricultural plots can be an important source of chromium, molybdenum, lead, zinc, manganese, arsenic, copper, mercury, uranium, and vanadium, copper, nickel, and lead to the soil [1, 10, 11].

Industrial activities such as mineral processing, refining, galvanisation, manufacturing of electric batteries, pigments and plastics are releasing large amounts of trace metals into the environment [13].

In road traffic, the wear of car tyres and exhaust gases are also sources of nickel and zinc emissions, and lead [12–14].

3. Behaviour of trace metals in soils

In soils, trace metals, depending on their speciation, can have several types of behaviour. Since this study aims to provide information on the toxicology of these metals, we will focus on the behaviour of metals in agricultural soils, which we consider to be the most important source of food for humans.

3.1 Cadmium

Cadmium is a relatively rare element in the earth's crust, with content of between 0.1 and 1 $mg.kg^{-1}$ [15]. In soils, the mobility of cadmium is strongly dependent on the pH and organic matter content of the soil. Thus, an acid pH favours cadmium phytoavailability [16], while a high soil organic matter content significantly reduces phytoavailability [17]. Indeed, soil organic matter easily forms complexes with cadmium and thus makes it less available to plants [17, 18]. According to European Union (EU) directives, the limit value for cadmium in soils should be between 1 and 3 $mg.kg^{-1}$ [19].

3.2 Chromium

Chromium is naturally present in soils. Its content depends on the content of the parent rock in which it is found. Generally speaking, the average content in the earth's continental crust is 35 $mg.kg^{-1}$. In soil, the migration and speciation of chromium are influenced by many factors such as the valence state of chromium ions, soil pH, redox potential, soil organic matter and the concentration of manganese dioxide in the soil [20–22]. The maximum allowable chromium content in agricultural soils is 100 $mg.kg^{-1}$ [22, 23].

3.3 Copper

Copper is a relatively abundant metal in the earth's crust. Its presence in the soil is therefore natural but can be enhanced by anthropogenic activities. The concentration of copper in the earth's crust is between 10 and 100 $mg.kg^{-1}$ [24]. In soil, the availability of copper to plants depends mainly on pH, cation exchange capacity (CEC), organic matter content, the presence of iron, manganese and aluminium oxides and redox potential [1]. Thus, in neutral or basic soil with a high CEC, copper will be adsorbed to the solid phase of the soil and therefore less available to the plant.

3.4 Manganese

The origin of manganese in soils and plants is mainly from rock decomposition and to a lesser extent from anthropogenic activities. Natural levels of manganese in soils are between 400 and 1500 ppm. In the soil, manganese is moderately mobile, compared to highly fixed elements such as cesium or lead. Its mobility depends on soil characteristics such as pH, cation exchange capacity, organic matter, and especially clay content.

3.5 Nickel

Nickel is naturally present in the soil from the weathering of rocks, which may contain about 0.009%, and from volcanic eruptions [25]. The maximum permissible nickel limit in agricultural soils is 75 $mg.kg^{-1}$ [19]. Nickel uptake by plant roots is highly dependent on the pH, CEC, soil texture, water content, redox potential, organic matter content, as well as on the concentrations of competing ions such as Ca2+, Cu2+, Mg2+ and Zn2+ [25, 26].

3.6 Plomb

Natural lead levels in the soil range from 5 to 20 mg.kg^{-1}. The maximum lead content in agricultural soils set by the European Union is 300 mg.kg^{-1}. Once in the soil, the behaviour of lead depends on its speciation and also on the characteristics of the soil [27–29]. As lead is generally very bound to soil colloids, it is one of the least mobile metallic micropollutants in the soil. However, it can accumulate in the roots with little diffusion to other plant organs [30]. Lead can also be delivered directly to plants through the discharge of lead-containing fuel from automobiles. This type of discharge usually occurs when plants (lettuce, cabbage) are grown on the roadside in many African countries.

3.7 Zinc

Zinc is a ubiquitous metal in the earth's crust. According to Taylor et al. 1964 in Ondo, 2011 [31], the average zinc content of the West African land crust is between 40 and 100 mg.kg^{-1}. In soil, the important factors controlling zinc mobility are clay and organic matter contents and pH. liming, the addition of high clay content soil, iron or phosphorus reduces the transfer of zinc to plants. Thus, clays and organic matter retain zinc, while an acid pH favours its release into the soil solution [24, 32].

4. Toxicological profile of metallic trace elements through dietary intake

4.1 Cadmium

Food is one of the main sources of cadmium exposure [29]. After absorption from the gastrointestinal tract, cadmium is transported into the blood plasma, initially bound to albumin [33, 34]. Albumin-bound cadmium is preferentially absorbed by the liver.

In the liver, cadmium induces the synthesis of metallothionein and a few days after exposure, cadmium bound to metallothionein appears in the blood plasma. Due to the low molecular weight of metallothionein, this protein transports cadmium to the tubules via the glomerulus of the kidney. Cadmium then accumulates in the human kidney throughout life [35–37]. The accumulation of cadmium in the kidneys leads to the most serious chronic effect of oral cadmium exposure, which is renal toxicity. This critical effect is characterised by tubular proteinuria resulting from renal tubular dysfunction [38]. In addition, the fixation of cadmium to albumin can lead to the disruption of calcium, zinc and iron homeostasis [39]. This lack of stability of calcium, zinc and iron concentration is capable of causing liver damage.

In addition, the disruption of calcium homeostasis due to the decrease in serum parathyroid hormone (PTH) concentration induces the release of calcium from bone tissue [40, 41]. This leads to loss of strength and bone fracture. Also, having the same oxidation states as zinc, cadmium can replace the zinc present in metallothionein (MT), thus preventing this protein from acting as a free radical scavenger in the cell [42].

According to Andujar, et al., 2010 [43], cadmium also has cardiovascular, hematological and hepatic effects. Inaba et al., 2005 [44], showed that cadmium was responsible for Itaï-Itaï disease, which occurred after long exposure to a concentration of up to 1 ppm. All these health effects have led to a very low tolerable daily intake of

0.36 μg.kg^{-1} is proposed by the National Agency for Food, Environmental and Health Safety [45]. Note that acute cadmium toxicity is very rare and requires very high concentrations.

4.2 Chromium

Depending on its degree of oxidation, chromium can be a trace element or a toxic element. According to Cotte and Duret, 2011 [46], trivalent chromium (III) is implicated in the action of insulin. Although, the human body is highly exposed to chromium through ingestion, a small percentage of ingested chromium enters the body through the digestive tract [47]. In fact, chromium (VI) is more absorbed in the small intestine than chromium (III) because of the structural similarity between chromium VI and sulphates. In humans, the adsorption of chromium III does not exceed 1%, whereas that of chromium VI can be around 10% [48, 49]. Moreover, once absorbed, chromium VI represents the real danger for the human body. It can enter many cells and be reduced by hydrogen peroxide (H2O2), glutathione (GSH) reductase and ascorbic acid to produce reactive intermediates including chromium (V), chromium (IV), thiyl radicals, hydroxyl radicals, which can disrupt cellular functions by attacking DNA, membrane proteins and lipids [50, 51]. This ability to produce oxidants makes chromium VI responsible, according to the French National Institute for Occupational Safety and Health, for gastric corrosion and renal failure [52, 53]. Also, according to the Agency for Toxic Substances and Disease Registry, chromium (VI) is responsible for ulcer and anaemia. These different actions of chromium VI on the body make chromium one of the eight metals present in the top 50 toxic substances in the world [47]. The World Health Organization (WHO) has classified chromium as carcinogenic to humans [54].

4.3 Copper

Copper is an essential element for good health and the proper functioning of certain biological processes [55]. Copper in food can be in monovalent Cu (I) or divalent (Cu (II)) form [56]. The predominantly active copper uptake involves the copper transporter 1 (Ctr1) which is specific for the transport of monovalent copper (CuI) into cells (including gastrointestinal cells). Copper absorption occurs mainly in the small intestine and is likely to be inhibited by transition metals such as iron or zinc [57–59]. Copper absorbed by the small intestine is transported in the blood by binding mainly to albumin, but also transcuprein [60]. Copper is transported to the liver and can be stored in hepatocytes. Copper present in hepatocytes is mainly linked to metallothionein or transcuprein [61].

Once absorbed into the body, plays a particularly important role in seed production, disease resistance and water regulation in plants [62, 63]. As a result, it participates in various metabolic processes and maintains the functions of organisms. However, the transition of copper from its oxidised to its reduced form can lead to the production of superoxide and hydroxyl radicals which cause damage to the body [60]. Indeed, Myers and al, 1993; Sokol and al 1933 [64, 65] have shown in studies on rats that at high concentrations of copper, these radicals can attack the cell's membrane lipids. As a result, copper disrupts the total antioxidant capacity of the body [63, 66]. Free radicals from copper reduction also tend to be responsible for amyotrophic lateral sclerosis, which results in progressive muscle paralysis [67].

According to Ellingsen and al, 2015 [68], nausea is the most frequently observed symptom of acute copper toxicity. These authors showed that the minimum concentration that can cause nausea is 4 $mg.L^{-1}$. In addition, Araya and al, 2007 [69], have shown that acute effects from a single, short-term exposure to copper result in gastrointestinal manifestations.

4.4 Manganese

After ingestion manganese is absorbed in the gastrointestinal (GI) tract by passive diffusion or by active transport by divalent metal transporter 1 (DMT1), which transports other metals such as iron, copper, zinc and calcium [70]. Manganese is then distributed through the bloodstream to the liver, pancreas, bones, kidneys, brain, colon, urinary system and erythrocytes [71]. The amount of manganese absorbed from the gastrointestinal tract in humans is variable, but generally averages around 3–5% [72].

As an essential nutrient, absorbed manganese plays many physiological roles. Manganese is required for the formation of cartilage and healthy bones and for the urea cycle, and also plays a key role in wound healing [73, 74].

However, once absorbed at high concentrations, manganese can exhibit various toxic effects, of which neurotoxicity is a prominent one. Mn neurotoxicity may be associated with the interaction with other essential trace elements, including iron [75–77]. Indeed, according to the work of Olanow [78], when neurons are exposed to a high concentration of manganese, the cellular regulation of iron by the divalent metal transporter 1 (DMT1) decreases, in favour of that of manganese. This leads to an accumulation of iron in neurons and can consequently produce cellular oxidative stress that leads to neuronal damage [77, 79]. In addition, in studies on rats, Mohammad [80] found a delay in the development of the skeleton and fetal organs in pups born to pregnant rats exposed to manganese by gavage at a dose of 33 $mg.kg^{-1}.d^{-1}$. Also, Bouabid et al. in 2016 [81], showed that during ingestion of high concentrations of manganese, a decrease in neurological activity was observed in rats.

4.5 Nickel

Once absorbed into the bloodstream, nickel is bound to albumin. It can therefore go to all organs, such as the thyroid and adrenal glands, brain, kidneys, heart, liver, spleen and pancreas [82, 83]. This mobility confers beneficial effects on the body. In humans, nickel is involved in the metabolism of methionine, an amino acid involved in protein synthesis [84].

Although, easily eliminated from the body in faeces and urine, nickel can also have adverse health effects. Indeed, at high concentrations, much of the toxicity of nickel may be associated with its interference with the physiological processes of zinc, calcium and magnesium [85]. Nickel can thus replace magnesium in certain stages of complement activation. For example, replacing nickel with magnesium can increase the formation of the C3b enzyme by 40-fold, which amplifies the activation of the complement pathway [86]. Therefore, various disease states such as myocardial infarction and stroke are associated with altered transport and serum concentrations of nickel [86].

Aleksandra and Urszula in 2011 [87], reported that an accidental ingestion of 570 mg of nickel had caused cardiovascular effects and the death of a child who had 2 years old. It should be noted that the acute toxicity of nickel after oral exposure depends on the chemical form of nickel. For example, a death due to nickel-induced adult respiratory distress syndrome was reported in a worker spraying nickel using a thermal arc process [88]. The death occurred 13 days after a 90-minute exposure to an estimated nickel concentration of 382.1 mg/m3; the total nickel intake was estimated to be nearly one gram. Furthermore, Das et al. in 2002 [89], in a study on rats, demonstrated a decrease in body weight in rats after daily intakes of 8.6 $mg.kg^{-1}.d^{-1}$ for 91 days. According to some authors [85, 89], gastrointestinal disorders consisting of nausea, abdominal cramps, diarrhoea, and vomiting have been reported in workers who consumed water contaminated with nickel sulphate. To our knowledge, no study has demonstrated a carcinogenic effect of nickel, nor chronic toxicity of nickel on human health.

4.6 Lead

In contrast to manganese or nickel, lead is not a trace element and is well known to be toxic [90]. In general, absorption by ingestion is the predominant route of exposure to lead. After ingestion, lead absorbed from the gastrointestinal tract enters the bloodstream by attaching to red blood cells, which transport it to various tissues or organs in the body [91]. This distribution of Pb in the body is independent of the route of absorption. As it cannot be destroyed in the body, lead accumulates in the bones. In fact, in adults, more than 90% of the lead present in the body is stored in the adult bones, compared with 70% in children. However, certain phenomena such as pregnancy, breastfeeding, menopause and osteoporosis increase the passage of lead from the bones to the blood [92, 93].

The mechanism of lead toxicity is manifested by the ability of this metal to replace cations such as Ca2+, Mg2+, Fe2+ Na + that have important functions in the cell [94, 95]. This disrupts the metabolism of the cell and leads to significant changes in various biological processes such as cell adhesion, intra- and intercellular signalling, protein folding, ion transport, enzyme regulation and neurotransmitter release. Furthermore, this substitution may also affect protein kinase C, which regulates neuronal excitation and memory storage [96]. These phenomena will therefore lead to adverse effects on human health regardless of the age group, even if infants and young children are more at risk [96, 97]. Organic forms are more toxic to humans than inorganic forms of lead. These reach humans through the food chain [93]. The pathologies resulting from lead poisoning are numerous and can be separated into two categories: physiological disorders and neurological disorders [53]. About physiological disorders [98], demonstrated that an average concentration of 29 $\mu g.L^{-1}$ caused arterial hypertension in men. Studies have also shown that blood lead concentrations below 100 $\mu g.L^{-1}$ are associated with kidney failure [98]. Moreover, according to Robert and et al., in 2004 [99] prolonged exposure to lead can cause sterility or serious problems for the fetus in the case of a pregnant woman. There are numerous studies demonstrating the existence of neurotoxic effects of lead in adults and children. According to Oscar and al, 2017 and Sanders and al, 2009 [53, 101], lead is believed to cause a decrease in intelligence quotient in children. Also, in their studies, Hsiang and Díaz in 2011, [102] showed that this metal was the basis of neurological dysfunctions and neurodegenerative effects. According to the same authors, these disorders generally follow chronic exposure to lead. In addition, other studies have shown disturbances in cognitive and behavioural functions, resulting from changes in the brain caused by lead poisoning [100]. According to these authors, children were more affected by these disorders than adults. Also, lead poisoning leads to lead poisoning, which manifests itself by anaemia, digestive disorders and damage to the nervous system with memory loss and disturbances in cognitive and behavioural functions [103].

4.7 Zinc

The absorption of zinc after ingestion takes place in the central part of the small intestine (jejunum). Zinc is transported by metallothionein from the enterocytes to the blood. In the blood, zinc is bound to albumin which distributes it throughout the body [104]. As an essential element for living beings, it plays a major role in cellular metabolism. It is involved in enzymatic systems either as an integral part of the active site of numerous enzymes or as a cofactor regulating the activity of so-called "zinc-dependent" enzymes [32]. Zinc is therefore an essential micronutrient for human health [105]. This metal is involved in major metabolic pathways through its role in enzyme systems. It is also essential in the structure and function of a large number of macromolecules. It is implicated in gene expression and stabilises the structure of proteins [106]. Zinc also plays a role in cell signalling, hormone release and nerve transmission.

However, at high concentrations of zinc in the body, the concentration of metallothionein increases to regulate zinc. This leads to a decrease in the concentration of certain metals such as copper, whose homeostasis is ensured by metallothionein. This leads to a malfunction in the metabolism of copper, which can have several adverse effects. It is true that the acute toxicity of Zn is found in rare abnormal food conditions (poisoning). According to studies, several cases of gastrointestinal disturbances and diarrhea have been caused by high zinc ingestion [107, 108]. In a study by Samman and Roberts in 1989, and reported by the US Environmental Protection Agency [109] symptoms such as abdominal cramps, vomiting and nausea appeared in 26 of 47 healthy volunteers after six-week ingestion of zinc sulphate tablets, containing 150 $mg.kg^{-1}$ of elemental zinc, for six weeks.

In addition, Gary in 1990 [110], stated that an ingestion of 1–2 g of zinc sulphate would have resulted in a concentration of nausea and vomiting, epigastric pain, abdominal cramps and diarrhoea (often bloody), while a young boy who ingested 12 g of elemental zinc over two days suffered only lethargy, dizziness, a slight shift in gait and difficulty in writing. These studies also show that the acute effects of zinc also depend on the form of zinc ingested.

In addition, chronic toxicity can manifest itself in bone marrow effects and polyneuropathy due to concomitant copper deficiency. It may also manifest itself as anaemia resulting from the malfunction of copper metabolism. Also, excessive zinc intake over a prolonged period of time increases the risk of prostate cancer and prostate cancer-related mortality [111].

5. Conclusion

The study aimed to document the toxicity of trace metals on human health via the food chain. At the end of this work, we can retain that the trace metals retained in our study have various sources and can all be present in the soil. In the soil, some trace metals are more phytoavailable than others. Also, we can retain that the metals characterized by strict pollutants such as cadmium and lead cause serious damage to health at low concentrations due to their accumulation in the body. Elements and also easily removable, it takes high concentrations to cause more or less significant effects on health.

Author details

Bamba Massa Ismaël* and Sorho Siaka
National Polytechnic Institute Félix Houphouët-Boigny (INPHB), Yamoussoukro, Côte d'Ivoire

*Address all correspondence to: bambamassaismael2014@gmail.com

References

[1] Adriano DC. Trace elements in the terrestrial environment. 2nd ed. New York: Springer; 2001

[2] Golan A, Ben G, Jacob B, Albert K, Boqer S. Soil and Water Pollution Monitoring, Protection and Remediation. Netherlands: Springer; 2006. DOI: 10.1007/978-1-4020-4728-2

[3] Temgoua E, Ntangmo H, Tsafack H-RP, Njine T. Teneurs en éléments majeurs et oligoéléments dans un sol et quelques cultures maraîchères de la ville de dschang, cameroun. African Crop Science Journal. 2015;**23**(1):35-44

[4] Baize D. Éléments traces dans les sols Fonds géochimiques, fonds pédogéochimiques naturels et teneurs agricoles habituelles: dé fi nitions et utilités. Courr. l'environnement l'INRA. 2009;**57**:63-72

[5] Ilyinskaya E, Mason E, Wieser PE, Holland L, Liu EJ, Mather TA, et al. Rapid metal pollutant deposition from the volcanic plume of Kīlauea, Hawai'i. Communications Earth and Environment. 2021;**2**(1):1-15. DOI: 10.1038/s43247-021-00146-2

[6] Ma Q, Han L, Zhang J, Zhang Y, Lang Q, Li F, et al. Environmental risk assessment of metals in the volcanic soil of Changbai mountain. International Journal of Environmental Research and Public Health. 2019;**16**(11):2047. DOI: 10.3390/ijerph16112047

[7] Mudimbi KJK, D, Kabamba TA, Fridolin K, Kasongo B, Kisunka BY, Musola CH. Profil des métaux lourds contenus dans les plantes vivrières consommées couramment dans quelques zones minières de la province du Katanga. Journal of Applied Biosciences. 2015;**96**:9049-9054

[8] Issaka S. Phytoextraction du cadmium, du cuivre, du plomb et du zinc par cinq espèces végétales (Vetiveria nigritana (Benth.)), Oxytenanthera abyssinica (A. Rich.) Munro, Barleria repens (Ness), Cymbopogon citratus (DC.) Stapf et Lantana camara Linn. Cultivées sur d. Bobo-Dioulasso: Universite Polytechnique De Bobo-Dioulasso (UPB); 2014

[9] Franklin RE, Duis L, Brown R, Kemp T. Trace element content of selected fertilizers and micronutrient source materials. Communications in Soil Science and Plant Analysis. 2005;**36**(11-12):1591-1609. DOI: 10.1081/CSS-200059091

[10] Adjia R, Fezeu WML, Tchatchueng JB, Sorho S, Echevarria G, Ngassoum MB. Long term effect of municipal solid waste amendment on soil heavy metal content of sites used for periurban agriculture in Ngaoundere, Cameroon. African Journal of Environmental Science and Technology. 2008;**2**(12):412-421

[11] Semadi F. Faisabilté du traitement des eaux d'un oued chargé en éléments traces métalliques (ETM) par filtres plantés de macrophytes (Phragmites australis): Cas de l'Oued Meboudja-Annaba-Algérie. Annaba, Algeria: Université Badji Mokhtar Annaba; 2010

[12] Yang Z, Zhang S, Liao Y, Li Q, Wu B, Wu R. Remediation of heavy metal contamination in calcareous soil by washing with reagents: A column washing. Procedia Environmental Sciences. 2012;**16**:778-785. DOI: 10.1016/j.proenv.2012.10.106

[13] Baize D. Teneurs totales en métaux lourds dans les sols français. Le Courrier de l'environnement. l'INRA. 2010;**22**:16

[14] Chafaa M, Maatoug M, Roman T, Hellal B, Ait Hammou M. Bio-Surveillance des métaux lourds (Pb, Zn, Cu) a La Sortie De La Station d'épuration de Tiaret (Algerie) au moyen des végétaux Aquatiques: Plante Lemna Minor, Algue Spyrogyra Link Sp Et Broyophyte Fontinalis Antipyretica. European Scientific Journal. [Internet]. 2015;**11**(3):155-174. Available from: file:///C:/Users/TOSHIBA/Downloads/4995-14531-1-PB (2).pdf

[15] Bril H, Bollinger J. Comprendre les pollutions par les métaux To cite this version: les pollutions par les métaux. Actualite Chimique. 2006;**298**:54-62

[16] Barbier O, Jacquillet G, Tauc M, Cougnon M, Poujeol P. Effect of heavy metals on, and handling by, the kidney. Nephron. Physiology. 2005;**99**(4):105-110. DOI: 10.1159/000083981

[17] Quenea K, Lamy I, Winterton P, Bermond A, Dumat C. Interactions between metals and soil organic matter in various particle size fractions of soil contaminated with waste water. Geoderma. 2009;**149**(3-4):217-223. DOI: 10.1016/j.geoderma.2008.11.037

[18] Sterckeman T, Thomine S. Mechanisms of Cadmium accumulation in Plants. CRC. Critical Reviews in Plant Sciences. 2020;**39**(4):322-359. DOI: 10.1080/07352689.2020.1792179

[19] Hudcová H, Vymazal J, Rozkošný M. Present restrictions of sewage sludge application in agriculture within the European Union. Soil Water Research. 2019;**14**(2):104-120. DOI: 10.17221/36/2018-SWR

[20] Dhal B, Thatoi HN, Das NN, Pandey BD. Chemical and microbial remediation of hexavalent chromium from contaminated soil and mining/metallurgical solid waste: A review Journal of Hazardous Materials. 2013;**250-251**:272-291. DOI: 10.1016/j.jhazmat.2013.01.048

[21] Zayed AM, Terry N. Chromium in the environment: Factors affecting biological remediation. Plant and Soil. 2003;**249**:139-156

[22] Keumean KN, Bamba SB, Soro G, Soro N, Soro B, Biemi J. Concentration en métaux lourds des sédiments de l' estuaire du fleuve Comoé à Grand-Bassam (Sud-Est de la Côte d' Ivoire). Journal of Applied Biosciences. 2013;**61**:4530-4539

[23] Hans Wedepohl K. The composition of the continental crust. Geochimica et Cosmochimica Acta. 1995;**59**(7):1217-1232. DOI: 10.1016/0016-7037(95)00038-2

[24] Kabata-pendias A, Pendias H. Trace Elements in Soils and Plants. 4th ed. Boca Raton: CRC Press; 2001

[25] Tamponnet C, Gonze MA, Santucci P. Fiche radionucléide: Nickel 63 et environnement. IRSN. Direction de l'environnement et de l'intervention. Service d'étude du Comportement des radionucléides dans les écosystèmes. 2002. p. 11

[26] Morris JW, Scheckel KG, McNear DH. Biogeochemistry of nickel in soils plants, and the Rhizosphere. In: Christos DT, Jö R, Selim HM, editors. Nickel in Soils and Plants. Boca Raton: CRC Press; 2018. p. 51-80. DOI: 10.1201/9781315154664-3

[27] McKenzie RM. The adsorption of lead and other heavy metals on oxides of manganese and iron. Australian Journal of Soil Research. 1980;**18**(1):61-73. DOI: 10.1071/SR9800061

[28] Sivakumar KK, Balamurugan C, Ramakrishnan D, Bhai LH. Assessment studies on wastewater pollution by textile dyeing and bleaching industries at Karur, Tamil Nadu. Rasayan Journal of Chemistry. 2011;**4**(2):264-269

[29] Soudek P, Kotyza J, Lenikusová I, Petrová Š, Benešová D, Vaněk T. Accumulation of heavy metals in hydroponically cultivated garlic (Allium sativum L.), onion (Allium cepa L.), leek (Allium porrum L.) and chive (Allium schoenoprasum L.). Journal of Food, Agriculture and Environment. 2009;7(3-4):761-769

[30] Tahar K. Étude de contamination, d'accumulation et de mobilité de quelques métaux lourds dans des légumes, des fruits et des sols agricoles situes près d'une décharge industrielle de l'usine Alzinc de la ville de Ghazaouet [thèse]. Tlemcen: Université Abou Bekr Belkaid; 2012

[31] Ondo JA. Vulnérabilité des sols maraîchers du Gabon (région de Libreville): Acidification et mobilité des éléments métalliques [thèse]. Marseille: Université de Provence Spécialité Sciences de l'Environnement Terrestre. École doctorale des Sciences de l'Environnement; 2011

[32] Finney LA, O'Halloran TV. Transition metal speciation in the cell: Insights from the chemistry of metal ion receptors. Science. 2003;**300**(5621):931-936. DOI: 10.1126/science.1085049

[33] Kjellstrom T, Nordberg GF. Model of Cadmium in the Human Being. Environmental Research. 1978;**16**:248-269

[34] Cherian MG, Goyer RA, Valberg LS. Gastrointestinal absorption and organ distribution of oral cadmium chloride and cadmium-metallothionein in mice. Journal of Toxicology and Environmental Health. 1978;**4**(5-6):861-868. DOI: 10.1080/15287397809529707

[35] Nordberg GF, Nogawa K, Nordberg M. Cadmium. 4th ed. Vol. 1. Academic Press Inc.(London) Ltd. 2014

[36] Perama YMI, Rashid NSA, Fadzil SM, Siong KK. Absorption, distribution and elimination behaviours of cadmium treated by in vitro DIN from WLP residue using SAAM II modeling. Sains Malaysiana. 2018;**47**(3):611-618. DOI: 10.17576/jsm-2018-4703-23

[37] Agency for Toxic Substances and Disease Registry. Toxicological Profile for Cadmium. Agency for Toxic Substances and Disease Registry; 2012. DOI: 10.1016/s1090-3798(09)70033-9

[38] Nordberg GF et al. Risk assessment of effects of cadmium on human health (IUPAC Technical Report). Pure and Applied Chemistry. 2018;**90**:1-54

[39] Schaefer HR, Dennis S, Fitzpatrick S. Cadmium: Mitigation strategies to reduce dietary exposure. Journal of Food Science. 2020;**85**(2):260-267. DOI: 10.1111/1750-3841.14997

[40] Schutte R et al. Bone resorption and environmental exposure to cadmium in women: A population study. Environmental Health Perspectives. 2008;**116**(6):777-783. DOI: 10.1289/ehp.11167

[41] Chen X, Wang Z, Zhu G, Nordberg GF, Jin T, Ding X. The association between cumulative cadmium intake and osteoporosis and risk of fracture in a Chinese population. Journal of Exposure Science & Environmental Epidemiology. 2019;**29**(3):435-443. DOI: 10.1038/s41370-018-0057-6

[42] McNeill RV, Mason AS, Hodson ME, Catto JWF, Southgate J. Specificity of the metallothionein-1 response by cadmium-exposed normal human urothelial cells. International Journal of Molecular Sciences. 2019;**20**(6):1344. DOI: 10.3390/ijms20061344

[43] Andujar P, Bensefa-colas L, Descatha A, Andujar P, Bensefa-colas L, Acute AD. Acute and chronic cadmium poisoning. La Rev de Médecine Interne. 2010;**31**(2):107-115

[44] Inaba T et al. Estimation of cumulative cadmium intake causing Itai – itai disease. Toxicology Letters. 2005;**159**:192-201. DOI: 10.1016/j.toxlet.2005.05.011

[45] Agence nationale de sécurité sanitaire de l'alimentation de l'environnement et du travail (ANSES). Exposition au cadmium: Propositions de valeurs toxicologiques de référence par ingestion, de valeurs sanitaires repères dans les milieux biologiques (sang, urines, ...) [rapport]. Illzach. 2017:1-77

[46] Cotte A, Duret A. Le chrome trivalent : intérêts et limites des supplémentations [thèse]. Grenoble: Université Joseph Fourier; 2011

[47] Agency for Toxic Substances and Disease Registry (ATSDR). Toxicological Profile for Manganese. Atlanta: United States Department of Health and Human Services. Agency for Toxic Substances and Disease Registry. 2012. DOI: 10.1201/9781420061888_ch4

[48] Paine AJ. Mechanisms of chromium toxicity, carcinogenicity and allergenicity: Review of the literature from 1985 to 2000. Human & Experimental Toxicology. 2001;**20**(9):439-451. DOI: 10.1191/096032701682693062

[49] Vincent JB, Edwards KC. The absorption and transport of chromium in the body. In: John Vincent editors. The Nutritional Biochemistry of Chromium (III). 2nd ed. 5. Elsevier B.V; 2018

[50] Dianyi YMD, Charlton C, John D, Bruce F, Kimberly G, Hall SL, Hatcher M, Kimberly J et al. Chromium (Cr) Toxicity. United States Department of Health and Human Services Agency for Toxic Substances and Disease Registry. Division of Toxicology and Environmental Medicine and Educational Services Branch. 2008. pp. 1-67. Available from: https://www.atsdr.cdc.gov/csem/chromium/docs/chromium.pdf

[51] A. for T. S. and D. R. (ATSDR). Toxicological Profile for Chromium2002. DOI: 10.1201/9781420061888_ch63

[52] Ma Y, Hooda PS. Chromium, Nickel and Cobalt. In: Peter H, editors. Trace Elements in Soils. London: Wiley; 2010. pp. 461-479

[53] Oscar T, John D, and Cronin D. "Lead Toxicity Case Studies in Environmental Medicine", 2017. Available from: https://www.atsdr.cdc.gov/csem/lead/docs/CSEM-Lead_toxicity_508.pdf

[54] Achmad RT, Budiawan, Auerkari EI. Effects of chromium on human body. Annual Research and Review in Biology. 2017;**13**(2):1-8. DOI: 10.9734/ARRB/2017/33462

[55] Peter GJ, Stephen N. Soil conditions and plant growth. 1st ed. Oxford: Wiley Blackwell; 2013

[56] Ceko MJ, Aitken JB, Harris HH. Speciation of copper in a range of food types by X-ray absorption spectroscopy. Food Chemistry. 2014;**164**(May):50-54. DOI: 10.1016/j.foodchem.2014.05.018

[57] WHO. Copper in Drinking-Water. 3rd ed. Geneva: World Health Organisation; 2004. DOI: 10.1111/1467-8292.00035

[58] Llanos RM, Mercer JFB. The molecular basis of copper homeostasis and copper-related disorders. DNA and Cell Biology. 2002;**21**(4):259-270. DOI: 10.1089/104454902753759681

[59] Taylor AA et al. Critical Review of Exposure and Effects: Implications for Setting Regulatory Health Criteria for Ingested Copper. Environmental Management. 2020;**65**(1):131-159. DOI: 10.1007/s00267-019-01234-y

[60] Turnlund JR, Keyes WR, Peiffer GL, Scott KC. Copper absorption, excretion, and retention by young men consuming low dietary copper determined by using the stable isotope 65Cu. The American Journal of Clinical Nutrition. 1998;**67**(6):1219-1225. DOI: 10.1093/ajcn/67.6.1219

[61] Gaetke LM, Chow-Johnson HS, Chow CK. Copper: toxicological relevance and mechanisms. Archives of Toxicology. 2014;**88**(11):1929-1938. DOI: 10.1007/s00204-014-1355-y

[62] Georgopoulos PG, Roy A, Yonone-Lioy MJ, Opiekun RE, Lioy PJ. Environmental copper: Its dynamics and human exposure issues. Journal of Toxicology and Environmental Health, Part B. 2001;**4**(4):341-394. DOI: 10.1080/109374001753146207

[63] Husak V. Copper and Copper-Containing Pesticides: Metabolism, Toxicity and Oxidative Stress. Journal of Vasyl Stefanyk Precarpathian National University. 2015;**2**(1):38-50. DOI: 10.15330/jpnu.2.1.38-50

[64] Myers BM, Prendergast FG, Holman R, Kuntz SM, Larusso NF. Alterations in hepatocyte lysosomes in experimental hepatic copper overload in rats. Gastroenterology. 1993;**105**(6):1814-1823. DOI: 10.1016/0016-5085(93) 91080-2

[65] Sokol RJ, Deverbaux MW, O'Brien K, Khandwala RA, Loehr JP. Abnormal hepatic mitochondrial respiration and cytochrome C oxidase activity in rats with long-term copper overload. Gastroenterology. 1993;**105**(1):178-187. DOI: 10.1016/0016-5085(93)90024-7

[66] Janet UA, Y and Keen CL. "Copper, oxidative stress, and human health". Molecular Aspects of Medicine. 2005:**26**(4-5 SPEC. ISS):268-298. DOI: 10.1016/j.mam.2005.07.015

[67] Monnot AD, Zheng G, Zheng W. Mechanism of copper transport at the blood-cerebrospinal fluid barrier: Influence of iron deficiency in an in vitro model. Experimental Biology and Medicine. 2012;**237**(3):327-333. DOI: 10.1258/ebm.2011.011170

[68] Ellingsen DG, Møller LB, Aaseth J. Copper. Handb. Toxicol. Met. Fourth Ed. 2015;**1**(29):765-786. DOI: 10.1016/B978-0-444-59453-2.00035-4

[69] Araya M, Olivares M, Pizarro F. Copper in human health. International Journal of Environmental Health Research. 2007;**1**(4):608-620. DOI: 10.1504/IJENVH.2007.018578

[70] Chen P, Bornhorst J, Aschner M. Manganese metabolism in humans. Frontiers in Bioscience-Landmark. 2018;**23**(9):1655-1679. DOI: 10.2741/4665

[71] Leggett RW. A biokinetic model for manganese. Science of the Total Environment. 2011;**409**(20):4179-4186. DOI: 10.1016/j.scitotenv.2011.07.003

[72] A. for T. S. and D. R. (ATSDR). Toxicological Profile for

2-Hexanone2012. DOI: 10.1201/9781420061888_ch4

[73] Beaugelin-Seiller K, Colle C, Adam C, Henner P. Fiche radionucléide: Manganèse 54 et environnement. IRSN. Direction de l'environnement et de l'intervention. Service d'étude du Comportement des radionucléides dans les écosystème. 2001. 20p

[74] Li L, Yang X. The essential element manganese, oxidative stress, and metabolic diseases: Links and interactions. Oxidative Medicine and Cellular Longevity. 2018;**2018**:7580707. DOI: 10.1155/2018/7580707

[75] Iqbal M, Monaghan T, Redmond J. Manganese toxicity with ephedrone abuse manifesting as parkinsonism: A case report. Journal of Medical Case Reports. 2012;**6**:2-5. DOI: 10.1186/1752-1947-6-52

[76] Zheng W, Crossgrave J. Manganese toxicity upon overexposure. NMR in Biomedicine. 2004;**17**(8):544-553. DOI: 10.1002/nbm.931.Manganese

[77] Zheng W, Zhao Q. Iron overload following manganese exposure in cultured neuronal, but not neuroglial cells. Brain Research. 2001;**897**(1-2):175-179. DOI: 10.1016/S0006-8993(01)02049-2

[78] Olanow WC et al. Manganese intoxication in the rhesus monkey. Neurology. 1996;**46**:492-498

[79] Lai JCK, Chan AWK, Leung TKC, Minski MJ, Lim L. Neurochemical changes in rats chronically treated with a high concentration of manganese chloride. Neurochemical Research. 1992;**17**(9):841-847. DOI: 10.1007/BF00993259

[80] Mohammad FK, Faris GAM. Behavioral effects of acute manganese chloride administration in chickens. Biological Trace Element Research. 2006;**110**(3):265-273. DOI: 10.1385/BTER:110:3:265

[81] Bouabid S, Tinakoua A, Lakhdar-Ghazal N, Benazzouz A. Manganese neurotoxicity: Behavioral disorders associated with dysfunctions in the basal ganglia and neurochemical transmission. Journal of Neurochemistry. 2016;**136**(4):677-691. DOI: 10.1111/jnc.13442

[82] European Chemicals Agency (ECHA). "ANNEX 1 Background document in support of the Committee for Risk Assessment (RAC) evaluation of limit values for benzene in the workplace. Helsinki. European Chemicals Agency. 2018. ECHA/RAC/A77-0- 0000001412-86-187/F". 2018

[83] Buxton S et al. Concise review of nickel human health toxicology and ecotoxicology. Inorganics. 2019;**7**(7):89. DOI: 10.3390/inorganics7070089

[84] Leblanc JC, Guérin T, Noël L, Calamassi-Tran G, Volatier JL, Verger P. Étude de l'alimentation totale en France. Les minéraux et oligoéléments -2e partie: Nickel, sélénium, sodium, zinc. Sciences des Aliments. 2005;**25**(4):259-267. DOI: 10.3166/sda.25.259-267

[85] Genchi G, Carocci A, Lauria G, Sinicropi MS, Catalano A. Nickel: Human health and environmental toxicology. International Journal of Environmental Research and Public Health. 2020;**17**(3):679. DOI: 10.3390/ijerph17030679

[86] Agency for Toxic Substances and Disease Registry (ATSDR). Toxicological Profile for Nickel. Atalanta: United States Department of Health and Human Services. Agency for Toxic Substances

and Disease Registry. 2005. DOI: 10.1201/9781420061888_ch163

[87] Aleksandra D-C, Urszula B. Secondary hypertension manifests renal artery stenosis and weakened kidney. Journal of Mechanics in Medicine and Biology. 2011;**11**(1):73-100. DOI: 10.1142/S021951941000371X

[88] Rendall REG, Phillips JI, Renton KA. Death following exposure to fine particulate nickel from a metal arc process. The Annals of Occupational Hygiene. 1994;**38**(6):921-930. DOI: 10.1093/annhyg/38.6.921

[89] Das KK, Dasgupta S. Effect of nickel sulfate on testicular steroidogenesis in rats during protein restriction. Environmental Health Perspectives. 2002;**110**(9):923-926. DOI: 10.1289/ehp.02110923

[90] Aranguren MMS. Contamination en métaux lourds des eaux de surface et des sédiments du Val de Milluni (Andes Boliviennes) par des déchets miniers. Approches géochimique, minéralogique et hydrochimique. Toulouse: Université de Toulouse; 2008

[91] Brian G, Fred S. Distribution and Effects of Lead. Lead Action News. 1993;**1**(2):1-2

[92] Jaishankar M, Tseten T, Anbalagan N, Mathew BB, Beeregowda KN. Toxicity, mechanism and health effects of some heavy metals. Interdisciplinary Toxicology. 2014;**7**(2):60-72. DOI: 10.2478/intox-2014-0009

[93] A. for toxic sunstance and disease registry (ATSDR). Toxicological Profile for Lead. 2020. DOI: 10.1201/9781420061888_ch106

[94] Wani AL, Ara A, Usmani JA. Lead toxicity: A review. Interdisciplinary Toxicology. 2015;**8**(2):55-64. DOI: 10.1515/intox-2015-0009

[95] Kirberger M. Defining a Molecular Mechanism for Lead Toxicity via Calcium- Binding Proteins. Atlanta: Georgia State University; 2011

[96] Flora SJS, Mittal M, Mehta A. Heavy metal induced oxidative stress & its possible reversal by chelation therapy. The Indian Journal of Medical Research. 2008;**128**(4):501-523

[97] Cecchi M. Devenir du plomb dans le système sol-plante: Cas d'un sol contaminé par une usine de recyclage du plomb et de deux plantes potagères (Fève et Tomate). Toulouse: These Dr. l'ecole Dr. des Sci. Ecol. Vétérinaires Agron. Bioingénieries, Spécialité Agrosystèmes, Ecosystèmes Environ. l'Institut Natl. Polytech; 2008. p. 226

[98] Jessie M. Évaluation des risques toxicologiques et écotoxicologues autour du lieu d'enfouissement technique à Saint-Nicéphore [Mémoire]. Sherbrooke: Université de Sherbrooke; 2013

[99] Weaver V et al. Blood cadmium and lead and chronic kidney disease in US adults: A joint analysis. American Journal of Epidemiology. 2009;**170**(9):1156-1164. DOI: 10.1093/aje/kwp248

[100] Goyer R, Golub M, Choudhury H, Hughes M, Kenyon E, Stifelman M. Issue paper on the human health effects of metals. [report]: Washington, DC: U.S. Environmental Protection Agency; 2004

[101] Sanders T, Lui Y, Buchner V, Tchounwou P. Neurotics Effects and Biomarkers of Lead Exposure. Reviews on Environmental Health. 2009;**1**(24):15-45. Available from: https://www.ncbi.nlm.nih.gov/pmc/articles/PMC2858639/pdf/nihms190515.pdf

[102] Hsiang J, Díaz E. Lead and developmental neurotoxicity of the central nervous system. Current Neurobiology. 2011;**2**(1):35-42

[103] Lamprea-Maldonado DK. Caractérisation et origine des métaux traces, hydrocarbures aromatiques polycycliques et pesticides transportés par les retombées atmosphériques et les eaux de ruissellement dans les bassins versants séparatifs péri-urbains [Thèse]. Nantes : École Doctorale Sciences Pour l'Ingénieur, Geosciences, Architecture. 2009. Available from: https://tel.archives-ouvertes.fr/tel-00596847

[104] Maares M, Haase H. A guide to human zinc absorption: General overview and recent advances of in vitro intestinal models. Nutrients. 2020;**12**(3):762. DOI: 10.3390/nu12030762

[105] Temple VJ, Masta A. Zinc in human health. Papua and New Guinea Medical Journal. 2004;**47**(3-4):146-158. DOI: 10.9790/0853-13721823

[106] Virginie C. Les oligoéléments: Rôle et conseils du pharmacien d'officine [thèse]. Marseille : Université d'Aix-Marseille; 2017

[107] Simon-Hertich B, Wibbertmann A, Wagner D, Tomaska L, Malcolm H. Environmental Health criteria [report]. Geneva; 2001:221. DOI: 10.1016/s0031-3025(16)36534-5

[108] Agency for Toxic Substances and Disease Registry (ATSDR). Toxicological Profile for Zinc. Atalanta: United States Department of Health and Human Services. Agency for Toxic Substances and Disease Registry. 2005. DOI: 10.1201/9781420061888_ch163

[109] U. S. E. P. A. (EPA). Toxicological Review of Zinc and Compounds. Rev. Lit. Arts Am. 2010;**39**(110):759-786. DOI: doi http://www.epa.gov/iris/toxreviews/0070tr.pdf

[110] Gary FJ. Zinc toxicity. The American Journal of Clinical Nutrition. 1990;**51**(7):225-227

[111] Ulrika AM, Todd SL. Zinc toxicity. Pediatrics. 1982;**70**(4):660-661. DOI: 10.1542/peds.70.4.660a

Chapter 4

Boron and Boron-Containing Compounds Toxicity

Çiğdem Sevim and Mehtap Kara

Abstract

Boron is an important element found in limited resources on earth, especially in Turkey, and is essential for living organisms. Boron plays key roles in human and animal systems. While boron shows its important effects as an essential element at low concentrations in the organism, it causes different toxic effects to occur at high concentrations. There are different studies on boron and boron-containing compounds effects on organisms, toxic effects mechanisms need to be detailed. Boron and its compounds can cause toxic effects in oral, dermal, and inhalation exposure and even deadly effects at very high concentrations. The use of disinfectant and cleaning products containing boron as sprays, fertilizers, etc., during the Covid-19 pandemic also increases the interest in this issue. Boron exposure could cause lung irritation, dermal irritation, genotoxicity in male reproductive system, teratogenicity in concentration-dependent manner. In vitro studies have tried to explain the toxic effects mechanisms. The aim of the current work is to explain the toxic effect mechanisms of boron and boron compounds on body systems.

Keywords: boron, boric acid, bortezomib, toxicity

1. Introduction

Boron (B) is an essential element for living organisms. B has different physiological effects on living organisms at low concentrations, whereas it has toxic effects at higher concentrations. Generally, B is not found as an element in nature and is commonly found in the form of boric acid, borax, and other complex forms. People are affected by boron:

- By contacting boron minerals in air and water
- Drinking and using the underground and surface waters in the basins rich in boron deposits
- Taking foods and drinks with high boron concentrations
- Working in quarries and factories
- Working in places that make cleaners and whiteners such as soap, detergent, beauty products, and similar products, or using such products

Since boron is ubiquitous, it will be accepted that no limit can be drawn for being under the influence of boron [1].

Animals and humans could be ingested higher levels of B through foods or may be exposed to boron due to occupational conditions as inhalation, dermal or oral exposure. During the exposure, damaged and injured absorption sites can lead to increased absorption. In some cases, dermal higher exposures to B could result in death. Boric acid could be fatal after higher ingestion [2, 3]. More studies are needed about the cellular toxicity mechanisms of B and B compounds at tissue level. Higher B exposure could cause:

- Mortality risk increase
- Osteoporosis
- Cognitive dysfunctions
- Cell injury
- Inflammation tendency
- Congestion
- Dermatitis
- Renal cells degeneration
- Edema
- Eye irritation
- Intestinal apoptosis
- Developmental toxic effects
- Reproductive dysfunctions
- Cardiovascular dysfunctions
- Data on carcinogenicity are unclear. There were not sufficient data about carcinogenic effects of B and B compounds (**Table 1**) [4].

As a normal consequence of boron uptake from food and drinking water, human tissues and body fluids contain B. Boron found in soft tissues is close to the blood level. B can accumulate in bones. Muscle tissue, heart, lung, and intestine contain lesser amounts of boron [6, 7]. The World Health Organization compared the blood levels of ingesting boron through drinking water and diet in humans and rats. The distribution of boron in blood and tissue samples for human and rat species, boron kinetics may be the same for both species [8].

Compound	Dose/concentration	Toxic effect
Boric acid	3–6 gr-infants 15–20 g-adults	Nausea, vomiting, greenish diarrhea, dehydration, hypotension, metabolic acidosis, oliguric renal failure, erythematous rash
Sodium borate	10 mg/kg day and > 15 mg/kg	Sex hormone decrease, globulin binding (SHGB) decrease, irritability, disturbed sleeping, vomiting, severe diarrhea, seizures, anemia and death
Bortezomib	>1.3 mg/ day	Peripheral neurotoxicity and lung toxicity
Dimethylamine borane	"occupational exposure"	Dizziness, nausea, diarrhea, cognitive dysfunction, slurred speech, irritability, ataxia, peripheral neuropathy, cerebellar damage and parkinsonism. Myelin and axonal degeneration
Boromycin	"in vitro study"	Hemolysis

Adopted from [5].

Table 1.
Boron compounds and toxic effects.

Numerous studies on humans and laboratory animals have revealed that more than 90% of borates taken into the organism are removed from the organism in the form of boric acid. It has been reported that boric acid can form complexes with different biological molecules depending on the dose [9].

Regardless of the route of its uptake into the organism, the elimination of boron mainly occurs by glomerular filtration. Glomerular filtration is 3–4 times faster in rats than in humans, and it has been reported that more than 90% of boron, which is taken into the organism by various ways in humans, is removed through urine within the first 24 hours [10, 11].

The data obtained from animal studies are not enough for determining the Bor's potential of causing cancer to human [12]. Boron was not evaluated as a carcinogen by EPA (US Environmental Protection Agency) and NTP (US National Toxicology Program), IARC (International Agency for Research on Cancer) [8]. The studies about boron and its compounds mainly focus on their toxicologies. In the studies about boron exposure, data are stated as equivalent of boron for providing compared data. Under the physiological pH conditions, borate salts are completely converted to boric acid; based on this, it was stated that boric acid and borate salts have similar toxicological properties [13].

In this chapter, we aimed to review current toxicity data of B, and B compounds.

2. Boron and boron compounds

Boron (B) as a metalloid belongs to third group of periodic table. Boron has an interesting unique and complex chemical structure like metal and nonmetal. It has very small atomic size as 4.39cm^3/mol. B includes three valance electrons, and its ionization energy is very high. B's p-orbital includes vacant electron at B^{+3} state. B has high potential to make anionic complexes than cationic complexes. B occurs in the nature as borates (such as borax $Na_2B_4O_7 \cdot 10H_2O$), boric acid [$B(OH)_3$ or H_3BO_3], and BF4 (not very common). In living cells, B occurs in the cytoplasm as H_3BO_3 and borate forms. Boric acid and borate interact with several different molecules very easily and form different esters and generate mono-, d, poly hydroxyl forms. Boric acid has affinity to furanoid rings of sugars, which are very important for life. These complex compounds are very important during evolution because of providing organisms stability and very strong defense mechanisms.

B's inorganic form is originated from anthropogenic sources in the nature and could found elsewhere in soil, water, and atmosphere. Also it circulates in the air, volcanos, ocean, geothermal water sources, etc. According to EPA (1987), boron compounds are released into the air as anthropogenic sources. Generally, because of boron dust, people are exposed to boron via the air in boron mines. A dose of 14 mg of boron per cubic meter of air has been reported in boron mines where boric acid and refined products are produced. Boron can be found in soil, especially in the form of bonk JMI or borate, absorbed on soil particles, or in soil solution as a free anion. In the research studies, it has been shown that the amount of boron in the plant is primarily related to the soil pH. Other important factors are the plant type, the boron content of the soil, the type of ions that can change in the soil, the amount and type of other minerals in the soil, the amount of organic matter in the soil, the temperature of the soil, the wetting and drying conditions of the soil, the soil-water ratio, the light intensity, and genetic factors. Low-boron soils contain up to 0.7 ppm boron and do not pose a problem for any plant. Medium-boron soils contain 0.7–15 ppm boron, and it has been determined that it does not cause problems for some plants. Soils with high boron contain 15–75 ppm boron and are mostly dangerous for plants, while soils with very high boron contain more than 75 ppm boron, and these are dangerous for plants. Boron has important metabolic functions in plants and plant growth stops in the absence of boron in the soil. Boron shows its effects on drinking water and agricultural water. In 1968, the Water Quality Criteria Committee set the limit value as 1 mg/l; in 1971, as a result of the investigations of the Drinking Water Standards Technical Review Committee, it was decided that there was no evidence to require the 1 mg/l limit, and that 0.3 mg/l was a reliable limit for human health. According to research studies, it is important for human health that drinking water does not contain high levels of boron [14, 15].

The negative effects of boron products on the environment are much lower than in other industrial sectors. In fact, with the effect of radioactive substances after chemotherapy, it is one of the elements that can be considered environmentally friendly due to its necessity for human and living creatures [16].

Depending on the technological developments, the economic grades of the ores are reduced with the development of new methods and equipment, and many stored heaps in the form of waste are evaluated in this way. Accordingly, possible evaluation possibilities in the future should be considered in the disposal of waste. For these reasons, it is necessary to pay maximum attention to the storage of boron wastes. It is possible to list the advantages to be obtained as follows [16].

- The problems arising from the stocking of wastes and the cost of stocking will decrease.
- Environmental pollution will be minimized.
- An additional income will be obtained with the new product produced.
- It will be prevented that the wastes pollute the underground and surface waters.

Predominant mineral sources of B are found in Australia, China, Turkey, Russia, and Argentina. B and B compounds could not naturally occur as volatile compounds; however, minimal volatile B compounds release to atmosphere via volcanic activities and different industrial places. B is an essential for several body organs and systems, and 1–13 mg/kg consumption is acceptable. High exposure could cause several health disorders in neurological, urogenital, skeleton, and cardiovascular systems [17].

3. Respiratory system

There are few studies on the effects of boron and its compounds on the lung. In some studies, it has been reported that exposure to boron may cause damage to the lung cellular layer. It causes symptoms such as irritation in the nasal epithelium, nosebleeds, cough, and shortness of breath in people working in boron mines [18]. Boron nitride nanoparticles (BNNTs) appear as a nanotechnological product with a wide range of applications in engineering and biomedical fields. Therefore, there is an increasing interest in studies on the risks these products may pose for health. It has been demonstrated that BNTTs cause cytotoxicity in human lung adenocarcinoma epithelial (A549) cells and murine alveolar macrophage cells (RAW 264.7), being concentration dependent (0.02, 0.2, and 2 μg/mL concentrations). In addition, cytomorphological examinations revealed serious cell morphology disorders in both cell types [19]. In another study, it was shown that high boron application may cause an increase in the capacity to transform in non-tumorogenic cells. In total, 5–50,000 μM concentration range of boric acid is applied to human nontumorigenic lung epithelial (BEAS-2B) cells and human lung epithelial carcinoma (A549) cells. It has been determined that 5000–50,000 μM concentrations significantly suppressed the anchorage-dependent growth of cells. This effect could have occurred via an important pathway that plays key role in cell transformation such as SRC and PI3K/AKT and MEK/ERK signaling pathway [20]. Diborane gas (B2H4) is a strong toxic substance for the respiratory tract. Mice were exposed to diborane gas at a concentration of 5 ppm diborane (1.7 mg boron/m3) for 2 weeks, which caused severe damage to their lungs, including pulmonary congestion, hemorrhage, and edema. Mild changes such as infiltration of polymorphous neutrophils in the peribronchiolar region were observed in the group given 0.7 ppm diborane (0.2 mg boron/m3). Case reports have stated that boron can be lethal after short-term oral exposure at high doses and can be quite large despite variability in human responses to acute exposure. It has been reported that the minimum lethal dose of boron (as boric acid) taken is 2–3 g in infants, 5–6 g in children, and 15–20 g in adults. However, 784 cases with boric acid (10–88 g) reported no deaths, of which 88% of the reviewed cases were asymptomatic. Liver, kidney, central nervous system and gastrointestinal effects, and skin lesions have been found in fatal cases following boron ingestion, but death has been attributed to respiratory failure [21].

4. Immune system

If boron levels decrease in body, this decrease causes immune deficiency. However, higher and/or chronical exposure could have negative effects on immune system homeostasis [4].

Jin et al. conducted a study that showed that the effect of boron on the immune system in vivo is dose-dependent. They supplemented 0, 20, 40, 80, 160, 320, and 640 mg/L B in drinking water of rats (1.5, 3, 6, 12, 24, 48, and 96 mg/kg/bw) for 70 days. It was demonstrated that 20 and 40 mg/kg doses of B improved immune functions in the rats and increased the concentrations of serum IgG levels, splenic IFN-γ and IL-4 expressions, and the expression levels of CD3+, CD4+, and that they also proliferated cell nuclear antigen (PCNA) + cells. However, at such high concentrations as >48 mg/kg/bw, toxic effects on immune system were detected and immune activities were suppressed. At higher concentrations of IgG, IL10 levels and CD8+ cells were significantly found as decreasing. This is a good example of U-shaped dose–response effect. Both very low and very high concentrations could be associated with harmful effects on immune system [22].

Boron nitride nanotubes (BNNTs) engineered nanomaterials have superior electrical, chemical, and thermal properties, and they were planned to be used in the area of engineering applications such as lightweight and high-temperature ceramic components, flame retardants, etc. BNNTs' size could be <100 nm in diameter and microns of length. Effects of mixture of BNNTs (BNNT-M) in vitro in THP-1 cells (human peripheral blood monocyte cell line) and in vivo pathogen-free, male C57BL/6J mice were evaluated by Kodali et al. The range of in vitro concentrations was 0–100 mg/ml and in vivo dose was 40 μg/mouse. BNNT induced cytotoxicity and cellular oxidative stress in THP-1 cells, being concentration-dependent. These results were in accordance with in vivo in the same study as increased lactate dehydrogenase levels in bronchoalveolar lavage, mitochondrial membrane potential loss. They demonstrated that cathepsin B, caspase 1, protein levels of IL-1b and IL-18 increased both in vitro and in vivo. These results indicated that BNNTs could increase acute inflammation and toxicity in vitro and in vivo [23].

The use of borax (Na2B4O2(H2O)10) as a food additive and its excessive consumption in recent years could result in serious toxic effects such as kidney damage. Higher borax exposure decreased immune cell numbers and increased sister chromatid exchange in blood immune lymphocyte cells [24].

5. Nervous system

Bortezomib (C19H25BN4O4), or dipeptidyl boronic acid, is a proteasome inhibitor drug used in chemotherapy against hematologic malignancy. It has an anticancer activity. However, bortezomib often causes severe peripheral neuropathy. This condition has a special name such as "bortezomib-induced peripheral neuropathy (BIPN)." BIPN includes numbness and painful paraesthesia. Bortezomib has toxic effects on dorsal root ganglia via endoplasmic reticulum stress, protein carbonylation, and oxidative stress inducing. It also causes morphological changes in nervous system cells such as microglia [25, 26].

It was determined that infants exposed to 5–14 g boric acid or sodium tetraborate exerted such serious neuronal symptoms such as headache, tremor, convulsions, and even death after coma. These symptoms were associated with neuron degeneration, edema, and hemorrhage in the brain. However, chronical B deficiency causes such mental disorders as focusing problems, electroencephalogram changes, vigilance and psychomotor activity problems. B deficiency is strongly related to nervous system action potential problems [27]. In another study, Ozansoy et al. demonstrated that sodium borate decahydrate and boric acid administrations improved amyloid-beta toxicity in SH-SY5Y cells in vitro via increased expression levels of Sirt1 and regulated GSK-3α/β expressions [28].

Thus, this information suggested that B and B compounds could have U-shaped effects in the nervous system. Excessive B and B compounds exposure causes toxicity, and deficiency causes neuron metabolic pathway problems, and even B and B compounds could be possible therapy options for neurological diseases.

6. Reproductive system

It is well known that boron has negative effects on male and female reproductive system. It causes atrophy in seminifer tubulus, germ cell loss, sperm mobility impairment, altered follicle stimulating hormone and testosterone, reduction of ovulation processes [4]. Exposure to a range of boric acid concentrations between 1000 and 9000 ppm causes serious male fertility problems such as testicular atrophy and decreased sperm motility in experimental animals. With the studies on different species of animals, these toxic effects were confirmed with different doses. Human studies with occupational workers in Turkey and in China did not confirm these results [29, 30]. As a result of a study conducted in Russia, it was determined that sexual activity decreased in boron workers (n = 28). In addition, interestingly, in the study conducted on boron workers in the United States, it was determined that there was an increase in the birth of girls compared with boys [7].

According to animal studies, it was reported that boron, boric acid, and sodium borate compounds could be toxic to reproductive system and also developmental system. For reproductive system, NOAEL levels of boron were 17.5 mg /kg/day and for developmental issue NOAEL levels of boron were 9.6 mg/kg/day. Duydu et al. reported that daily 14.45 ± 6.57 mg/day boron exposure in boron workers did not lead to any change in reproduction-related hormone levels (FSH, LH) and sperm cells morphology and count [31].

In different studies, it was shown that low levels of boron compounds caused developmental problems. Low levels disrupted developmental processes of chicken (400 mg B/L drinking water), rat (640 mg B/L drinking water), and African ostrich (640 mg boric acid/L) experimentally. In another study, boric acid exposure higher than 0.5 mmol/L in male rats' Sertoli cells triggered necrosis and apoptosis and caused a decrease in cell viability rate. At 40 and 80 mmol/L boric acid levels, it was reported that sertoli cell viability was arrested at G0/G1 phase [32].

In one lineage study, male rats were exposed to boron via oral gavage with different concentrations. Then they mated with unexposed female rats. It was observed that fetus viability rate decreased at higher exposure levels (100 mg B/kg/day) and fetus malformations increased at higher concentration. Additionally, testicular enzyme levels (MDH, SDH, G3PDH) and FSH levels changed. These changes were associated with lipid metabolism changes that play a key role in hormone and enzyme activities via metabolomic assays [33].

7. Cardiovascular system

There are many studies showing that the inclusion of boron and boron compounds as food supplements has a positive effect on the cardiovascular system. It has been reported that it will reduce especially cardiovascular risk factors. Today, however, the production and use of boron-containing compounds for the treatment of various diseases are popular. Some of these compounds have been reported to cause cardiovascular toxicity in toxicity studies. Boron nitride (BN) nanoparticles and different formulations could be good candidates for biomedicines. Liu et al. reported that BN nanoparticles coated by PEG (BN-PEG) highly were distributed in the heart tissue and caused high toxic effects histopathologically [34–36].

Hexagonal boron nitride nanoparticles (hBNNPs) are nanomaterials that have special chemical properties and candidate therapeutics in medical applications. In Wistar albino rats, it has been determined that hBNNPs increased oxidative stress. In the cardiac tissues, 3200 μg/kg dose of hBNNPs caused a statistically more significant increase in LOOH levels than the controls [37].

It is known that Bortezomib leads to neurological disorders as peripheral neuropathy; however, a study conducted with Bortezomib showed that it decreased the left ventricular ejection fraction, led to cardiomyocyte abnormalities, damaged the cardiomyocyte contraction through decreased ATP [38]. In another study that compared Boronic acid and Epoxyketone Proteasomal-Targeted Drugs found that boronic acid was much more damaging to myocyte [39].

8. Anticancer boron compounds

Cancer is the disease that reduces the life quality of patients the most and causes the highest rate of death in the world. For this reason, intensive scientific research continues on strategies that will both improve the quality of life of patients and treat the disease. Boronic acid, bortezomib, talabostat, and boron nitride capture therapy are important boron-containing candidates for anticancer therapy. Bortezomib is a 26S proteosoma inhibitor and activates NF-κB. This process enhances apoptotic mechanism in the cells. Boronic acid is used as an anticancer agent via ROS modulation in the cells. It has been demonstrated that boronic acid prodrugs significantly induce apoptosis in primary leukemic lymphocytes [40]. Bortezomib was approved by US Food and Drug Administration (FDA) in 2003, and at the present time, it is used for chemotherapy of multiple myeloma and mantle cell lymphoma, but peripheral neuropathy is one of the common adverse effects of Bortezomib [41].

9. Conclusions

Boron is a vital element for living organisms. Boron and several types of its compounds have different beneficial effects in humans at sufficient doses. However, too little or too much intake in the required amount causes serious health problems. Its use as a food supplement to prevent boron deficiency in the body has become popular today. In addition, the use of boron and its compounds in many fields such as cosmetics, cleaning, medicine, electronics, war industry, and the development of new products for these fields are increasing day by day. Such reasons cause an increase in exposure not only to individuals working in boron mines, but also in daily life. Besides, boron and its compounds appear as candidate molecules in the treatment of various diseases. All of these factors indicate that there will be more exposure to boron and its compounds today and in the future. For this reason, it is a fact that these compounds, which are mentioned as having many benefits under normal conditions, will also encounter toxic effects due to the increased exposure over time.

DOI: http://dx.doi.org/10.5772/intechopen.103179

It is also possible that some boron-containing compounds can be candidates for cancer treatment through their structural effects and cytotoxic effects on cellular mechanisms. This shows the importance of toxicity studies of these compounds at all times. However, developing scientific technologies will also enable these effects to be minimized.

Conflict of interest

The authors declare no conflict of interest.

Author details

Çiğdem Sevim[1]* and Mehtap Kara[2]

1 Faculty of Medicine, Department of Medical Pharmacology, Kastamonu University, Kastamonu, Turkey

2 Faculty of Pharmacy, Department of Pharmaceutical Toxicology, Istanbul University, Istanbul, Turkey

*Address all correspondence to: cigdemsevim@kastamonu.edu.tr

References

[1] Demirtaş A. Bor'un insan beslenmesi ve sağlığı açısından önemi. Atatürk Üniversitesi Ziraat Fakültesi Dergisi. 2010;**41**(1):75-80

[2] Hadrup N, Frederiksen M, Sharma AK. Toxicity of boric acid, borax and other boron containing compounds: A review. Regulatory Toxicology and Pharmacology. Apr 2021;**121**:104873. DOI: 10.1016/j.yrtph.2021.104873. Epub 22 Jan 2021. PMID: 33485927

[3] Uluisik I, Karakaya HC, Koc A. The importance of boron in biological systems. Journal of Trace Elements in Medicine and Biology. 2018;**45**:156-162

[4] Khaliq H, Juming Z, Ke-Mei P. The physiological role of boron on health. Biological Trace Element Research. 2018;**186**(1):31-51

[5] Farfán-García E et al. Current data regarding the structure-toxicity relationship of boron-containing compounds. Toxicology Letters. 2016;**258**:115-125

[6] Naghii M, Samman S. The effect of boron supplementation on the distribution of boron in selected tissues and on testosterone synthesis in rats. The Journal of Nutritional Biochemistry. 1996;**7**(9):507-512

[7] Kocatürk P. Rat Testis Dokusu Üzerine Akut Borik Asit Uygulamasının Fizyopatolojik ve Histopatolojik Etkileri [thesis]. Ankara Üniversitesi, Sağlık Bilimleri Enstitüsü, Doktora Tezi, Ankara; 1998

[8] Becking GC, Chen B-H. International programme on chemical safety (IPCS) environmental health criteria on boron human health risk assessment. Biological Trace Element Research. 1998;**66**(1):439-452

[9] Güven EAC. and Hacimüftüoğlu A. Borik Asitin Yeni Doğan Siçan Beyin Hücre Kültürlerinde Glutamatla Oluşturulan Nörotoksisiteye Etkisi

[10] Nielsen FH et al. Dietary magnesium, manganese and boron affect the response of rats to high dietary aluminum. Magnesium. 1988;**7**(3):133-147

[11] Litovitz TL et al. Clinical manifestations of toxicity in a series of 784 boric acid ingestions. The American Journal of Emergency Medicine. 1988;**6**(3):209-213

[12] Eckhert C, Barranco W, Kim D. Boron and prostate cancer a model for understanding boron biology. In: Advances in Plant and Animal Boron Nutrition. Springer; 2007. pp. 291-297

[13] Duydu Y, Başaran N, Ustundag A, Aydın S, Undeger U, Ataman OY et al. Is boric acid toxic to reproduction in humans? Assessment of the animal reproductive toxicity data and epidemiological study results. Current Drug Delivery (CDD). 2016;**13**:324-329

[14] Parks JL, Edwards M. Boron in the environment. Critical Reviews in Environmental Science and Technology. 2005;**35**(2):81-114

[15] Doğan G, Sabah E, Erkal T. Borun çevresel etkileri üzerine Türkiye'de yapılan bilimsel araştırmalar. Türkiye. 2005;**19**:9-12

[16] Miçillioğlu S. Lactuca sativa bitkisi kullanılarak bor konsantrasyonu yüksek suların arıtılabilirliğinin araştırılması [thesis]. Fen Bilimleri Enstitüsü; 2010

[17] Princi MP, Lupini A, Araniti F, Longo C, Mauceri A, Sunseri F et al. Chapter 5 – boron toxicity and tolerance in plants: Recent advances and future perspectives A2 – ahmad, parvaiz. Plant Metal Interaction. Elsevier; 2016. pp. 115-147

[18] Oil WM. Provisional Peer-Reviewed Toxicity Values for

[19] Horvath L et al. In vitro investigation of the cellular toxicity of boron nitride nanotubes. ACS Nano. 2011;**5**(5):3800-3810

[20] Xu H et al. High levels of boron promote anchorage-independent growth of nontumorigenic cells. Environmental Pollution. 2020;**266**:115094

[21] Lumpkin M. and Williams MD. Toxicological Profile for Boron. 2010: US Department of Health and Human Services, Public Health Service, Agency

[22] Jin E et al. Boron affects immune function through modulation of splenic T lymphocyte subsets, cytokine secretion, and lymphocyte proliferation and apoptosis in rats. Biological Trace Element Research. 2017;**178**(2): 261-275

[23] Kodali VK et al. Acute in vitro and in vivo toxicity of a commercial grade boron nitride nanotube mixture. Nanotoxicology. 2017;**11**(8):1040-1058

[24] Pongsavee M. Effect of borax on immune cell proliferation and sister chromatid exchange in human chromosomes. Journal of Occupational Medicine and Toxicology. 2009;**4**(1):1-6

[25] Yamamoto S, Egashira N. Pathological mechanisms of Bortezomib-induced peripheral neuropathy. International Journal of Molecular Sciences. 2021;**22**(2):888

[26] Robak P, Robak T. Bortezomib for the treatment of hematologic malignancies: 15 years later. Drugs in R&D. 2019;**19**(2):73-92

[27] Białek M et al. Selected physiological effects of boron compounds for animals and humans. A review. Journal of Animal and Feed Sciences. 2019;**28**(4):307-320

[28] Ozansoy M et al. Two boron-containing compounds affect the cellular viability of SH-SY5Y cells in an in vitro amyloid-beta toxicity model. Turkish Journal of Biology. 2020;**44**(4):208-214

[29] Bolt HM, Başaran N, Duydu Y. Effects of boron compounds on human reproduction. Archives of Toxicology. 2020;**94**(3):717-724

[30] Başaran N et al. Evaluation of the DNA damage in lymphocytes, sperm and buccal cells of workers under environmental and occupational boron exposure conditions. Mutation Research, Genetic Toxicology and Environmental Mutagenesis. 2019;**843**:33-39

[31] Duydu Y et al. Reproductive toxicity parameters and biological monitoring in occupationally and environmentally boron-exposed persons in Bandırma, Turkey. Archives of Toxicology. 2011;**85**(6):589-600

[32] Lu L et al. Effects of boron on cytotoxicity, apoptosis, and cell cycle of cultured rat Sertoli cells in vitro. Biological Trace Element Research. 2020;**196**(1):223-230

[33] Wang C et al. Reproductive toxicity and metabolic perturbations in male rats exposed to boron. Science of the Total Environment. 2021;**785**:147370

[34] Donoiu I et al. Effects of boron-containing compounds on cardiovascular disease risk factors–a review. Journal of

Trace Elements in Medicine and Biology. 2018;**50**:47-56

[35] Liu B et al. In vivo biodistribution and toxicity of highly soluble PEG-coated boron nitride in mice. Nanoscale Research Letters. 2015;**10**(1):1-7

[36] Kharkovskaya EE, Osipov GV, Mukhina IV. Ventricular fibrillation induced by 2-aminoethoxydiphenyl borate under conditions of hypoxia/reoxygenation. Minerva Cardioangiologica. Dec 2020;**68**(6):619-628. DOI: 10.23736/S0026-4725.20.05376-1. Epub 15 Oct 2020. PMID: 33059404

[37] Kar F, Söğüt I, Hacıoğlu C, Göncü Y, Şenturk H, Şenat A et al. Hexagonal boron nitride nanoparticles trigger oxidative stress by modulating thiol/disulfide homeostasis. Human & Experimental Toxicology. Sep 2021;**40**(9):1572-1583. DOI: 10.1177/09603271211002892. Epub 23 Mar 2021. PMID: 33754873

[38] Nowis D et al. Cardiotoxicity of the anticancer therapeutic agent bortezomib. The American Journal of Pathology. 2010;**176**(6):2658-2668

[39] Hasinoff BB, Patel D. Myocyte-damaging effects and binding kinetics of Boronic acid and Epoxyketone proteasomal-targeted drugs. Cardiovascular Toxicology. 2018;**18**(6):557-568

[40] Song S, Gao P, Sun L, Kang D, Kongsted J, Poongavanam V et al. Recent developments in the medicinal chemistry of single boron atom-containing compounds. Acta Pharmaceutica Sinica B. Oct 2021;**11**(10):3035-3059. DOI: 10.1016/j.apsb.2021.01.010. Epub 20 Jan 2021. PMID: 34729302; PMCID: PMC8546671

[41] Park SB et al. Chemotherapy-induced peripheral neurotoxicity: A critical analysis. CA: A Cancer Journal for Clinicians. 2013;**63**(6):419-437

Chapter 5

Environmental Pollution Originated by the Excessive Use of Agrochemicals in the Production of Granadilla (*Passiflora ligularis*) Oxapampa District, Pasco, Perú

Benito Buendía Quispe and Raymundo Erazo Erazo

Abstract

The purpose of this research was to evaluate the environmental pollution originated by the excessive use of agrochemicals in the production of granadilla *(Passiflora ligularis)* in the Oxapampa district, Pasco – Peru. The crops of this fruit were chosen in the sectors named: Abra (Ab), Chacos (Ch), Quillazú (Qll), Acuzazú (Ac), Cañera (Ca), San Alberto (SA), Alto Río Pisco (ARP), and Paradise (Pa), where applying the nonexperimental and comparative design, the soil, water, and fruit samples were taken, which were analyzed in the specialized laboratory of the Faculty of Chemistry and Chemical Engineering, of the Universidad Nacional Mayor de San Marcos (UNMSM). A survey was also carried out by the farmers to form groups (ABC), and the results obtained were statistically analyzed by means of the comparative difference of concentration of heavy metals in three groups selected according to intensity of use of agrochemicals, which were between 0.26 and 0.36 mg of Cu/kg of fruit, between 0.001 and 0.003 mg of Cd and Pb/kg of fruit, between 0.0012 and 0.0006 mg As and Hg/kg of fruit, between 19 and 25 mg of Cu/kg of soil, between 0.02 and 0.08 mg of Cd and Pb/kg of soil, between 0.05 and 0.08 mg of As and Hg/kg of soil; between 1 and 1.12 mg of Cu/l of water, between 0.002 and 0.003 mg of Cd and Pb/l of water, between 0.002 and 0.005 mg of As and Hg/l of water; being observed high averages in some heavy metals and whose comparisons were not significant for As, Hg, Pb, Cd, Cu in fruits, soil, and water, and significant only the Cd in fruits and Hg in soils, concluding that there is a potential risk of toxicity due to ingestion of granadilla (*P. ligularis*).

Keywords: heavy metals, soil, water, fruits, toxicity

1. Introduction

In the agricultural fields of some sectors of the district of Oxapampa, it has been detected that farmers are applying agrochemicals in excess during the production process of granadilla fruit (*Passiflora ligularis*), generating environmental contamination, which must be evaluated and made known community-wide to take corrective measures regarding the concentration of possible heavy metals that would be found in the soil, runoff water from rainfall, and fruits. Everyone's concern is to contribute to the knowledge of environmental contamination in the agricultural sectors. The most important environmental and social consequences of the use of agrochemicals are: persistence of the agrochemical, bioaccumulation, soil and water pollution by agrochemical residues [1].

Under this evidence found in the agricultural activity, human health is put at risk due to the consumption of fruits contaminated with toxic residues of heavy metals. Pesticides cause damage to the environment, to the cultivation soil, and to the water so it is inadmissible that the same practices continue to be carried out in agricultural management [2]. One of the main characteristics of heavy metals is their level of toxicity according to their concentration in the habitat they are found. This has been the subject of many studies in order to evaluate the mechanisms involved in their toxicity and their harmful effects on human beings. For example, mercury is one of the environmental contaminants with the greatest negative impact [3].

There are studies in many countries of the world on the negative effects caused by agrochemicals. They report that vegetable species presented concentrations of lead and arsenic that did not exceed the reference regulations; however, in the case of medicinal plants, arsenic was found in 0.2 mg/kg, so it is recommended that it is necessary to monitor whether the content of this heavy metal is due to the use of chemical substances in soil where it was cultivated [4]. Studies carried out on samples of *Tessaria integrifolia* leaves from Trujillo, La Libertad, found concentrations of lead at 2.022 mg/kg, cadmium at 0.155 mg/kg, mercury at 0.073 mg/kg, and arsenic at 0.308645 mg/kg [5]. This is evidence that contamination exists in different places and under different conditions.

The purpose of the research was to determine the comparative difference in concentration of heavy metals between the sampling groups according to the intensity of application of agrochemicals during the agricultural management of the granadilla fruit crop, so it raises the hypothesis that "the different agrochemical application intensities during the management of the granadilla (*P. ligularis*) crop in three sampling groups (A, B and C), generate significant differences in the content of heavy metals in the fruit, soil and runoff water, in the district of Oxapampa."

For this, surveys were planned and carried out among the farmers to select according to the frequency of application of agrochemicals the sample size of the geographical area that was 55 Ha in full production of granadilla, from where soil, runoff water, and fruit samples were taken, based on the protocols defined by the Chemical Analysis Laboratory (USAQ) of the Faculty of Chemistry and Chemical Engineering of the National University of San Marcos (UNMSM) Lima, Peru, and for the chemical analysis of heavy metals, an atomic absorption spectrophotometer was used.

Codes were defined (see appendices) that identify the origin of the different samples, achieving the study of three groups of farmers who apply agrochemicals in the granadilla fruit production process at different frequencies in various sectors.

2. Methodology, results, and discussion

2.1 Methodology

The research carried out, due to its purpose, falls within the type of basic research, since it was analyzed what metallic elements the fruits, soil, and runoff water contain in the granadilla fruit production process. On the other hand, social information is obtained that allows determining the cause of contamination under three dimensions of groups selected according to the intensity of use of agrochemicals, which is considered as a process of environmental contamination by human intervention (anthropic) and, likewise, allows to determine how the soil-water interaction influences the contamination of granadilla fruit [6].

2.1.1 Population and sample

The population was of the finite type that was made up of all granadilla fruit crop fields (*P. ligularis*) in full production in the district of Oxapampa, with 1463 Ha [7].

The sample size consisted of 55 Ha of granadilla fruit in production and was determined using the following equation:

$$n = \frac{Z^2pqN}{E^2(N-1) + Z^2pq} \tag{1}$$

Where: Z = 1.65, P = 0.70, q = 0.30, N = 1463 y E = 0.10.

From the 55 Ha of granadilla fruit crop in full production, corresponding to several owners with diverse extensions of granadilla fruit crop, they were geographically distributed in rural sectors within the district of Oxapampa, such as: Alto Rio Pisco, Cañera, Abra, Chacos, San Alberto, Acuzazú, Quillazú, Paradise.

The production fields were taken randomly in each sector, then a survey was carried out on each owner (farmer) through a questionnaire, information was collected on the surface of their granadilla fruit production fields, types of agrochemicals that are generally used, and with what frequency they are applied during the year of crop management. Three groups were then selected and formed according to the intensity of agrochemicals application per year. Group "A" includes those who apply agrochemicals with high frequency; group "B," with medium frequency; and group "C," with low frequency.

From these groups, samples were taken in different sectors already classified and duly coded for each production area. Fruit sampling was randomly selected, taking six fruits/sample; in the same way, soil samples were extracted from the field, also at random points, following a zigzag scheme at a depth of 20 cm, homogenizing the subsamples and obtaining a single representative sample in the amount of 0.5 kg. Runoff water samples were also taken from the production fields in an amount of 1 liter/sample; for this last case, it was necessary to previously prepare collectors, which were holes prepared on the ground surfaces covered at the base or bottom with plastic to ensure the accumulation of runoff water on rainy days, distributed at various points in the study area.

The period of extraction and transport of the samples from the field to the laboratory was 2 days. Water was collected in a white polyethylene bottle with a capacity of 1 liter as a representative sample; the fruit and soil samples were collected in hermetic polyethylene bags for the appropriate capacity. All the collected samples, 15 fruit samples, 15 soil samples, and 15 water samples were transported from the study fields to the UNMSM laboratory, following strict quality control, for the corresponding analyses.

2.1.2 Design of the investigation

Due to the nature of the research, the nonexperimental and comparative design was applied; defined as a schematized structure, which consists of determining the significance between two or more variables of interest in one or more samples, comparing the observations obtained and analyzing the inferences between two or more different populations, the scheme of which is as follows (see **Figure 1**):

The techniques used during the investigation were: identification, observation, data collection, and samples in field and laboratory phases. For the social component, the interview and dialogue technique was used. For the assessment of heavy metals: As, Pb, Hg, Cd, and Cu present in the samples, an atomic absorption spectrophotometer was used, and the results were measured in mg of contaminant/kg of sample.

The instruments used in the research were: predesigned formats and questionnaires, to record the data obtained during the evaluation process. The questionnaire for the interview was validated with professionals and research experts in the social area, using the DELPHI method, which is a method of structuring a communication process that is effective in allowing a group of individuals, such as a whole in dealing with a complex [8].

The data obtained in the study area were processed in the cabinet, SPSS and Excel software were used, descriptive and inferential statistics, ANOVA for the comparison between sectors comprising three ABC groups, the analysis was carried out based on the processing and interpretation of the data.

2.2 Results

The results of the environmental pollutants analysis in the laboratory of the samples of fruits, soil, and runoff water show that, with respect to the fruits: in the sectors of AcAf SA1Bf, PaCf, average values between 0.26 and 0.36 mg of Cu/kg of sample; (Ch2Af, Ab3Bf ARP3Cf, QllAf, Ch3Bf, SA2Cf) average values between 0.001 and 0.003 mg of Cd and Pb/kg; (Ab1Af, CaBf, ARP1Cf, Ch1Af, Ab2Bf, ARP2Cf) average values between 0.0012 and 0.0006 mg of As and Hg/kg. Soils: in the sectors of (AcAs SA1Bs, PaCs) average values between 19 and 25 mg of Cu/kg; (Ch2As, Ab3Bs ARP3Cs, QllAs, Ch3Bs, SA2Cs) average values between 0.02 and 0.08 mg of Cd and Pb/kg; (Ab1As, CaBs, ARP1Cs, Ch1As, Ab2Bs, ARP2Cs) average values between 0.05 and 0.08 mg of As and Hg/kg. Runoff water: (AcAa SA1Ba, PaCa) average values between 1 and 1.12 mg of Cu/kg; (Ch2Aa, Ab3Ba ARP3Ca, QllAa, Ch3Ba, SA2Ca) average

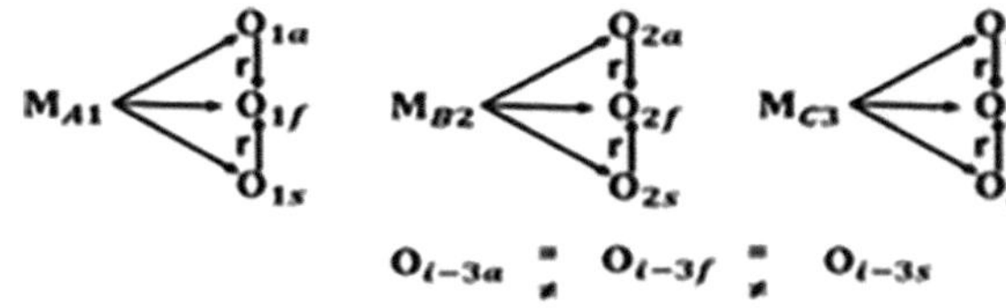

Figure 1.
Scheme of the research design derived from reference [6]. Where: M_{A_1} *= Sample of areas with low pesticide application.* M_{B2} *= Sample of areas with medium pesticide application.* M_{C_3} *= Sample of areas with high pesticide application.* Oi_{-3a} *= Observation of metal variables in contaminated water.* Oi_{-3s} *= Observation of metal variables in contaminated soil.* Oi_{-3f} *= Observation of metal variables in contaminated granadilla fruits. R = relationship between variables (*$Oi_{-3a} - Oi_{-3f}$*) and (*$Oi_{-3s} - Oi_{-3f}$*). =, ≠: comparisons between samples of the variables between three different populations (a = water, s = soil, f = fruits).*

values between 0.002 and 0.003 mg of Cd and Pb/kg; (Ab1Aa, CaBa, ARP1Ca, Ch1Aa, Ab2Ba, ARP2Ca) average values between 0.002 and 0.005 mg of As and Hg/kg.

High values were found in the average content of arsenic, mercury, lead, cadmium, and copper, which constitute a risk to human health. However, through ANOVA, it was found that there is no significance for the comparison of concentration of heavy metals for As, Hg, Pb, and Cu in the fruit, and it was significant for Cd. In the case of the comparison of concentration of metals As, Pb, Cd, and Cu in the soil, it was not significant, and for Hg it was significant. The comparison of the concentration of heavy metals in the runoff water was not significant for the metals As, Hg. Pb, Cd, and Cu. This corresponds to a reality observed in the study area in the granadilla fruit production systems and is dependent on chemical inputs with inappropriate management for the farmers and coupled with this the minimum commitment by the institutions to the respective control.

The following figures show average content of heavy metals in fruits, soil, and runoff water of the granadilla crop (*Passiflora ligularis*).

Figure 2 shows that in the sectors of Abra, Chacos, Quillazú, and Acuzazú, belonging to group A; in the Cañera, the Abra, Chacos, and San Alberto sectors, for group B and from the Alto Río Pisco, San Alberto, and El Paraíso sectors for group C, which are within the jurisdiction of the Oxapampa district, were found fruits with high average values of arsenic, mercury, lead, cadmium, and copper content. Thus, in the sectors of (AcAf SA1Bf, PaCf), they have averages between 0.26 and 0.36 mg of Cu/kg. Other samples taken in the sectors such as Ch2Af, Ab3Bf ARP3Cf, QllAf, Ch3Bf, SA2Cf have averages between 0.001 and 0.003 mg of Cd and Pb/kg and in the sectors of Ab1Af, CaBf, ARP1Cf, Ch1Af, Ab2Bf, ARP2Cf, they have averages between 0.0012 and 0.0006 mg of As and Hg/kg.

From **Figure 3** it can be seen that in the sectors of Abra, Chacos, Quillazú, and Acuzazú, for group A; from the Cañera, El Abra, Chacos, and San Alberto sectors, for group B and from the Alto Río Pisco, San Alberto, and El Paraíso sectors for group C, which are within the jurisdiction of the Oxapampa district, were found soils with average values of arsenic, mercury, lead, cadmium, and copper high content. Thus, in the sectors of AcAs SA1Bs, PaCs, have averages between 19 and 25 mg of Cu/kg. Other samples taken in the sectors such as Ch2As, Ab3Bs ARP3Cs, QllAs, Ch3Bs, SA2Cs have

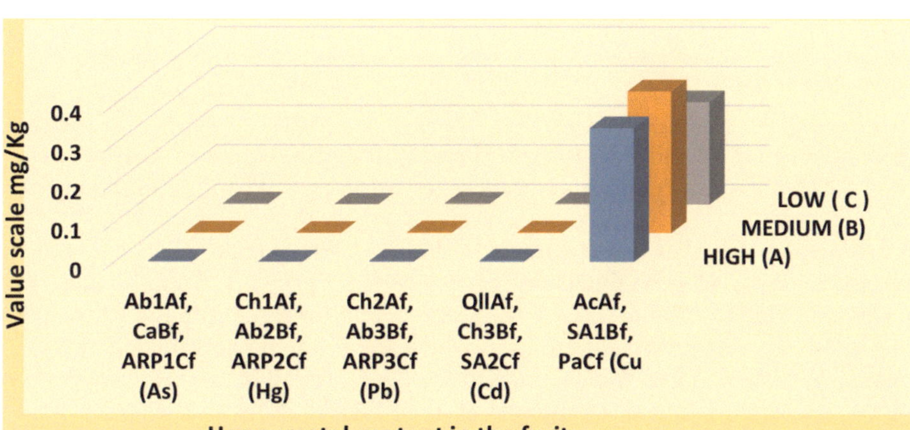

Figure 2.
*Average content of heavy metals in granadilla fruit (*Passiflora ligularis*) fruits in mg of contaminant/kg of sample.*

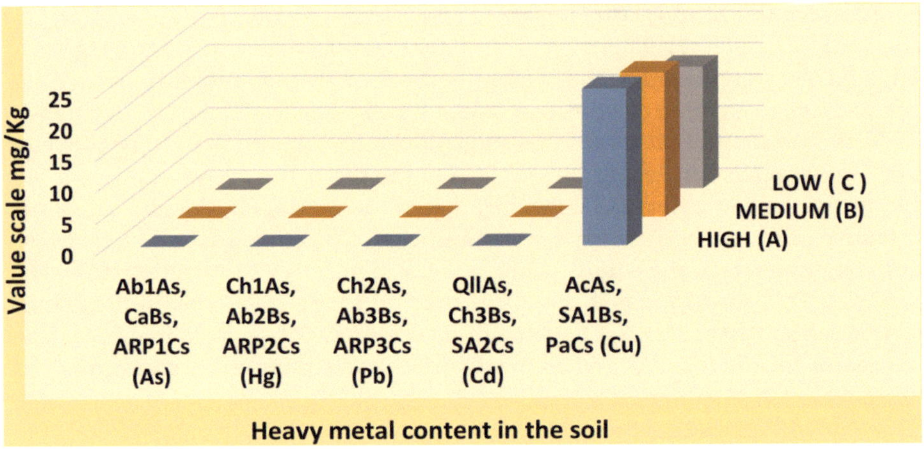

Figure 3.
*Average content of heavy metals in granadilla fruit (*Passiflora ligularis*) crop soils in mg of contaminant/kg of sample.*

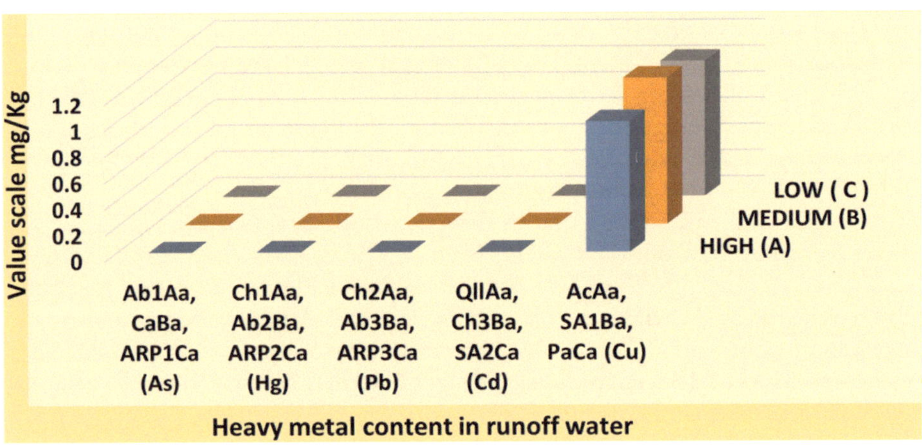

Figure 4.
*Average content of heavy metals in the runoff water of the granadilla fruit crop (*Passiflora ligularis*) in mg of contaminant/kg of sample.*

averages between 0.02 and 0.08 mg of Cd and Pb/kg, the sectors of Ab1As, CaBs, ARP1Cs, Ch1As, Ab2Bs, ARP2Cs have averages between 0.05 and 0.08 mg of As and Hg/kg.

In the samples of runoff water extracted from the fields of fruit-producing granadilla sectors, such as Abra, Chacos, Quillazú, and Acuzazú, for group A; from the Cañera, El Abra, Chacos, and San Alberto sectors, for group B; and from the Alto Río Pisco, San Alberto, and El Paraíso sectors for group C, which are within the jurisdiction of the Oxapampa district, high values of average content were found of arsenic, mercury, lead, cadmium, and copper. Thus, in the sectors of AcAa SA1Ba, PaCa, they have averages between 1 and 1.12 mg of Cu/kg. Other samples taken in the sectors such as Ch2Aa, Ab3Ba ARP3Ca, QllAa, Ch3Ba, SA2Ca have averages between 0.002 and 0.003 mg of Cd and Pb/kg, and the sectors of Ab1Aa, CaBa, ARP1Ca, Ch1Aa, Ab2Ba, ARP2Ca have averages between 0.002 and 0.005 mg of As and Hg/kg, (see **Figure 4**).

A statistical analysis was carried considering the different intensities of application of agrochemicals during the management of the granadilla (*P. ligularis*) crop in three sampling groups and considering that there are significant differences in the content of heavy metals in the fruit, soil, and runoff water in the Oxapampa district.

2.2.1 Analysis of results in relation to the concentration of arsenic and mercury in the fruits (mg/kg)

Ho: There are no differences in As and Hg between sampling groups.

H1: There are differences in As and Hg between sampling groups.

In the ANOVA, it is observed that the significance values are 0.062 (As) and 0.626 (Hg), a result that is obtained when comparing the selected groups A, B, and C, respectively, according to the heavy metal of arsenic and mercury and according to the intensity of use of agrochemicals. Said value is greater than the significance of $\alpha = 0.05$; therefore, the statistical decision in this regard is to accept the null hypothesis; consequently, the alternative hypothesis is rejected, concluding that here there is enough evidence to affirm that there are no significant differences in the concentration of arsenic and mercury in the fruits at different intensity of application of agrochemicals with a confidence level of 95% (see **Table 1**).

2.2.2 Analysis of results in relation to the concentration of lead and cadmium in fruits (mg/kg)

In **Table 2**, it is observed from ANOVA that the significance values are 0.475 (Pb) and 0.042 (Cd), a result obtained from comparing selected groups A, B, and C, respectively, according to the heavy metals of lead and cadmium, according to the intensity of use of agrochemicals. Said value with respect to Pb is greater than the significance of $\alpha = 0.05$; therefore, the statistical decision in this regard is to accept the null hypothesis; consequently, the alternative hypothesis is rejected. However, the value with respect to cadmium is less than the significance of $\alpha = 0.05$; the alternative hypothesis is accepted and the null one is rejected, concluding that there is sufficient evidence that affirms the existence or not of significant differences in the concentration of lead and cadmium in fruits at different intensity of application of agrochemicals with a confidence level of 95%.

Ho: There are no differences in Pb and Cd between sampling groups.

H1: There are differences in Pb and Cd between sampling groups.

Variation Source	SC	gl	CMe	F		Sig.	
				As	Hg	As	Hg
Between groups (ABC)	0.000	2	0.000	3545	0.488	0.062	0.626
within groups	0.000	12	0.000				
Total	0.000	14					

Source: Data processed from chemical analysis Laboratory UNMSM 2019.

Table 1.
*ANOVA of comparison between groups of concentration of arsenic and mercury in granadilla fruits (*Passiflora ligularis*), according to the intensity of use of agrochemicals.*

Variation Source	SC	gl	CMe	F		Sig.	
				Pb	Cd	Pb	Cd
Between groups (ABC)	0.000	2	0.000	0.792	4174	0.475	0.042
within groups	0.000	12	0.000				
Total	0.000	14					

Source: Data processed from chemical analysis Laboratory UNMSM 2019.

Table 2.
*ANOVA of comparison between groups of concentration of lead and cadmium in granadilla fruits (*Passiflora ligularis*), according to the intensity of use of agrochemicals.*

2.2.3 Analysis of results in relation to the concentration of copper in fruits (mg/kg)

Ho: There are no differences in Cu between sampling groups.

H1: There are differences in Cu between sampling groups.

In the ANOVA, it is observed that the significance value is 0.371, a result that is obtained from comparing selected groups A, B, and C, respectively, in accordance with the heavy metal of copper according to intensity of use of agrochemicals. Said value is greater than the significance of $\alpha = 0.05$; therefore, the statistical decision in this regard is to accept the null hypothesis; consequently, the alternative hypothesis is rejected, concluding that there is sufficient evidence to affirm that there are no significant differences in copper concentration in fruits at different intensity of application of agrochemicals with a confidence level of 95% (see **Table 3**).

2.2.4 Analysis of results in relation to the content of arsenic and lead in the soil (mg/kg)

Ho: There are no differences in As and Pb between sampling groups.

H1: There are differences in As and Pb between sampling groups.

In the ANOVA, the significance values are of 0.863 (As) and 0.579 (Pb), results obtained from comparing selected groups A, B, and C, respectively, according to the heavy metal content of arsenic and lead in the soil from the fields of granadilla fruit production (*P. ligularis*) according to intensity of use of agrochemicals. These values are greater than the significance of $\alpha = 0.05$; therefore the statistical decision in this regard is to accept the null hypothesis; consequently, the alternative hypothesis is rejected. In this way, it is concluded that there is sufficient evidence to affirm that there are no significant differences in the content of arsenic and lead in the soil samples at different intensity of application of agrochemicals at a confidence level of 95% (see **Table 4**).

Variation Source	Sum of squares	gl	Root mean square	F	Sig.
Between groups	0.028	2	0.014	1077	0.371
within groups	0.156	12	0.013		
Total	0.184	14			

Source: Data processed from chemical analysis Laboratory UNMSM 2019.

Table 3.
*ANOVA of comparison between groups of copper concentration in passion fruit (*Passiflora ligularis*), according to the intensity of use of agrochemicals.*

Variation Source	SC	gl	CMe	F		Sig.	
				As	Pb	As	Pb
Between groups (ABC)	0.000	2	0.000	0.149	0.571	0.863	0.579
within groups	0.000	12	0.000				
Total	0.000	14					

Source: Data processed from chemical analysis Laboratory UNMSM 2019.

Table 4.
*ANOVA of comparison between groups of arsenic and lead content in the soil of the granadilla fruit crop (*Passiflora ligularis*), according to the intensity of use of agrochemicals.*

2.2.5 Analysis of results in relation to the mercury content in the soil (mg/kg)

Ho: There are no differences in Hg between sampling groups.

H1: There are differences in Hg between sampling groups.

From the ANOVA analysis, the significance value is 0.012, whose result has been obtained after comparing between selected groups A, B, and C, respectively, in accordance with the heavy metal content of mercury in the soil from the granadilla fruit production fields (*P. ligularis*) according to intensity of use of agrochemicals. As can be seen, such value is less than the significance of $\alpha = 0.05$; therefore the statistical decision in this regard is to reject the null hypothesis; consequently, the alternative hypothesis is accepted. In this way, it is concluded that there is sufficient evidence to affirm that there are significant differences in mercury content in the soil samples at different intensity of application of agrochemicals at a confidence level of 95% (see **Table 5**).

2.2.6 Analysis of results in relation to the content of cadmium in the soil (mg/kg)

Ho: There are no differences in Cd between sampling groups.

H1: There are differences in Cd between sampling groups.

From the ANOVA analysis in **Table 6**, it is observed that the significance value is 0.331, a result obtained from comparing selected groups A, B, and C, respectively, in accordance with the heavy metal content of cadmium in the soil from fruit production fields granadilla (*P. ligularis*) according to intensity of use of agrochemicals. Said value is greater than the significance of $\alpha = 0.05$; therefore the statistical decision in this regard is to accept the null hypothesis; consequently, the alternative hypothesis is rejected, concluding that there is sufficient evidence to affirm that there are no

Variation Source	Sum of squares	gl	Root mean square	F	Sig.
Between groups	0.003	2	0.001	6576	0.012
within groups	0.003	12	0.000		
Total	0.006	14			

Source: Data processed from chemical analysis Laboratory UNMSM 2019.

Table 5.
*ANOVA of comparison between groups of mercury content in the soil of the granadilla fruit crop (*Passiflora ligularis*), according to the intensity of use of agrochemicals.*

Variation Source	Sum of squares	gl	Root mean square	F	Sig.
Between groups	0.012	2	0.006	1215	0.331
within groups	0.057	12	0.005		
Total	0.069	14			

Source: Data processed from chemical analysis Laboratory UNMSM 2019.

Table 6.
*ANOVA of comparison between groups of cadmium content in the soil of the granadilla fruit crop (*Passiflora ligularis*), according to the intensity of use of agrochemicals.*

significant differences in cadmium content in the soil samples at different intensity of application of agrochemicals at a confidence level of 95%.

2.2.7 Analysis of results in relation to the copper content in the soil (mg/kg)

Ho: There are no differences in Cu between sampling groups.

H1: There are differences in Cu between sampling groups.

In the ANOVA, the significance value is 0.317, a result that is obtained from comparing selected groups A, B, and C, respectively, in accordance with the heavy metal content of copper in the soil from granadilla fruit (*P. ligularis*) production fields according to intensity use of agrochemicals. Said value is greater than the significance of $\alpha = 0.05$; therefore the statistical decision in this regard is to accept the null hypothesis; consequently, the alternative hypothesis is rejected, concluding that there is sufficient evidence to affirm that there are no significant differences in copper content in the soil samples at different intensity of application of agrochemicals at a confidence level of 95% (see **Table** 7).

2.2.8 Analysis of results in relation to the content of arsenic and mercury in runoff water (mg/kg)

Ho: There are no differences in As and Hg between sampling groups.

H1: There are differences in As and Hg between sampling groups.

In the ANOVA, the significance values are of 0.469 (As) and 0.624 (Hg), a result obtained from comparing selected groups A, B, and C, respectively, according to the heavy metal content of arsenic and mercury in the runoff water of fields of production from granadilla fruit (*P. ligularis*) according to intensity of use of agrochemicals. These values are greater than the significance of $\alpha = 0.05$; therefore the statistical

Variation Source	Sum of squares	gl	Root mean square	F	Sig.
Between groups	80.,533	2	40.267	1268	0.317
within groups	381.200	12	31.767		
Total	461.733	14			

Source: Data processed from chemical analysis Laboratory UNMSM 2019.

Table 7.
*ANOVA of comparison between groups of copper content in the soil of the granadilla fruit crop (*Passiflora ligularis*), according to the intensity of use of agrochemicals.*

Variation Source	SC	gl	CMe	F		Sig.	
				As	**Hg**	**As**	**Hg**
Between groups (ABC)	0.000	2	0.000	0.808	0.491	0.469	0.624
within groups	0.000	12	0.000				
Total	0.000	14					

Source: Data processed from chemical analysis Laboratory UNMSM 2019.

Table 8.
*ANOVA of comparison between groups of arsenic and mercury content in runoff water in the granadilla fruit (*Passiflora ligularis*) crop, according to the intensity of use of agrochemicals.*

decision in this regard is to accept the null hypothesis; consequently, the alternative hypothesis is rejected, concluding that there is sufficient evidence to affirm that there are no significant differences in the content of arsenic and mercury in the runoff water samples at different intensity of application of agrochemicals at a confidence level of 95% (see **Table 8**).

2.2.9 Analysis of results in relation to the content of lead and cadmium in the runoff water (mg/kg)

Ho: There are no differences in Pb and Cd between sampling groups.
H1: There are differences in Pb and Cd between sampling groups.

In the ANOVA, the significance values are 0.887 (Pb) and 0.813 (Cd), a result obtained from comparing selected groups A, B, and C, respectively, according to the heavy metal content of lead and cadmium in the runoff water of fields of production from granadilla fruit (*P. ligularis*) according to intensity of use of agrochemicals. These values are greater than the significance of $\alpha = 0.05$; therefore the statistical decision in this regard is to accept the null hypothesis; consequently, the alternative hypothesis is rejected, concluding that there is sufficient evidence to affirm that there are no significant differences in lead and cadmium content in runoff water samples at different intensity of application of agrochemicals at a confidence level of 95% (see **Table 9**).

2.2.10 Analysis of results in relation to the copper content in the runoff water (mg/kg)

Ho: There are no differences in Cu between sampling groups.
H1: There are differences in Cu between sampling groups.

Variation Source	SC	gl	CMe	F		Sig.	
				Pb	**Cd**	**Pb**	**Cd**
Between groups	0.000	2	0.000	0.121	0.211	0.887	0.813
within groups	0.000	12	0.000				
Total	0.000	14					

Source: Data processed from chemical analysis Laboratory UNMSM 2019.

Table 9.
*ANOVA of comparison between groups of lead and cadmium content in runoff water in granadilla fruit (*Passiflora ligularis*) cultivation, according to the intensity of use of agrochemicals.*

Variation Source	Sum of squares	gl	Root mean square	F	Sig.
Between groups	0.038	2	0.019	0.494	0.622
within groups	0.465	12	0.039		
Total	0.503	14			

Source: Data processed from chemical analysis Laboratory UNMS 2019.

Table 10.
*ANOVA of comparison between groups of copper content in runoff water in the cultivation of granadilla (*Passiflora ligularis*), according to the intensity of use of agrochemicals.*

In the ANOVA, the significance value is 0.622, a result obtained from comparing selected groups A, B, and C, respectively, according to the heavy metal content of copper in the runoff water from the granadilla fruit production fields (*P. ligularis*) according to intensity of use of agrochemicals. Said value is greater than the significance of $\alpha = 0.05$; therefore the statistical decision in this regard is to accept the null hypothesis; consequently, the alternative hypothesis is rejected, concluding that there is sufficient evidence to affirm that there are no significant differences in copper content in runoff water samples at different intensity of application of agrochemicals at a confidence level of 95% (see **Table 10**).

2.3 Discussion

Next, you perform the comparison of the content and concentration of heavy metals between sampling groups (A, B, and C) according to intensity of application of agrochemicals in the agricultural management of granadilla (*P. ligularis*), Oxapampa district.

The average results obtained for heavy metals in the fruits were: in the sectors of AcAf SA1Bf, PaCf between 0.26 and 0.36 mg of Cu/kg; (Ch2Af, Ab3Bf ARP3Cf, QllAf, Ch3Bf, SA2Cf) between 0.001 and 0.003 mg of Cd and Pb/kg; (Ab1Af, CaBf, ARP1Cf, Ch1Af, Ab2Bf, ARP2Cf) between 0.0012 and 0.0006 mg of As and Hg/kg. In soils: in the sectors of AcAs SA1Bs, PaCs, between 19 and 25 mg of Cu/kg; (Ch2As, Ab3Bs ARP3Cs, QllAs, Ch3Bs, SA2Cs) between 0.02 and 0.08 mg of Cd and Pb/kg; (Ab1As, CaBs, ARP1Cs, Ch1As, Ab2Bs, ARP2Cs) between 0.05 and 0.08 mg of As and Hg/kg. For the runoff waters: in the sectors of AcAa SA1Ba, PaCa, between 1 and 1.12 mg of Cu/kg; (Ch2Aa, Ab3Ba ARP3Ca, QllAa, Ch3Ba, SA2Ca) between 0.002 and 0.003 mg of Cd and Pb/kg; (Ab1Aa, CaBa, ARP1Ca, Ch1Aa, Ab2Ba, ARP2Ca) between 0.002 and 0.005 mg of As and Hg/kg.

These results show high levels of risk in human health and the environmental contamination in the agroecosystems of the district of Oxapampa, whose main cause is lack of technical advice from state agencies and coupled with this a nontechnical dosage of pesticides and fertilizers, chemicals, agrochemicals, applied by farmers in the production of granadilla fruit.

The average results obtained for heavy metals in fruits are shown below in **Table 11**, where the Provisional Tolerable Weekly Intake (PTWI) values [9] are also shown, in mg/kg of body weight for the same heavy metals, in order to observe that there is a toxicological risk related to a weekly consumption of these fruits.

It has been preferred to use the PTWI and not the maximum levels (ML), since this toxicological result is appropriate for food contaminants, such as heavy metals, due to

Heavy metal in granadilla fruit (*Passiflora ligularis*)	Average results mg/kg sample	PTWI: Provisional Tolerable Weekly Intake in mg/kg body weight *
Arsenic, As	0.0012 to 0.0006	0.015
Mercury, Hg	0.0012 to 0.0006	0.005
Lead, Pb	0.001 to 0.003	0.025
Cadmium, Cd	0.001 to 0.003	0.007
Copper, Cu	0.26 to 0.36	1

* *Source: CODEX STAN 193–1995 Revision 2009 Mod. 2019.*

Table 11.
Comparison of the average experimental results with the PTWI of heavy metals in food.

their cumulative capacity. The PTWI by definition is a value that represents the permissible weekly human exposure to such contaminants.

These results are comparable with those obtained in other investigations such as the studies by Fang and Zhu, who showed concentrations of five heavy metals (chromium, copper, cadmium, mercury, and lead) in four fruits (pear, grape, peach-shaped plum, and orange), which exceeded safety standards. They state that the origin of these metals was mainly due to the application of foliar fertilizers, ripening agents, fungicides, and pesticides during flowering and ripening [10]. Shaheen et al. used inductively coupled plasma mass spectrometry (ICP-MS) and demonstrated the presence of toxic heavy metals such as As, Cd, Pb, Cr, Mn, Ni, Cu, and Zn in representative samples of fruits and vegetables in Bangladesh. These results exceeded the maximum permissible concentration (MAC) established by the FAO/WHO for Pb in mango and Cd in tomato among the fruits and vegetables analyzed, representing risks to human health [11].

Other researchers such as Abbasi et al. also evaluated the concentration of heavy metals and associated health risk in processed fruit products sold in local markets in northern Pakistan. They quantified seven metals: cadmium (Cd), chromium (Cr), cobalt (Co), copper (Cu), iron (Fe), lead (Pb), and zinc (Zn) in different food samples and showed that measured levels of these metals varied significantly and were relatively higher than their allowable limits. Univariate and multivariate analysis yielded a strong association between Cr, Co, Pb, and Fe and confirmed heavy metal contamination through natural and anthropogenic sources in processed foods [12].

Likewise, Marini et al. evaluated the daily intake in various foods of four heavy metals, such as cadmium, mercury, lead, and arsenic; and four minerals: chromium, nickel, selenium, and zinc. The risk of exceeding the provisional tolerable daily intake in the four proposed Danish dietary profiles was on average 60%, 17%, and 16% for cadmium, mercury, and lead, respectively. For total arsenic, the risk of exceeding the provisional daily intake was 33%, and they emphasize the importance of implementing measures to reduce the risk cycle of heavy metals that threaten environmental health and food safety [13], showing a relationship with the results obtained in this work.

As will be seen later, the results obtained in the investigation agree with other studies, in which they also demonstrated that the contaminated water used for growing vegetables has contaminated the soil and that the samples of water, soil, and vegetables were contaminated with Ni, Cd, Cr, Cu, Pb, and Zn, and the concentration trends of these metals were as follows: 0,613 > 0,316 > 0,162 > 0,065 > 0,041 >

Place	Lead, mg/kg	Arsenic mg/kg	Cadmium mg/kg	Copper mg/kg	Mercury mg/kg
Granadilla cultivation field	0.002 to 0.003	0.002 to 0.005	0.002 to 0.003	1 to 1.12	0.002 to 0.005
Oxapampa*	7.78475	ND	ND	ND	0.29675

NA = not detected.
**Source: Bernal Marcelo, A.R., 2019.*

Table 12.
Concentration of heavy metals: Pb, As. Cd, Cu, and Hg in runoff water and water collected in the cattle town of Chontabamba – Oxapampa [16].

0,028 mL/L for Ni, Cd, Pb, Cr, Cu, and Zn, respectively, in the contaminated water and 189,09 > 125 > 104,92 > 41,85 > 28,58 > 21,72 for Zn, Cr, Ni, Pb, Cu, and Cd mg/kg in the soil, which represents a risk to the health of the population [14, 15].

Table 12 shows the concentrations of heavy metals: Pb, As. Cd, Cu, and Hg, obtained by this research in runoff water in the granadilla fruit (*P. ligularis*) cultivation fields and the concentrations of water destined for livestock activity for dairy animal consumption in the location of Chontabamba [16].

Table 12 shows the results obtained by Bernal from the analysis of water from broken, rivulets that originate from wetlands, groundwater, and that are relatively protected by natural forest areas, and that correspond to areas dedicated only to livestock, where no As, Cd, and Cu are detected, while Hg and Pb present relatively low levels. Compared with the results of the study for this water factor, an impact on runoff water contamination is observed, which would be related to the use of agrochemicals in granadilla fruit (*P. ligularis*) crops and the consequent risk to human health.

Table 13 shows the contents of heavy metals in the grazing soil of the dairy herds analyzed in samples from the localities of Chontabamba and Oxàpampa [16] and the concentrations of these heavy metals obtained by the study in the soils intended for the cultivation of granadilla (*P. ligularis*).

In **Table 13** it can be seen how the concentrations of heavy metals present in the soils destined for livestock, downstream of the soils destined for the cultivation of granadilla show a higher concentration of heavy metals in arsenic, mercury, lead, and cadmium with the exception of copper, where its value is small compared with the soil for granadilla fruit that has a high concentration, which corroborates the hypothesis that the excessive use of agrochemicals would be the cause of these negative environmental impacts and that they represent a risk to human health.

Place	Lead, mg/Kg	Arsenic mg/Kg	Cadmium mg/Kg	Copper mg/Kg	Mercury mg/Kg
Granadilla cultivation soil localities	0.02 to 0.08	0.05 to 0.08	0.02 to 0.08	19 to 25	0.05 to 0.08
Chontabamba*	30.5638	12.847	0.1248	22.667	0.0486
Oxapampa*	22.3833	10.095	0.1153	22.995	0.0445

**Source: Bernal Marcelo, A.R., 2019.*

Table 13.
*Concentration of heavy metals: Pb, As, Cd, Cu, and Hg, in the soil of granadilla fruit (*Passiflora ligularis*) cultivation and soil of the cattle town of Chontabamba and Oxapampa [16].*

The studies carried out by other authors corroborate the results obtained in this investigation, agreeing when mentioning that there are differences between the different managements studied, evidencing that in those intensively used soils, the highest values were recorded for $Cu2^{+}$ and $Pb2^{+}$ while in the case of $Cd2^{+}$, the agricultural management system presented the highest content, reaching a value higher than the maximum permissible limit of several countries [17]. On the other hand, it is also mentioned that that the coefficient of variation of the analyzed metal content indicates that the values are dispersed in a range average: copper from 0.007 to 0.053, cadmium from 0.013 to 0.070, and lead from 0.010 to 0.064 [18].

From the results of the statistical analysis by ANOVA of comparison between groups according to intensity of use of agrochemicals (A, B, and C) for soil samples obtained from the production fields of *P. ligularis* of the selected farmers, it is found that the heavy metals found such as arsenic, lead, cadmium, and copper, according to hypothesis testing, it was shown that there is no significant difference in the concentrations of these heavy metals in soils. However, in the case of mercury concentration, it did show significant differences between the groups of samples that were analyzed. These results indicate that the contamination of the soil by these chemical elements is limiting the quality of the agricultural products of Oxapampa. In this regard, they point out that the high proportion of Pb is a potential bioavailable contaminant that can interfere with the development of crops and that can be incorporated into the different levels of the food chain until reaching human beings.

On the other hand, from the analysis by ANOVA of comparison between groups of samples selected according to intensity of use of agrochemicals, for heavy metals such as arsenic, mercury, lead, cadmium, and copper that were found and analyzed in the runoff water of the granadilla fruit (*P. ligularis*) production fields, the hypothesis that there is no significant difference in the concentration of these chemical elements was demonstrated, the same ones that agree with the results obtained by Pérez [18].

Finally, from the ANOVA analysis of comparison between groups according to the intensity of use of agrochemicals (A, B, and C) for samples of granadilla (*P. ligularis*) fruits from the fields of the selected farmers, the heavy metals found that such as arsenic, mercury, lead, and copper and according to the verification of hypotheses, it was shown that there is no significant difference in the concentrations of said heavy metals. However, in the case of the concentration of cadmium, it did show significant differences between the groups of samples analyzed. This statistical procedure carried out is reinforced by mentioning that through the analysis of variance of one factor (ANOVA), the comparison tests serve to evaluate the behavior of the experimental data obtained in the analysis [19].

3. Conclusions

From the results that have been obtained in the investigation related to the contamination of water, soil, and passion fruit (*P. ligularis*) in Oxapampa, due to the excessive use of agrochemicals in the agricultural fields, it is concluded that the fruits indeed have a content of metals As, Pb, Cd, Hg, and Cu, which when compared with the provisional tolerable weekly intake, PTWI, toxicological criteria for heavy metal intake in foods because they are cumulative, expressed in mg/kg of body weight for each heavy metal is evident that the risk of toxicity to human health is increasing if corrective measures are not taken to mitigate these future impacts.

The quality of runoff water in the agricultural sector was compared with water quality data from the livestock sector within the same area of study, observing that the levels of contamination by As, Cd, and Cu are increasing in the agricultural sector compared with nonpresence of the same in the cattle fields. Not so in relation to soil contamination, because when comparing the results of the study with others within the sector, it was observed that the livestock sector is more impacted by the five heavy metals compared with the agricultural sector. This accumulation of heavy metals in livestock soils would be due to the drag, transport, and diffusion mechanisms of agrochemical contaminants formulated with these metals, which are applied in excess in agricultural fields that occupy higher slopes, concluding that there is a process increasing environmental contamination in Oxapampa and that represents a potential risk to human health due to ingestion through fruits, and other foods that are consumed in the place and outside of it, as some of these are for export.

By an analysis of variance, with a probability of $\alpha = 0.05$ and a confidence level of 95%, for comparisons between three groups of farmers (A, B, and C), selected according to the intensity of application of agrochemicals in production of granadilla fruits, it was shown that in the case of the concentrations of heavy metals in fruits, such as arsenic, mercury, lead, and copper, there are no significant differences; not so for cadmium, which showed a significant existence. In the case of the content of heavy metals in soils, such as arsenic, lead, cadmium, and copper, it was also shown that there are no significant differences; however, mercury showed significant existence. In the case of the content of heavy metals in runoff waters such as arsenic, mercury, lead, cadmium, and copper, it was shown that there are no significant differences.

Therefore, considering the spatial and temporal environment of agricultural and livestock activities in the district of Oxapampa, it is concluded that there is a potential risk of toxicity to human health due to ingestion of granadilla (*P. ligularis*).

Acknowledgements

Our thanks to the authorities of the Universidad Nacional Mayor de San Marcos (UNMSM) and Daniel Alcides Carrión de Cerro de Pasco (UNDAC) for allowing us the use of their laboratories and facilities during the execution of this investigation.

Nomenclature

MLP	Maximum permissible limit of heavy metals, (mg/kg)
Ab1Af	Code (Abra, first sample, group A, fruit components)
CaBf	Code (Cane, group B, fruit component)
ARP1Cf	Code (Alto Rio pisco, first sample, group C, fruit component)
Ch1Af	Code (Chacos, first sample, group A, fruit component)
Ab2Bf	Code (Abra, second sample, group B, fruit component)
ARP2Cf	Code (Alto Rio Pisco, second sample, group C, fruit component)
Ch2Af	Code (Chacos, second sample, group A, fruit component)
Ab3Bf	Code (Abra, third sample, group B, fruit component)
ARP3Cf	Code (Alto Rio Pisco, third sample, group C, fruit component)

QllAf	Code (Quillazú, group A, fruit component)
Ch3Bf	Code (Chacos, third sample, group B, fruit component)
SA2Cf	Code (San Alberto, second sample, group C, fruit component)
AcAf	Code (Acuzazú, group A, fruit component)
SA1Bf	Code (San Alberto first sample, group B, fruit component)
PaCf	Code (Paraíso, group C, fruit component)
Ab1As	Code (Abra, first sample, group A, soil components)
CaBs	Code (Sugar cane, group B, soil component)
ARP1Cs	Code (Alto Rio Pisco, first sample, group C, soil component)
Ch1As	Code (Chacos, first sample, group A, soil component)
Ab2Bs	Code (Abra, second sample, group B, soil component)
ARP2Cs	Code (Alto Rio Pisco, second sample, group C, soil component)
Ch2As	Code (Chacos, second sample, group A, soil component)
Ab3Bs	Code (Abra, third sample, group B, soil component)
ARP3Cs	Code (Alto Rio Pisco, third sample, group C, soil component)
QllAs	Code (Quillazú, group A, soil component)
Ch3Bs	Code (Chacos, third sample, group B, soil component)
SA2Cs	Code (San Alberto, second sample, group C, soil component)
AcAs	Code (Acuzazú, group A, soil component)
SA1Bs	Code (San Alberto first sample, group B, soil component)
PaCs	Code (Paraíso group C soil component)
Ab1Aa	Code (Abra, first sample, group A, water component)
CaBa	Code (Sugar cane, group B, water component)
ARP1Ca	Code (Alto Rio Pisco, first sample, group C, water component)
Ch1Aa	Code (Chacos, first sample, group A, water component)
Ab2Ba	Code (Abra, second sample, group B, water component)
ARP2Ca	Code (Alto Rio Pisco, second sample, group C, water component)
Ch2Aa	Code (Chacos, second sample, group A, water component)
Ab3Ba	Code (Abra, third sample, group B, water component)
ARP3Ca	Code (Alto Rio Pisco, third sample, group C, water component)
QllAa	Code (Quillazú, group A, water component)
Ch3Ba	Code (Chacos, third sample, group B, water component)
SA2Ca	Code (San Alberto, second sample, group C, water component)
AcAa	Code (Acuzazú, group A, water component)
SA1Ba	Code (San Alberto first sample, group B, water component)
PaCa	Code (Paradise, group C, water component)

A. Appendices

Photographs of the sectors chosen for sampling
See (**Figures 5–8**).

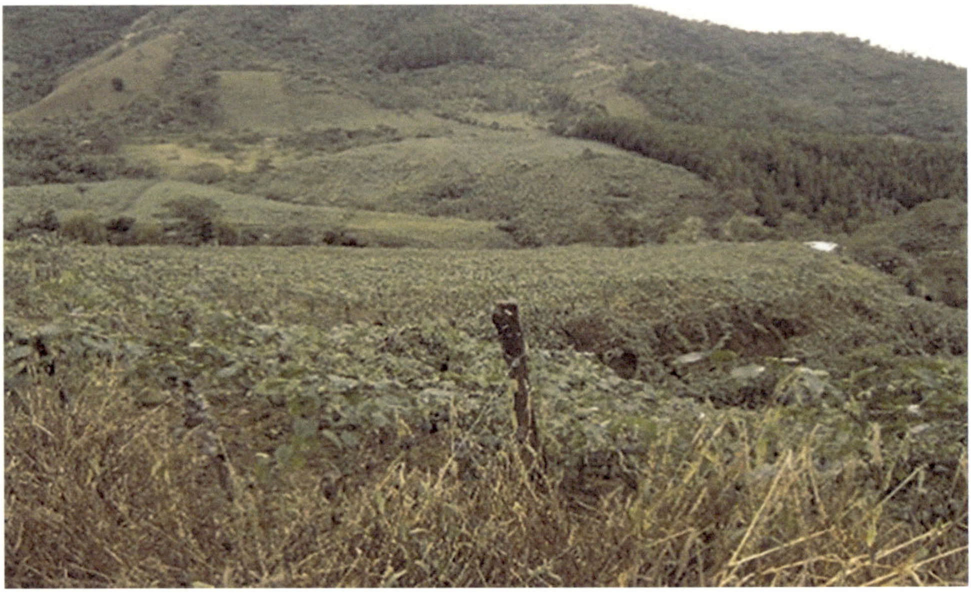

Figure 5.
Sectors of Chacos and the Abra.

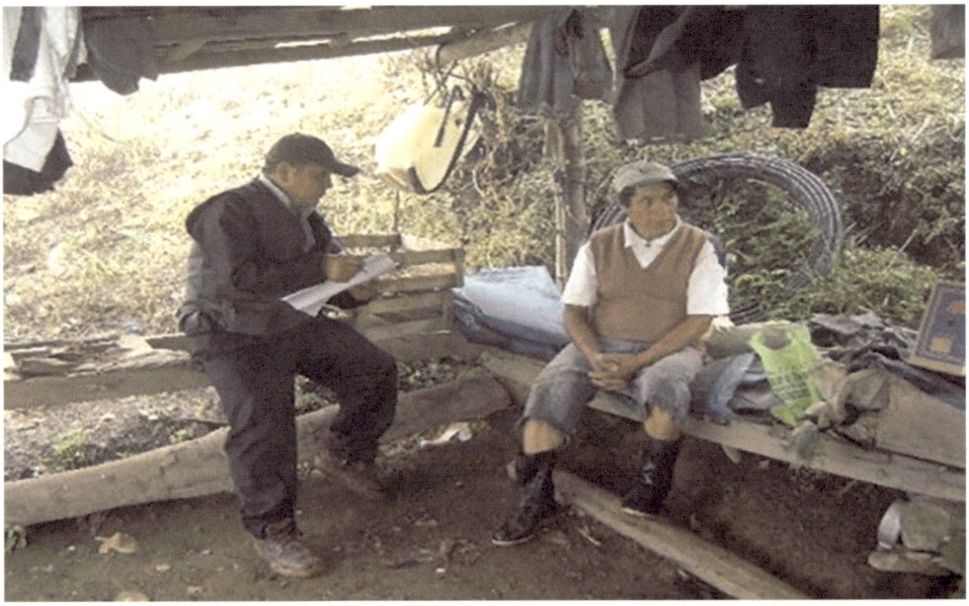

Figure 6.
Interview with a farmer.

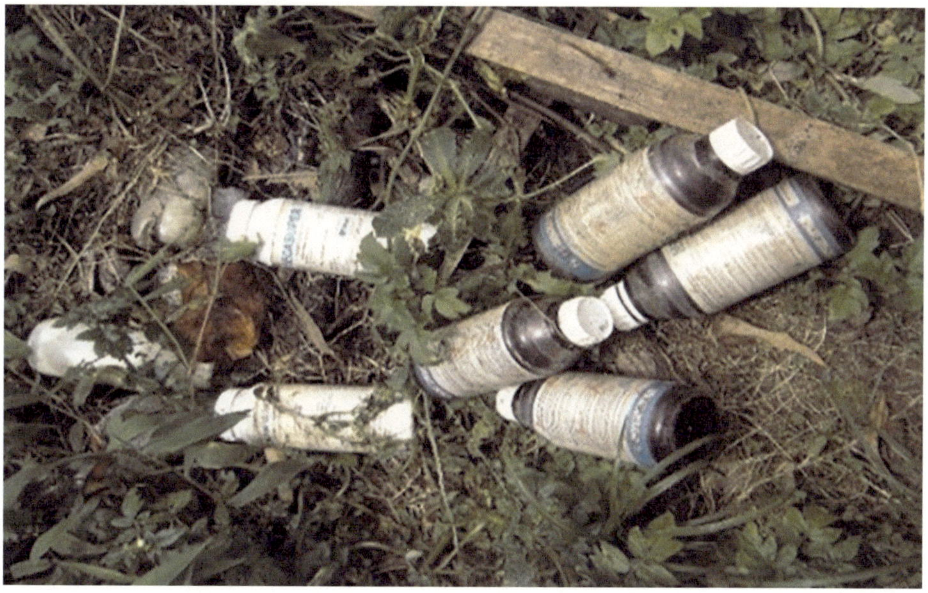

Figure 7.
Agrochemical residues.

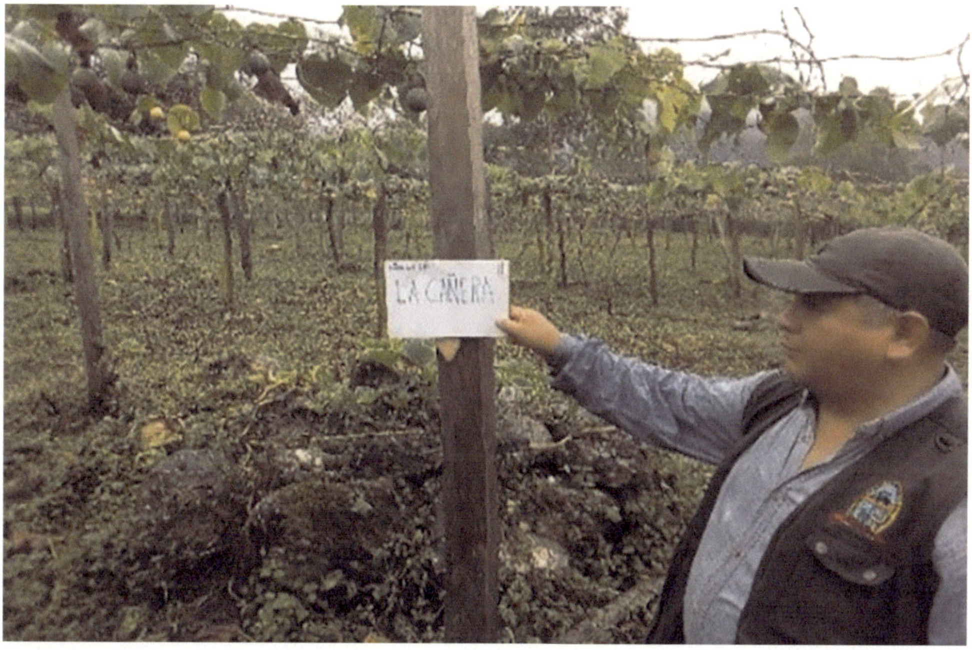

Figure 8.
Fields of study duly codified.

Author details

Benito Buendía Quispe[1] and Raymundo Erazo Erazo[2*]

1 Daniel Alcides Carrión National University (UNDAC), Pasco, Perú

2 Major National University of San Marcos (UNMSM), Lima, Perú

*Address all correspondence to: rerazoe@unmsm.edu.pe

References

[1] Goycochea Tocto T, Lozano C, Luiza M. Determination of the Environmental Impact Produced by the use of Agrochemicals in the Agricultural Production of the District of Jepelacio. National University of San Martin; 2016. Repository National University of San Martin. Collections: (Br.) Environmental Engineering. http://repositorio.unsm.edu.pe/handle/UNSM/245

[2] Freire G, Ernesto G. The Accumulation of Pesticide Containers and Their Impact on Environmental Pollution in the Quero canton [thesis]. 2014. http://repositorio.uta.edu.ec/jspui/handle/123456789/7549

[3] Lima F, Norma C, Francelino Valero T, Figueiredo Leite N, Alencar B, Beatriz L, et al. Protective action of Duguetia furfuracea (A. St.-Hil.) Saff against mercuric chloride toxicity in Escherichia coli. Cuban. Journal of Medicinal Plants. 2014;**19**(3):179-188

[4] Ulises GC, Hernández S, Morataya S, Núñez K, Carranza FA, Martínez ML et al. Determination of heavy metals, macro and trace elements in selected medicinal plants from Central Market of San Salvador, El Salvador. Open Journal of Chemistry. 2021;4(1)19-26. ISSN: 2618-0758 (Online) 2618-074X (Print). DOI: 10.30538/psrp-ojc2021.0021

[5] Rodríguez C, Karito E, Soto I, Patricia L. Quantification of Heavy Metals (Pb, As, Cd, Hg) in Tessaria Integrifolia Leaves from the Moche-Trujillo-La Libertad District. [thesis]. National university of Trujillo; 2017. Repository National University of Trujillo. Pharmacy Thesis Collections. http://dspace.unitru.edu.pe/handle/UNITRU/8056

[6] Sampieri R, Collado C, Baptista L. Investigation Methodology. 6th ed. Mexico: McGraw-Hill/Interamericana Editores, S.A. of C.V; 2014. p. 634. https://www.uca.ac.cr › 2017/10 › Research

[7] Bulletin of the agrarian agency of Oxapampa. 2016. Pasco Regional Agrarian Directorate. http://www.agropasco.gob.pe

[8] Landeta, Jon. Current validity of the Delphi method in social sciences. Technological Forecasting and Social Change Vol. 73, N° 5, 2006. pp. 467-482. DOI: 10.1016/j.techfore.2005.09.002

[9] Food and Agriculture Organization of the United Nations - World Health Organization (2019). GENERAL STANDARD FOR CONTAMINANTS AND TOXINS IN FOOD AND FEED CXS 193-1995 Adopted in 1995 Revised in 1997, 2006, 2008, 2009 Amended in 2010, 2012, 2013, 2014, 2015, 2016, 2017, 2018, 2019. 2019. https://www.fao.org/fao-who-codexalimentarius/codex-texts/list-standards/en/

[10] Fang B, y Zhu X. High content of five heavy metals in four fruits: Evidence from a case study of Pujiang County, Zhejiang Province, China. Food Control. 2014;**39**:62-67. DOI: 10.1016/j.foodcont.2013.10.039

[11] Shaheen N, Md. Irfan N, Nourin I, Islam S, Islam M. y Kawser M. Presence of heavy metals in fruits and vegetables: Health risk implications in Bangladesh. Chemosphere. 2017;**152**:431-438. DOI: 10.1016/j.chemosphere.2016.02.060

[12] Abbasi H et al. Quantification of heavy metals and health risk assessment in processed fruits' products. Arabian Journal of Chemistry. 2014;**13**(12): 8965-8978. DOI: 10.1016/j.arabjc.2020.10.020

[13] Marini M, Angouria-Tsorochidou E, Caro D, y Thomsen M. Daily intake of heavy metals and minerals in food – A case study of four Danish dietary profiles. Journal of Cleaner Production. 2021;**280**(1):1-12. DOI: 10.1016/j.jclepro.2020.124279

[14] Tariq F. Heavy metals concentration in vegetables irrigated with municipal wastewater and their human daily intake in Erbil city. Environmental Nanotechnology, Monitoring & Management. 2021;**16**:1-8. DOI: 10.1016/j.enmm.2021.100475

[15] Liu R, Xu Y, Zhang J, Wang W, y Elwardany R. Effects of heavy metal pollution on farmland soils and crops: A case study of the Xiaoqinling Gold Belt, China. China Geology. 2020;**3**(3): 402-410. DOI: 10.31035/cg2020024

[16] BERNAL MARCELO, A.R. Heavy Metal Levels in Dairy Herds in the Oxapampa Valley - Pasco. Thesis to opt for the Academic Degree of Doctor in Environmental Sciences and Sustainable Development. Huancayo – Peru: National University of the Center of Peru; 2019

[17] Reyes-Rodríguez R, Guridi-Izquierdo F, Valdes-Carmenate, R. Agricultural management modifies the properties and availability of heavy metals in Red Ferralitic soils. Rev Cie Téc Agr [online]. 2016;**25**(N° 4):23-31. DOI: 10.13140/G.2.2.15279.33448

[18] Pérez S, García M, Castro P, Duarte M. Total and exchangeable lead content in agricultural soil irrigated with wastewater and its accumulation in alfalfa. In: 2nd AMICA National Congress, Mexico; 2015. http://www.amica.com.mx

[19] Anaya R, Solano R. Determination of Heavy Metals (Lead and Arsenic) and Trace Elements (Iron, Copper and Zinc) in Crotalaria Longirostrata (Chipilin) Leaves by the Atomic Absorption Method. [thesis]. University of El Salvador Faculty of Chemistry and Pharmacy 2016. Institutional Repository of the University of El Salvador. http://ri.ues.edu.sv

Chapter 6

Application of Lead Transport through Brain Capillary for Determination of Weight, Brain Damage, and Encephalization Quotient in Humans

Saganuwan Alhaji Saganuwan

Abstract

The ability of lead to cause brain damage and reduce intelligence quotient has been established. However, transport of lead through brain capillary has not been elucidated. Hence, plasma and brain tissue kinetics of lead was studied mathematically. Literatures were searched for formulas that could be used for the determination of relationship between plasma and brain tissue kinetics of lead with an interest to discovering the residence time of lead residues in brain. Findings have shown that 5 $\mu g/dl$ of lead in plasma permeates the brain of human weighing 20 kg faster than that of 40 kg and 70 kg body weight, respectively. The surface area of permeability of brain cell is higher, in low body weight human than in high body weight human. Time of exposure and concentration of lead are higher in low body weight human as compared to high body weight human. Hence, neonates and children are more vulnerable to brain damage than adult human.

Keywords: encephalopathy, lead, brain capillary, toxicokinetics, encephalization quotient, transport

1. Introduction

Plasma concentration (>5 to >100 μg/dl) of lead can cause neurological, cardiovascular, hematological, reproductive, renal, immunological, and respiratory problems [1]. The reported lead concentrations of surface sample of soil was 23–35 mg/kg soil, whereas the concentration of the lead elute from soil was 0.6 mg/L, respectively [2]. Lead has the ability to penetrate brain having molecular weight of 207.28 g [3] and elimination half-life of 18 months. Highly contaminated soil could have the concentration of lead 3.03 times higher than the maximum limit for agricultural soil and 1.97 times higher than the value limit for fodder [4], suggesting that lead is very stable in soil and toxic to human [5]. However, soil concentration of lead (11.42 mg/L) could decrease during rainy season relative to dry season [6]. Lead exerts opposite effects on antibody response and phagocytosis [7]. Some plants such as *Cyamopsis tetragonoloba* and *Sesamum indicum* could tolerate lead concentration of up to 1000 mg/kg; hence, they could be used for bioremediation of soil heavily contaminated by lead [8]. The factors responsible for penetration of central nervous system acting agents are lipid solubility, pH, and molecular weight [9]. Hence, toxicological study of chemicals is necessary for the identification of potential toxicants [10]. Severe lead poisoning in young children and neonatal rats may cross microvessel endothelium of the brain. There is evidence that lead can cause brain damage, and lead uptake in the endothelium is reduced by calcium adenosine triphosphatase (ATPase) pump [11]. In view of this, transport of lead through brain capillary was mathematically assessed with a view to identifying pathogenesis of brain injury caused by lead in humans.

2. Materials and methods

2.1 Calculation of blood and plasma lead concentration

Literatures were assessed with a view to obtaining formulas that could be used for the calculation of lead transport through brain capillaries and its pathogenesis of causing brain damage and low intelligence quotient. Measurement of red blood cell (RBC) partitioning of lead is done as follows:

$$Plasma\ Imax,u - fup\left(Plasma\ Imax + \frac{F_a \times F_g \times K_a \times Dose}{\frac{Qh}{Rb}}\right) \quad (1)$$

where $Imax = C_{max}\,(\mu mol), Dose\,(\mu mol), fup$ = fraction of unbound drug in plasma (lower limit, 0.01), K_a= absorption rate constant (0.1 min^{-1}), F_a= fraction absorbed (1), F_g= fraction escaping gut metabolism (1), Qh= hepatic blood flow (1.6 L/min), and Rb= blood–plasma concentration ratio [12].

$$\text{Distribution of lead to red blood cells (\%)} = \left(1 - \frac{Plasma\ conc \times (100 - HC)}{Blood\ conc \times 100}\right) \times 100 \quad (2)$$

$$\text{Blood to plasma ratio} = \frac{Blood\ Conc}{Plasma\ Conc} \quad (3)$$

$$Hb = PV - \left(\frac{CrCl \times D \times Scr \times 72}{K \times (140 - Age)}\right) \times 12.5 \times \frac{1}{0.33} \quad (4)$$

$$D = \frac{Pcr}{Scr} \times 144. \quad (5)$$

$$RDB = RRW \times 80\ ml\ 1kg \times \frac{Desired\ PCV - Recipient\ PCV}{Donor\ PCV} \quad (6)$$

2.2 Blood and tissue kinetics of lead

$$Cl = {}^{DR}/_{Css} \quad (7)$$

$$LD = Css \times Vd \quad (8)$$

The first-order equation that describes the release of lead from biological system is concentration-dependent and can be expressed as [13]:

$$\log C_t = \frac{\log C_o - K_t}{2.303} \tag{9}$$

where C_o= initial concentration of lead and C_t= concentration of lead in solution at time t. slope equals $-K/2.303$ [14]. The elimination rate constant (1.16 h^{-1}) terminal half-life (0.6 h^{-1}) and volume of distribution (1.03 L/kg) have been reported for 60 kg weighted man.

Hence, terminal half-life

$$\left(t\frac{1}{2}\beta\right) = \frac{Vd}{PCl} \times 0.693 \tag{10}$$

where PCl = plasma clearance. However, initial concentration (C_o) is calculated as:

$$C_o = \frac{D}{V_{app}} \tag{11}$$

where D = dose of lead; V_{app} = apparent volume of distribution, when renal function is not impaired the serum concentration:

$$(C_s) = \frac{observed\ concentration}{0.2\,x\ Albumin\ (g/dl) + 0.1} \tag{12}$$

When there is end-stage renal failure, the serum concentration is calculated as:

$$C_s = \frac{observed\ concentration}{0.1\,x\ Albumin\ (g/dl) + 0.1} \tag{13}$$

Integration of exposure time with toxic dose of lead is presented as:

$$D = \frac{T^n}{K} \tag{14}$$

where D = dose, T = time of exposure, and K = concentration of toxicant causing toxicity [15].

2.3 Translation of lead dose in animals to human

$$HED = \frac{Animal\ dose \times Km}{Human\ Km} \tag{15}$$

Animal dose and animal Km are substituted with 40 and 20 kg as well as 31.3 and 25.0, respectively [16].

2.4 Transport of lead through brain capillary

Lead can be transported through brain capillary having the rate constant:

$$(\text{Kin}) = \frac{QE}{Vbrain} \tag{16}$$

$$E = 1 - e^{\frac{-PSA}{Q}} \tag{17}$$

$$\text{Alternatively } E_r = \frac{Cin - Cout}{Cin} \tag{18}$$

where Q = brain capillary blood flow, E = fraction of lead that flow into the brain, V_{brain} = volume of brain, E_r = extraction ratio of lead, PSA = permeability surface area ($(MS^{-1}m^2)$ of blood-brain barier, C_{in} = concentration of lead entering the brain capillary $(mol\ L^{-1})$, and C_{out} = concentration of lead leaving the brain capillary [17, 18].

The passive flux (QPas) of lead across blood-brain barrier between plasma and the brain extracellular fluid (ECF) is given as:

$$QPas = P\left(C_{pl} - C_{(ECF)}\right) \tag{19}$$

where QPas = passive flow rate $(mol\ m^{-2}s^{-1})$, P = permeability of the BBB (MS^{-1}), C_{pl}=concentration of the lead in the plasma $(mol\ m^{-3})$, and C_{ECF}= concentration of lead in the ECF [19]:

$$\frac{\Delta C_{ECF}}{\Delta t} = kBBB\ \left(C_{pl} - C_{ECF}\right) \tag{20}$$

$$V_{ECF} = \frac{\Delta(ECF)}{\Delta t} = CLBBB\ \left(C_{pl} - C_{ECF}\right) \tag{21}$$

$$C_{ECF} = \frac{A_{ECF}}{V_{ECF}} \tag{22}$$

Cerebral metabolic rate (CMR) scales with brain volume, hence:

$$\frac{CMR}{V} = \alpha\ V^{0.167} \tag{23}$$

$$\text{Density of neuron } (\mathrm{D}_n) = \alpha\ V^{0.167} \tag{24}$$

$$\text{The capillary length density } (\mathrm{C}_n) = \alpha\ V^{0.167} \tag{25}$$

Total length of capillary is proportional to the number of neurons [20].

$$\text{Capillary diameter } (\mathrm{C}_d) = \alpha\ V^{0.08} \tag{26}$$

It is 7 μm diameter in human brain [21]. The flow rate of blood to the brain is 800 mL/min [22]where ΔC_{ECF} = change in lead concentration of extracellular fluid, KBBB = rate constant of lead transport across the BBB (S^{-1}), CL BBB = transfer clearance of lead transport across the BBB (m^3S^{-1}), A_{ECF} = molar amount of lead in the brain ECF (mol), and V_{ECF}= volume of the brain ECF (m^3) [23–25].

$$\text{Passive permeability } (p) = Ptrans + \frac{D_{para}}{W_{TJ}} \tag{27}$$

where Pt = passive transcellular permeability (ms^{-1}), D_{para} = diffusity of lead through the BBB intercellular space (m^2s^{-1}), and W_{TJ} = width of tight junction (m) [24].

$$\text{Total flux }(\mathrm{Q_{total}}) = \mathrm{P_{tot}}\left(C_{pl} - C_{ECF}\right) \tag{28}$$

$$\mathrm{Q_{total}} = PAF_{in}\left(C_{pl}\right) - PAF_{out}(C_{ECF}) \tag{29}$$

where P_{total} = rate of active and passive transport across BBB, PAF_{in} = affinity of lead to active transport into the brain, and PAF_{out} = affinity of lead to active transport out of the brain [25].

$$P_{tot} = P_{pas} \times C_{part} \tag{30}$$

P_{pas} = passive permeability to BBB; C_{part}= coefficient of partition [26].

$$\text{Active clearance }(Cl_{act}) = \frac{Tm}{Km + C} \tag{31}$$

where Tm = maximum rate of lead transport across the BBB $(\left(\mu mol\ L^{-1}S^{-1}\right)$, K$m$ = concentration of free lead $\left(\mu mol\ L^{-1}\right)$ at which half of Tm is attained, and C = concentration of lead in plasma [27].

Change in lead concentration within the cells of the brain is given as follows:

$$\frac{\Delta C_{ICF}}{\Delta t} = K_{cell}(C_{ECF} - C_{ICF}) \tag{32}$$

$$V_{ICF}\frac{\Delta C_{ICF}}{\Delta t} = C_{cell}(C_{ECF} - C_{ICF}) \tag{33}$$

$$C_{ICF}\frac{A_{ICF}}{V_{ICF}} \tag{34}$$

where C_{ICF} = concentration of lead in the brain ICF $\left(\mu mol\ L^{-1}\right)$, K_{cell}= rate constant of lead transport across the cell membrane $\left(S^{-1}\right)$, and V_{ICF}= apparent volume of distribution in the brain ICF [28].

$$\text{Dissociation constant }(kd) = \frac{k_{on}}{k_{off}} \tag{35}$$

where $kd = 45.62\ nM\ (0.91\ \mu g/dL)$ that has been reported for on-site lead detection using a biosensor device [29].

2.5 Michaelis-Menten kinetics of lead

Clearance of lead by Michaelis-Menten kinetics is given as follows:

$$CLact - cell = \frac{Tm - cell}{\propto(Km - cell + C)} \tag{36}$$

where $CLact - cell$ = active transfer clearance of free lead across the cell membrane, C = concentration of lead in the brain ECF or ICF, $Tm - cell$= maximal veolocity of the transporter, and $Km - cell$= Michaelis –Menten constant [30].

Enzyme metabolic clearance (φmet) is given as follows:

$$\varphi met = V_{max} \frac{C}{Km + C} \tag{37}$$

where φmet = flux of the enzymatic metabolic reaction $\left(mmol\, L^{-1} min^{-1}\right)$, V_{max} = maximum flux of the reaction $\left(mmol\, L^{-1}\right)$, C = concentration of substrate in ECF or ICF ($\left(mmol\, L^{-1}\right)$, and Km = affinity of coefficient of the enzyme substrate $\left(mmol\, L^{-1}\right)$ [31]. Three-dimensional model that integrates lead transport through BBB and lead binding within the brain could predict lead distribution in the brain [32]. One kilogram equals 1000 mililiters [33].

2.6 Relationship between brain mass and encephalization quotient

$$\text{Encephalization quotient (EQ)} = \frac{Brain\ mass}{0.14 \times Body\ weight^{0.528}} \tag{38}$$

$$\text{Brain mass (E)} = k_p \beta \tag{39}$$

where k = 0.14, p = body weight, and β = 0.528 [34, 35].

$$\text{Brain volume } \left(\log_{10}(B)\right) = 3.015 + 0.986 \log_{10} C \tag{40}$$

where B = brain size (mm^3) and C = internal cranial capacity (mm^3).

$$\text{Also brain volume } (V_{brain}) = 4/3 \times \pi \times r^3 \tag{41}$$

where

$$\pi = 3.14159 \text{ and } r = \text{radius} = \frac{diammeter}{2} \tag{42}$$

$$T\frac{1}{2}\beta = \frac{0.693}{\beta} \tag{43}$$

Lead concentration (Ct), plasma clearance (Pcl), calculated administered lead and time of exposure to lead were extrapolated to 60, 40, and 20 kg weighed human, using human equivalent dose formula.

2.7 Parameters for the determination of therapeutic and toxic agents across brain cells

The relevant parameters that can be used for the determination of therapeutic and toxic agents across brain cells are as follows: capillary radius (3–5 $\times 10^{-6}\, m$), capillary surface area (15–25 m^2), intercapillary distance (40–60 $\times 10^{-6} m$), capillary blood flow rate (0.3–200 $\times 10^{-1}\, L\, min^{-1}$), BBB passive permeability $\left(6 \times 10^{-8} - 10^{-6}\, ms^{-1}\right)$, BBB rate constant ($1.4 \times 10^{-4} - 1.4 \times 10^{-2} S^{-1}$), BBB transfer clearance $\left(113 - 850 \times 10^{-5}\, LS^{-1}\right)$, BBB trancellular permeability $\left(0.6 - 10 \times 10^{-7} ms^{-1}\right)$, BBB paracellular diffusity $\left(550 - 767 \times 10^{-12} m^2 s^{-1}\right)$, width tight junction $\left(0.3 - 0.5 \times 10^{-6}\, m\right)$, active transport velocity $\left(22 - 167\, \mu mol\, L^{-1} S^{-1}\right)$, concentration to reach half of Tm $\left(4.5 - 5 \times 10^3 \mu mol\, L^{-1}\right)$, BBB surface area $(12 - 18167 m^2)$, blood cebrospinal fluid barrier (BCSFB) surface area $(6 - 9\, m^2)$, cerebrospinal fluid (CSF) flow rate $\left(50 - 67 \times 10^{-7} LS^{-1}\right)$, brain ECF flow velocity $\left(2 - 8 \times 10^{-7} ms^{-1}\right)$, brain ECF volume fraction (0.23–0.49), tortuosity (1.5–1.7), effective diffusion constant $\left(0.1 - 15 \times 10^{-10} m^{-2} s^{-1}\right)$, cellular uptake rate $(0.22 - 304.3\, s^{-1})$, cellular transfer clearance $\left(4.2 \times 10^3 - 3 \times 10^5\, LS^{-1}\right)$, ICF volume (960 L), association rate constant $\left(2.8 \times 10^{-5} - 2.8 \times 10^2\, \mu mol\, L^{-1} S^{-1}\right)$, binding site concentration $\left(1 \times 10^{-3} - 5 \times 10^{-1}\, \mu mol\, L^{-1}\right)$, affinity constant $\left(0.003 - 528 \times 10^3 \mu mol\, L^{-1}\right)$, maximum reaction flux $\left(5.76 \times 10^2 - 1 \times 10^9 \mu mol\, L^{-1}\, min^{-1}\right)$, and elimination rate constant $\left(1.1 \times 10^{-7} - 6.8 \times 10^4 S^{-1}\right)$ have been reported for human brain [12].

3. Results

Table 1 shows kinetic parameters of lead in various compartments of brain of 20, 40, and 60 kg weighted adult humans.

Parameters	Value		
Weight (kg)	**60**	**40**	**20**
Volume of brain (mm^3)	4400	3000	1500
Fraction of blood flowed into the brain (μg/dl)	5.0	5.0	5.0
Rate constant of brain transport through capillary (kin) (L/min)	3.4×10^{-4} to 2.3×10^{-1}	5×10^{-4} to 3.3×10^{-1}	1.0×10^{-3} to 6.7×10^{-1}
Permeability surface area (m^2)	0.064	0.25	1.13
Concentration at time (Ct) (mol/s)	1.87	2.24	2.81
Plasma clearance (Pcl) (L/S)	1.19	1.43	1.78
Dose of administered lead CD	5.15	6.17	7.73
Time of exposure (T) (h)	5.20	6.23	7.80
Brain diameter (mm)	20.4	17.9	14.2
Brain radius (mm)	10.2	8.9	7.1
Brain elimination half-life (S^{-1})	6.3×10^{-8}–1.0×10^{-3}	6.3×10^{-8}–1.0×10^{-3}	6.3×10^{-8}–1.0×10^{-3}
Blood lead level (μg/dl)	0.52–8.38	131–7.29	2.1–6.2
Blood-to-plasma ratio	0.1–1.7	0.3–1.5	0.4–1.2
Erythrocytes lead level (μg/dl)	3.38	2.29	1.2
Brain mass (kg)	4.4	3.0	1.5
Encephalization quotient	3.6	3.1	2.2

Table 1.
Kinetic parameters of lead in the brain of humans of varying weights.

4. Discussion

The increased rate constant of lead transport through brain capillary, permeability surface area, concentration of lead in the brain, and time of exposure to lead in 20 kg weighed human as compared to 40 and 60 kg weighed humans agree with the report of Nicholson [35] indicating that young humans are more vulnerable to plumbism. The increased plasma clearance of lead in the human of 20 kg body weight as compared to 40 and 60 kg body weight human agrees with the report indicating that children have the ability to eliminate lead faster than adult [35]. Absorption of lead by bone and teeth is 94% in adult as compared to 70% in children [36]. Half-life of blood lead is 40 days in human. Renal insufficiency caused by plumbism could delay lead elimination. Lead concentration lower than 5 μg/dL is associated with reduced academic performance. Tyrosine and phenylalaine are the two main binding sites in albumin. The binding site is Tyr_{84} and Cys_{34} [37]. The allowable lead limit in drinking water is 15 *Ppb* (73 *nM*) [38, 39]. Serum albumin consists of 585 amino acids which have three structural domains stabilized in disulfide bonds with binding sites for fatty acids, glycerol, and metal ions. The ability of lead to bind serum albumin is used to detect micromolar concentration of lead ions in biological solution [40–42]. Centre for disease control's (CDC's) limit of 5 μg/dl in blood is contrary to revised limit of 3.5 μg/dl, but even 3 μg/dl has caused diminished cognitive function [43]. Protein kinases regulate the development of brain capillaries and expression of blood-brain barrier. Lead could stimulate protein kinase, disrupting BBB development at the regulation of neuronal development. More so, low doses of lead can stimulate protein kinase C that may enhance the release of neurotransmitters [44]. Protein kinase C is most sensitive to lead followed by calmodulin-protein kinase C and cyclic adenosine monosphosphate protein kinase [45]. Toxic action of lead is influenced by the interaction between endothelial cells and astrocytes [46]. Genetic and environmental factors could make some particular children more vulnerable to lead neurotoxicity [47]. Human brain is made up of 100 billion neurons, which consumes 15–20 W power. Brain consumes 15–20% of consumed glucose [48]. Utilization of adenosine triphosphate (ATP) in gray matter and white matter are 9.5 $\mu mol\, g^{-1}S^{-1}$ and 3 $\mu mol\, g^{-1}S^{-1}$, respectively, signifying that 77% energy is consumed by cortical gray matter, which is 50% of brain volume. Components of gray matter are dendrites, neurons, glial cells, unmyelinated axons, and capillaries, but components of white matter are glial cells, myelinated axons, and capillaries. The density of brain capillary is 2–4 times more in gray matter [49]. Adult human brain weighs 1500 g and occupies 1200 cm^3, with surface area of microvessels (100–200 $cm^2 g^{-1}$) [50]. Brain extracellular space constitutes 15–30% of the brain volume and brain vasculature 3% of the brain volume [51]. Increased size of human brain from 400 cm^3 to 1200 cm^3 [52] indicates increased cognition capacity of modern human. Serum creatinine($0.88 \pm 0.2\, mg/dl$) has been reported for human with blood lead level of $2.36 - 2.54\, \mu g/dl$ [53]. Blood level of $24.43 \pm 5.31\, \mu g/dl$ has been reported for traffic policeman in Taiwan [54]. Less than 1.5 min cerebral perfusion of labeled lead chloride was fast, providing a space of 9.7 mol/100 g of frontal cortex at 1 min. The influx was linear with concentration of 4 μM. Albumin (5%), cistern (200 Mm), and ethylene diamine tetraacetate (EDTA) (1 μm) slipped lead uptake. Potassium reduces lead 203 uptakes [55]. Concentration of lead in blood ($2.1 - 6.2\, \mu g/dl$) has been reported for children [56] and 0.52–8.38 $\mu g/dl$ in adults [57]. Brain weight of man decreases by 2.7 g and that of human by 2.2 g per year with increasing age. Also brain weight increase of 3.7 g is independent of sex [58].

However brain weight increased by 0.78 g/year for 80 years between 1860 and 1940, amounting to 62.4 g [59]. Cognitive ability is dependent on number of neurons [60]. White matter decreases in old (75–85 years) as compared to young by 11% [61]. Hence, there is a need to revise the toxic reference value of lead in children. The reference value of 3.5 μg/dl should be revised to guide clinical and public intervention for individual children [62], because the relationship between encephalization and intelligence could be affected by low allometric value, when linear regression line was used [63]. Brain size, different regions of the brain including cerebral cortex, cortical thickness, frontal cortex, parietal cortex, cerebellum, and experience correlated positively with intelligence. Therefore, gene and environmental influence plays a key role in intelligence quotient [64], as such brain size based on cognitive equivalence is preferred to the encephalization quotient in empirical cognitive studies [65]. Environment could affect the development of neural tissues [66].

5. Conclusion

Lead fragments permeate blood–brain barrier of a young human weighing 20 kg body weight faster than those of humans weighing 40 and 60 kg body weights. However, rate constant of brain transport, permeability surface area, lead concentration in the brain, and exposure time of lead are higher in children leading to low encephalization quotient.

Abbreviations

Hb	haemoglobin
PV	plasma volume
D	depuration
Scr	serum creatinine
K	constant
Pcr	plasma creatinine
RDB	required donor blood
RRW	recipient real weight
PCV	packed cell volume
Cl	clearance
DR	dose rate
Css	steady state concentration
LD	loading dose
Vd	volume of distribution
HED	human equivalent dose
Km	metabolism consant
Kin	rate constant of lead transport through brain capillary
V_{ECF}	extracellular fluid volume
α	flow rate of blood to the brain
A_{ICF}	molar amount of lead in intracellular fluid
Kon	dissociated lead
Koff	original lead
β	elimination rate constant of lead

Author details

Saganuwan Alhaji Saganuwan
Department of Veterinary Pharmacology and Toxicology, College of Veterinary Medicine, Federal University of Agriculture, Makurdi, Benue State, Nigeria

*Address all correspondence to: pharm_saga2006@yahoo.com

References

[1] Hayes AW. Principles and Methods of Toxicology. 5th ed. Boca Raton, FL: CRC Press; 2008. p. 2270

[2] Thi LanBinh N, Hoang NT, Thi Thanih Truc N, Khang VD, Anh Le H. Estimating the possibility of lead contamination in soil surface due to lead deposition in atmosphere. Journal of Nanomaterials. 2021;**2021**:ID5586951

[3] Winecker RE, Rofero-Miller JD, Broussard LA, Hammett-Stabler CA. The toxicology of heavy metalal: Getting the lead out. Laboratory Medicine. 2002;**33**: 934

[4] Castro-Bedrinana J, Chirinos-Peinado D, Garcia-Olarte E, Quispe-Ramos R. Lead transfer in the soil-root-plant system in a highly contaminated Andean area. Peer Journal. 2021;**2021**:10624

[5] Lima FDS, Nascimento CND, da Silva FBV, de Carvalho VGB, Fillio MRR. Lead concentration and allocation in vegetable crops grown in a soil contaminated by battery residues. Horticultura Brasileira. 2009;**29**(3): 362-365

[6] Obasi PN, Akudinobi BB. Potential health risk and levels of heavy metals in water resources of lead-zinc communities of Abakaliki, Southeast Nigeria. Applied Water Research. 2020; **10**(184):1-23

[7] Laschi-Loquerie A, Eyraud A, Morisset D, Samai A, Tachon P, Veysscyre C, et al. Influence of heavy metals on the resistance of mice toward infection. Immunopharmacology and Immunotoxicology. 1987;**9**(2&3): 235-241

[8] Amin H, Arain BA, Jahangor TM, Abbasi MS, Amin F. Accumulation and distribution of lead (pb) in plant tissues to guar (*Cyamopsis tetragonolosis* L) and sesame (*Sesamum indiaim* L.): Profitable phytoremediation with biofuel crops. Geological Ecology Landscape. 2018; **2**(1):51-60

[9] Saganuwan SA. Piroxicam: Source for synthesis of central nervous system (cns) acting drugs. Central Nervous Agent Medicine Chemistry. 2017; **17**:1-6

[10] Saganuwan SA. Toxicity studies of drugs and chemicals in animals: An overview. Bork Journal of Veterinary Medicine. 2016;**10**:983

[11] Bradbury NW, Deane R. Permeability of the blood-brain barrier to lead. Neurotoxicology. 1993;**14**(2-3):131-136

[12] Saganuwan SA. In: Erkekogh P, Ogawa T, editors. Toxicosis of snake, scorpion, honeybees, spider, and wasp venoms: Part 2, Medical Toxicology. Hund: Intech Open; 2021. p. 335

[13] Saganuwan SA. Application of modified Michaclis-Menten equations for determination of enzyme inducing and inhibiting drugs. BMC Pharmacology and Toxicology. 2021; **22**(57):1-15

[14] Suvakanta D, Nhurthy PN, Lilakanta N, Prasanta C. Kinetic modeling on drug release from controlled drug delivery systems. Act Polori Pharmaceutic. 2010;**67**(3):217-223

[15] Saganuwan SA. Comparatives therapeutic index, lethal time and safety margin of various toxicants and snake antivenins using newly derived and old formulas. BMC Research Notes. 2020; **13**(292):1-7

[16] Saganuwan SA. The paradox of human equivalent dose formula: A canonical case study of Abrus Precatorius aqueous leaf extract in monogastric animals. Macedonian Veterinary Review. 2016;**39**(1):23-32

[17] Renkin EM. Transport of potassium −42 from blood to tissue in isolated mammalian skeletal muscles. American Journal of Physiology. 1959;**197**(6): 1205-1210

[18] Crone C. The permeability of capillaries in various organs as determined by use of the indicator diffusion method. Acta Physiologica. 1963;**58**(4):292-305

[19] Calvetti D, Cheng Y, Somersalo E. A spatial distributed computational model of brain cellular metabolism. Journal of Theoretical Biology. 2015;**376**:48-65

[20] Karbowski J. Scaling of brain metabolism and blood flow in relation to capillary and neural scaling. PLoS One. 2011;**6**:e26709

[21] Wong AD, Ye M, Levy AF, Rothstein JD, Bergles JD, Searson PC. The blood-brain barrier: An engineering perspective. Frontiers in Neuroengergy. 2013;**6**(7):1-22

[22] Zlokovic BV. Neuromuscular mechanisms of Alzheimer's neurodegeneration. Trends in Neurosciences. 2005;**28**:202-208

[23] Ball K. A physiologically based modelling strategy during preclinical CNS drug development. Molecular Pharmaceutics. 2014;**11**:836-848

[24] Yamamoh Y, Valitalo PA, Huntjens DR, Proost JH, Vermenlen A, Krauwinkel W, et al. Predicting drug concentration – Time profiles in multiple CNS compartments using a comprehensive physiologically –based pharmacokinetic model. CPT Pharmacemetrics and System Pharmacology. 2017;**6**(11):765-777

[25] Yamamoto Y, Valitalo PA, van den Berg DJ, Hertran R, van den Brink W, Wong YC, et al. A generic multi-compartmental CNS distribution model structure for 9 drugs allows prediction of human brain target site concentrations. Pharmaceutical Research. 2017;**34**(2): 333-351

[26] Westerhout J, van den Berg DJ, Hartman R, Danhot M, De Lange ECM. Prediction of methotrexate CNS distribution in different species – Influence of disease conditions. European Journal of Pharmaceutical Sciences. 2014;**57**(1):11-24

[27] Syvanen S, Xie R, Sahin S, Hammarhind-Udenaes M. Pharmaco-kinetic consequences of active drug efflux at the blood-brain barrier. Pharmaceutical Research. 2006;**23**(4):705-7147

[28] Nhan T, Burgesb A, Lilge L, Hynynen K. Modelling localized delivery of doxorubicin to the brain following focused ultrasound enhanced blood-brain barrier permeability. Physics Medical Biology. 2014;**59**:5987-6004

[29] Lai WQ, Chang YF, Chou FN, Yang DM. Protable FRET- based biosensor device for on-site lead detection. Bios. 2022;**12**(157):1-17

[30] Nicholson C, Chen KC, Hrabetova S, Tao L. Diffusion of molecules in brain bitracellular space: Theory and experiment. Brain Research. 2000;**125**:129-154

[31] Saltzman WM, Radiomsky ML. Drugs released from polymers: Diffusion and elimination in brain tissue. Chemical Engineering Science. 1991;**46**(10): 2429-2444

[32] Vendel E, Rottschafer V, de Lange ECM. The new for mathematical modelling of spatial drug distribution within the brain. Fluid Barrier CNS. 2019;**16**(12):1-33

[33] Saganuwan SA. Mathematical determination of some oncological parameters and their therapeutic implications in dogs. Composite Clinical Pathology. 2019;**28**:1025-1030

[34] Saganuwan SA. Modified formulas for calculation of encephalization quotient in dogs. BMC Research. 2021; **14**(223):1-5

[35] Nicholson C. Diffusion and related transport mechanisms in brain tissue. Reports on Progress in Physics. 2001;**64**: 815-884

[36] Barbosa F Jr, Taruis-Santos JV, Gerlach RF, Parsons PJ. A critical review of biomarkers used for monitoring human exposure to lead: Advantages, limitations, and future needs. Environmental Health Perspectives. 2005;**113**:1569-1174

[37] Wani AL, Ara A, Usman JA. Lead toxicity: A review. Interdisciplinary Toxicology. 2015;**8**(2):55-64

[38] Saha A, Yakovlev VV. Applied Physics Letters. 2009;**95**:143704-143706

[39] Rossi E. Clinical Biochemistry. 2008; **29**:63-70

[40] He XM, Carter DC. Nature. 1992; **358**:209-215

[41] Yuan Y, Cai Y, Xie Q, Yao S. Analytical Sciences. 2002;**18**:967-771

[42] Peng L, Hongyu X, Xi L, Lifang R, Chaocan Z. Biological Trace Element Research. 2007;**118**:97-103

[43] Ruckart PZ, Jones RL, Courtney JG, LeBlanc TT, Jackson W, Karwowski MP, et al. Update of the blood leads reference value-United States, 2021. Morbidity and Mortality Weekly Report. 2021;**70**(43): 1509-1512

[44] Goldstein GW. Lead poisoning and brain cell function. Environmental Health and Protection, Brogan and Partners Available from: http://www.jstor.org/stable/3430903. [Accessed: June 17, 2014]

[45] Markovac J, Goldstein GW. Picomolar concentrations of lead stimulate brain protein kinase C. Nature. 1988;**334**:71-73

[46] Gebhart AM, Goldstein GW. Use of an in-vitro system to study the effects of lead on astrocyte-endothelial cell interactions: A model for studying toxic injury to the blood-brain barrier. Toxicology and Applied Pharmacology. 1988;**94**:191-206

[47] Lidsky TI, Schneider JS. Lead neurotoxicity in children: Basic mechanisms and clinical correlates. Brain. 2003;**126**:5-19

[48] Navarrete A, van Schaik CP, Isler K. Energetics and the evolution of human brain size. Nature. 2011;**480**:91-93

[49] Heinzer S, Kahn G, Krucker T, Meyer E, Ulmann-Schuler A. Novel three-dimensional analysis tool for vascular trees indicates complete micro-networks, not single capillaries, as the angiogaric and point in mice overexpressing human VEGF (65) in the brain. Neuroimag. 2008;**39**:1549-1558

[50] Gross PM, Sposito NM, Pettersen SE, Fenstermacher JD. Differences in function and structure of the capillary endothelium in gray matter, white matter and circumventricular

organ of rat brain. Blood Vessels. 1986; **23**:261-270

[51] Potts R. Evolution big brains explained. Nature. 2011;**480**:43-44

[52] Fang CW, Nimy HC, Huang YC, Chiang YS, Chuang CW, Wang IK, et al. Trend in blood lead levels in Taiwanese adults 2005 – 2007. PLoS One. 2021; **16**(12):e0260744

[53] Chiang HC, Chang PY. Lead exposure among Kaosiung traffic policemen. Gaoxiong Yi Xueke Xue Zazhi. 1989;**5**(6):314-319

[54] Deane R, Bradbury NWB. Transport of Lead – 203 at the Blood-Brain Barrier during Short Cerebrovascular Perfusion with Saline in the Rats. 1990

[55] Frndak L, Barg G, Canfield RL, Quierolo EL, Manay N, Kordas K. Behavioural signatures of lead and manganese exposed children. Available from: https://www.sciencedirect.2022

[56] Rocha A, Trujillo K. Neurotoxicity of low-level lead exposure: History, mechanisms of action, and behavioural effects in humans and prechemical models. Neurotoxicology. 2019;**73**: 58-80

[57] Kosnett MJ, Wedeen RP, Rothenberg SJ, Hipkins KL, Materna BL, Schwartz BS, et al. Recommendations for medical management of adult lead exposure. Environmental Health Perspectives. 2007;**15**(3):463-471

[58] Hartman P, Ramsier A, Gudat F, Mihatsch MJ. Normal weight of the brain in adults in relation to age, sex, body height and weight. Der Pathologe. 1994; **15**(3):165-170

[59] Miller AKH, Corsellis JAN. Evidence for a secular increase in human brain weight during the past century. Annals of Human Biology. 1973;**4**(3):253-257

[60] Herculano-Houzel S. The human brain numbers: A linearly scaled-up primate brain. Frontiers in Human Neuroscience. 2009;**3**(31):1-11

[61] Beason-Held LL, Horwitz B. Aging brain. In: Encyclopedia of the Human Brain. Amsterdam, Netherlands: Elsevier Science Limited; 2002

[62] Paulson JA, Brown MJ. The CDC blood lead reference value for children: Time for a change. Environmental Health. 2019;**18**(16):1-2

[63] Albo DM. Cognitive inferences in fossil apes (Primates, Hominoidea):Does encephalization reflect intelligence? Journal of Anthropological Sciences. 2010;**88**:11-48

[64] Cairo O. External measures of cognition. Frontiers in Human Neuroscience. 2011;**5**(108):1-9

[65] van Schaik CP, Triki Z, Bshary R, Heldstab SA. A farewell to the encephalization quotient: A new brain size measure for comparative primate cognition. Brain Behaviour and Evolution. 2021;**96**:1-12

[66] Worthy GA, Hickie JP. Relative brain size in marine mammals. American Nature. 1986;**128**:445-459

Chapter 7

Ecotoxicity Effects of Lead Bullets in Human and Wildlife: The Consequences of Environmental Pollution, Low Intelligence Quotient, Brain Damage and Brain Overclaim Syndrome

Saganuwan Alhaji Saganuwan

Abstract

Bullets from gunshots made of lead are used to kill and arrest criminals, as they are also used by criminals to intimidate or kill innocents for psychosocial gains. So the increased environmental pollution caused by lead from industries, firearms, gasoline, among others is a source of concern for environmental health specialists, clinical toxicologists, experimental toxicologists, industrial toxicologists and ecotoxicologists. Lead can get into body system accidentally via oral, inhalational, epidermal, dermal, intraperitoneal, and intravenous routes. The toxicokinetic data of lead disposition via various routes of administrations are quite inconsistent. Hence the set blood limit concentration has been considered to be incorrect. In view of this, toxicokinetic data analysis of lead was carried out with intent to determine toxic doses of lead in various organs, and its toxicological consequences. Findings have shown that at lower doses, kinetics of lead is linear (first order), and at higher doses the kinetics becomes non-linear (zero-order). Metabolic processes modulated by lead could be either rate limiting or non–rate-limiting causing induction and inhibition of a myriad of metabolizing enzymes in liver, brain, kidney, intestine and lung. The LD50 of lead bullet in human was 450 mg/kg, which caused death in 9.1 days, and penicillamine (18 mg/kg) can be used for treatment. Mean residence time (MRT) and elimination half-life ($\frac{T^1}{2^\beta}$) were 25.8 and 18 days, respectively.

Keywords: plumbism, toxicokinetic, Michaelis-Menten order, brain, half-life, tissue concentration, bullet, lead, overclaim syndrome, neurosis, pollution

1. Introduction

Bullets made from lead cause lead intoxication (plumbism), which may be fatal if left unremoved for a period of time [1]. Fragment of lead radiates in target animals [2]. The target doses of lead fragments in Andean condors, Turkey vulture and bald eagle are 45.5–58.2, 20.7–33.8 and 11.5–27.0 mg/kg, respectively [3–5]. Interference of lead with calcium metabolism can lead to neurological and neuromuscular disorders via signal transduction of protein kinases, neurotransmitter and calcium [6]. Behavioural and learning deficiencies have been linked to interference of lead with signalling of brain cells in human and birds [7, 8]. Bullet fragments can be lodged in body joints and cause anaemia, abdominal colic, nephropathy and neuropathy. The precipitating factors are infection, metabolic stress and alcoholism [2]. Mass spectrometric isotope dilution analysis with chelation therapy was used for the mobilization of lead from bone [1]. Violence can lead to the use of firearms causing lead poisoning characterized in part by changes in behaviour, neurological status and death. Clinical neuronal manifestations are fatigue, malaise, irritability, loss of libido, headache, encephalopathy, delirium, ataxia, convulsions and motor neuropathy [9]. As low as 10 μg/dl interferes with haem synthesis and increases aminolevulinic acid (ALA) that suppresses gamma aminobutyric acid (GABA) neurotransmission [10]. Lead concentration less than 4 μm causes acute encephalopathy [11]. Lead exposure (0.25 μg/g) of brain tissues for 50 days, starting on post-natal day 1, caused abnormal expression of glial-related genes [12]. Lead (19–31 μg/dl) caused decrease in the size of cortical column in somatosensory cortex [13]. Placental blood lead (10 μg/dl) caused cognitive impairment [14]. Bullet lodged in various parts of the body can stay in the body for 3 months to 40 years, and associated neurodiseases are alcoholism, delirium tremens, thyrotoxicosis and shock. Gunshot after 4 years caused depression with detected blood lead of 6.7 μg/dl [1]. Intracellular bullets may result in unwanted long-term complications [15]. After 4 years gunshot, caused malaise and weakness with blood level of lead 62 μg/dl, whereas gunshot after 3 years caused paroxysmal abdominal pain and post prandial emesis [16]. Clinical toxic threshold doses for lead fragments in blood (50–100 μg/dl), liver (6 mg/kg), Kidney (4–16 mg/kg) and bone (>20 mg/kg) have been reported for Anseriformes, Falconiformes and Accipitriformes, respectively [17]. Lead concentration of blood (<0.2 ppm), liver and kidney (>2 ppm) and bone (<10 ppm) have been reported for birds not exposed to lead [18], but the cost of antidotes has increased [19]. Therefore, poisoning severity score can be modified to assess the degree of bullet toxicity [20] in human and wildlife with a view to curtailing consequences of lead poisoning.

2. Materials and methods

Literatures were searched for information on acute and chronic effects of lead bullets in wildlife, young and adult humans, especially in relation to brain damage and criminology. Some established formulas for determination of LD_{50} were modified for determination of acute and chronic toxicity effects of lead in wildlife and human. The developed formulas were used to determine lethal time fifty (LT_{50}), chronicity factor (CF), dose of lead that can kill one man, toxic dose rate, target concentration, clearance, effective dose of antidote, volume of distribution, area under curve, mean residence time and elimination rate constant [21–23]. Up and down procedure (UPD) was used to estimate LD_{50} of bullets, as the initial estimate of the LD_{50} was within a factor of the authentic LD_{50} [24], and has been validated [25].

2.1 Kinetic energy of lead bullet

The velocity of bullet is proportionally more influential than the weight of the bullet. Therefore, the kinetic energy transferred to the target animal is presented by the equation given below [26]. Kinetic energy of bullet is the mass of bullet times squared velocity of the bullet.

$$\mathrm{KE} = \frac{1}{2}\mathrm{mv}^2 \tag{1}$$

KE = kinetic energy; m = mass of bullet; v = velocity.

Low velocity = 1200 ft./s; medium = 1200–2500 ft./s; high = >2500 ft./s [27]. Bullets from handguns have velocity of <1000 ft./s, rifles (<2500 ft./s) and bullets of 5.56 mm are small but relatively fast. Outer jacket of the bullet determines margin line of tissue injury which is responsible for bullet moving more than 2000 ft./s [28].

Air rifle pellet that weighed 8.25 grains and of 0.38 calibre received velocity of 101 m/s, but could damage the brain, whereas that of 113 grains of 58 m/s could damage brain matter [29]. An impactor (bullet) of 200–297 mm^2 could exert force of 980–1334 N on parietal bone [30]. Therefore Head Injury Criterion (HIC) is used as protective measure for skull. It is a function of the period of acceleration at the head centre of gravity, bearing in mind that head is a one-mass structure:

$$\mathrm{HIC} = \left\{ \left(t^2 - t^1\right) \left[\frac{1}{t^2 - t^1} \int_{t^2}^{t^1} a(t)\mathrm{d}t \right]^{2.5} \right\} \max \tag{2}$$

t_1 = initial time (s); t_2 = final time (s); $a(t)$ = acceleration at the centre of gravity of the head; t_2-t_1 = acceleration window (15–36 ms) [31].

2.2 Determination of calcium-lead concentration in erythrocytes

Erythrocyte volume $(V) = \frac{4}{3}\pi a^2 xb$, where a = larger axis; b = minor axis; π = 3.1415. Surface area and volume of a single red blood cell are 155 μm^2 and 87 μm^3 respectively [32]. Calcium concentration (mg/100 ml) to per cent decrease of lead erythrocytes content is equal to;

$$\frac{\%\ \text{decrease erythrocytes lead content}}{\text{concofCa}_2\ \text{mixture}} = \frac{40 - 10}{8 - 4} = 1:7.5 \tag{3}$$

2.3 Determination of acute toxicity of lead in rodents

The detection limit of lead (0.04 μg/dl) at 5% level of significance, blood level lead (0.2–37 μg/dl) and urine lead (9–930 μg/dl) as well as less than 1% of lead transport from sink to plasma have been considered for calculations [21–23, 33, 34].

$$\text{Chronicity factor (CF)} = \frac{\acute{\mathrm{LD}}_{50}}{90\mathrm{daysLD}_{50}} \tag{4}$$

$$\text{Dose rate (DR)} = \text{Target concentration (TC)} \times \text{Clearance (Cl)} \tag{5}$$

$$\text{Also median lethal time fifty(LT50)} = \frac{\text{LD}_{50}}{D^P} \text{ whereas } D = \text{LD}; \tag{6}$$

P = Power coefficient 1/3

$$\text{Note that ED50} = \frac{\text{LD}_{50}}{3} x W_a x 10^{-4} \tag{7}$$

$$\frac{\text{LD}_{50}}{3} = \frac{\text{ED}_{50}}{W_a \times 10^{-4}} \tag{8}$$

$$\text{LD}_{50} = \frac{3(\text{ED}_{50})}{W_a \times 10^{-4}} \tag{9}$$

$$\text{LD}_{50} = \text{LT}_{50} \times D^P = \frac{3(\text{ED}_{50})}{W_a \times 10^{-4}} \tag{10}$$

$$D^P = \frac{3(\text{ED}_{50})}{W_a \times 10^{-4}} \times \frac{1}{\text{LT}_{50}} \tag{11}$$

Therefore:

$$\text{ED}_{50} = \frac{D^P \times W_a \times 10^{-4} \times \text{LT}_{50}}{3} \tag{12}$$

$$\text{Also the volume of distribution (Vd)} = \frac{\text{Dose}}{\text{Concentration}} \tag{13}$$

$$\text{Clearance} = \frac{\text{Dose}}{\text{AUC}} \tag{14}$$

2.4 Calculation of pulmonary oxygen toxicity of lead

The cumulative pulmonary toxic dose (CPTD) of lead expressed as OTU (oxygen toxicity units) is calculated thus, partial pressure of oxygen (PO_2) remains constant [35].

$$\text{OTU} = t_x x \left(\frac{0.5}{\text{PO}_2 - 0.5}\right)^{\frac{-5}{6}}. \tag{15}$$

Where as t_x = time of exposure; PO_2 = constant; $\frac{-5}{6}$ = exponent (−0.8333).

$$\text{Exposure time } t_x = \text{Segmenttime x} \left(\frac{\text{MaxPO}_2 - \text{lowPO}_2}{\text{MaxPO}_2 - \text{MinPO}_2}\right) \tag{16}$$

2.5 Calculation of central nervous system oxygen toxicity of lead

CNS oxygen toxicity is calculated thus, PO_2 remains constants [36]. Therefore

$$\text{CNSfraction} = \frac{\text{TimeatPO}_2}{\text{TimelimitforPO}_2} = \frac{\text{TimeatPO}_2}{m\text{PO}_2 + b} \tag{17}$$

where as m = slope of the time; b = intercept for the given range of PO_2.

2.6 Calculation of exposure dose of lead from contaminated environment

The equation for calculation of exposure dose of lead from contaminated environment [35, 36] is given as follow:

$$D = C \times \text{IR} \times \text{AF} \times \frac{\text{EF}}{\text{BW}}, \tag{18}$$

whereas D = exposure dose; C = contaminated concentration; IR = intake rate of contaminated medium; AF = bioavailability factor; EF = exposure factor; BW = body weight, but the exposure factor is calculated as follow:

$$\text{EF} = \frac{(F \times \text{ED})}{\text{AT}}, \tag{19}$$

whereas F = frequency of exposure (days/year); ED = Exposure duration (years); AT = averaging time (ED × 365 days/year).

2.7 Calculation of water dermal contact dose of lead

Dose of water concentration of lead that can penetrate dermal layer of skin [35, 36] is calculated as follow:

$$D = \frac{(C \times P \times \text{BSA} \times \text{ET} \times \text{CF})}{\text{BW}}, \tag{20}$$

whereas D = dose (mg/kg); C = contaminant concentration (mg/l); P = permeability coefficient (cm/h); BSA = exposed body surface area (m^2); ET = exposure time; CF = conversion factor (1 l/1000 cm^3); BW = body weight.

2.8 Calculation of soil ingestion exposure time of lead

Dose of lead ingested via soil can be calculated [35, 36] using the following formula:

$$D = \frac{(C \times \text{IR} \times \text{ET} \times \text{CF})}{\text{BW}}, \tag{21}$$

where D = exposure dose (mg/kg); C = contaminant concentration (mg/kg); IR = intake rate of contaminated soil (mg/day); EF = exposure factor; CF = conversion factor (kg/mg); BW = body weight.

2.9 Calculation of dose of lead particles present in food

Quantity of lead fragments present in the ingested food can be calculated as follow:

$$D = \sum_{n=i}^{n} \frac{C \times \text{Cri} \times \text{EF}}{\text{BW}}, \tag{22}$$

whereas D = exposure dose (mg/kg/day); C = contaminant concentration (mg/g); Cri = consumption rate of incriminating food (g/day); EF = exposure factor; BW = body weight (kg); n = total number of incriminating food group [30].

2.10 Toxicokinetic scaling of lead fragments

Steady state volume of distribution (Vss) of lead fragments is calculated thus:

$$\text{Vss} = 1.22W^{0.68} \text{ where } W = \text{body weight of animal} \tag{23}$$

$$\text{Cl} = 0.91W^{0.5} \text{ where Cl} = \text{clearance} \tag{24}$$

Vss and Cl are based on plasma concentrations of blood and free lead. However, the Vss and Clu for plasma free concentration of lead are presented below.

$$\text{Vss} = 247W^{0.93} \tag{25}$$

$$\text{Clu} = 186W^{0.76} \tag{26}$$

Maximum tolerated dose (MTD) = $47.5e^{-0.51}$, e = 2.718 [37].

Relationship between respiratory minute volume and body weight is given by the equation.

$$V_m = 0.518W^{0.802} \tag{27}$$

A value of 15.6 l/min has been calculated for 70-kg weighed human [38].

Apparent volume of distribution (Vd) related to absolute oral bioavailability is given as follow:

$$\frac{\text{Vd}}{F} = \frac{\text{Dose}}{\text{AUC} \times \text{Kel}}, \tag{28}$$

where F = bioavailability; AUC = area under curve; Kel = elimination constant.

$$\text{Cl}/F \times \text{MLP} = \beta \times W^{a} \tag{29}$$

where Cl = clearance; MLP = maximum lifespan potential; W = body weight; a = exponent.

$$\text{Dose (mg)} = \text{Animal AUC} \times \text{Scaled Human } \frac{\text{Cl}}{F} \tag{30}$$

AUC = lowest value among species [39].

$$\text{Blood/Plasma concentration ratio (Pp)} = 1 + \text{H} \times (\text{fu}–1) \tag{31}$$

whereas fu = fraction unbound in plasma; H = hematocrit (human, 0.44; rat,0.46; mouse, 0.45; rabbit, 0.36; monkey, 0.36).

$$\text{Cl} = 33.35\text{ml}/\min x \frac{(a)^{0.77}}{\text{Rfu}} \tag{32}$$

Rfu = ratio of unbound fraction in plasma between rats and humans; a = coefficient of surface area.

$$\text{Conc.}H = \text{Conc.}Ax \frac{\text{Dose}_H}{\text{Dose}_A} x \left(\frac{W_A}{W_H}\right)^{c} \tag{33}$$

$$\text{Time}_H = \text{Time}_A x \left(\frac{W_A}{W_H}\right)^b \tag{34}$$

where b and c are exponents of simple allometry of Cl and Vd_{ss}, Percent (%) error between observed clinical concentration and predicted concentration of lead is calculated thus [40].

$$\%\text{error} = \frac{\text{Observed} - \text{Predicted}}{\text{Observed}} \times 100 \tag{35}$$

The experiment for elimination half-life has allometric exponent of 0.25 [41].

Error involved in prediction of clearance is in most cases >30% [42]. Since inhaled lead particles can be distributed immediately the following equation can be used to calculate lead concentration in the blood.

$$C_t = C_o e^{-kt} \tag{36}$$

C_t= lead concentration at time t; C_o= theoretical lead concentration obtained if it had been inhaled at time t = 0; k = elimination rate constant [43–45].

$$\text{Ratio of urinary clearance to total body clearance} = \frac{\text{Cl}_\text{u}}{\text{Cl}_\text{b}} \tag{37}$$

$$\text{Ratio of plasma free lead to total body lead} = \frac{PL}{Bl} \tag{38}$$

2.11 Application of the formulas for calculation of toxicokinetic parameters of lead

The reported LD50 of lead in human is 450 mg/kg body weight, but LD1 = 450/50 = 9 mg/kg body weight

i. $\text{LT}_{50}(\text{d})\ \frac{\text{LD}_{50}}{D^P} = \frac{450}{9\frac{1}{3}} = \frac{450}{2.06} = \frac{218.4}{24\ \text{h}}$ 9.1 days

   However, for an adult man weighing 60 kg, the ED50 for lead antidote is calculated as follows:

ii. $(\text{ED50})\ \frac{\text{LD}_{50}}{3} \times W_a \times 10^{-4}$

   $(\text{ED50})\ \frac{450}{3} \times 60,000 \times 10^{-4}$

   $(\text{ED50})\ 150 \times 6 = 900$

   $\text{ED}_1\ \frac{90}{50} = 18$ mg/kg of antidote

iii. Using dose rate (DR) = TC × Cl

   1080 = 0.037 × Cl

   Cl = $\frac{1080}{0.037}$ = 29189.2 kg/h.

   $\frac{29189.2}{1000} \times \frac{1}{24} = 1.24$ l/kg/h.

At concentration of lead = 525 μg/dl.

If LD_1 = 9 mg/kg.

Dose of lead for 60 kg man = $60 \times 9 = 540$ mg

iv. $(Vd=)\frac{Dose}{Concentration}$

$Vd = \frac{540}{525} = 1.028 = 1.03$ l/kg

v. $AUC = \frac{Dose}{Clearance}$

$\frac{450}{1.24} = 362.9$ mg/kg/h

vi. $\beta = \frac{Clb}{Vd} = \frac{1.24}{1.03} = 1.20$ h.

vii. $MRT = \frac{Vd}{Clb} = \frac{1.03}{1.24} = 0.83$ h.

viii. $T½\beta = \frac{0.693}{\beta} = \frac{0.693}{1.20} = 0.58$ h.

3. Results

LD_{50}, ED_{50}, clearance, LD_1, and volume of distribution of lead bullet in adult human, Red grouse, Mallard, Partridge, pheasant, Woodpigeon and Woodcock are presented in **Tables** 1 and 2. However indices of lead poisoning at various concentrations are presented in **Table** 3. Concentrations of lead ($\leq 5 - > 100$ mg/dl) are

Weight (kg)	LD_{50} (mg/kg)	ED_{50} (mg/kg)	CL (kg/h)	LD (mg/kg)	Vd (L/kg)	AUC (mg/kg/h)	β (h)	MRT (h)	T½β
60	450	18	1.24	9.0	1.03	0.01875	1.16	0.86	0.6

Keys: LD_{50} = Median lethal dose; ED_{50} = Effective dose fifty; Cl = Clearance; LD_1 = Lethal dose for 1 human; Vd = Volume of distribution; AUC = Area under curve; β = Elimination rate constant; MRT = Mean residence time; T½β = Elimination half-life.

Table 1.
Toxico-therapeutic and pharmacokinetic parameters of lead in adult human.

Name of bird	Weight (kg)	LD_{50} (μg/kg)	ED_{50} (μg/kg)	Cl (kg/h)	LD (μg/kg)	Vd (I/kg)
Red grouse	0.600	384	7.6	5.49	8	0.07
Mallard	1.063	274	9.7	4.65	5	0.06
Partridge	0.488	267	4.3	4.85	5	006
Pheasant	1.163	360	14	3.68	7	0.10
Woodpigeon	0.453	120	1.8	6.16	2	0.02
Woodcock	0.300	126	1.3	1.23	3	0.10

Keys: LD_{50} = Median lethal dose, ED_{50} = Effective dose fifty; Cl = Clearance; LD_1 = Lethal dose for 1 human; Vd = Volume of distribution.

Table 2.
Toxicokinetic parameters of lead bullet fragments in birds.

DOI: http://dx.doi.org/10.5772/intechopen.105850

Systemic	Range of toxic doses of plasma blood lead (μg/dl) and their toxicity signs						
	≤5–14	15–24	25–34	35–44	45–54	55–100	>100
Neurological	Depression, loss of 4–7 IQ, damage D_1 receptors, Reduction of glutamine synthetase, positioning range, bad mood, headache, memory loss, drowsiness, trembling, tingling of limbs, penetration of brain by lead, Kills birds and humans or birds and humans are severely poisoned, 10 μg/dl exceeds EU limit	Reduction of glutamine synthetase	—	Abnormal oligodendrocytes	Increased D_1 in T = striatum, decreased D_1 in nucleus accumbens	Acute encephalopathy neurological signs Acute death	Epilepsy death
Cardiovascular	Hypertension	—	—	—	—	—	Death
Haematological	Ratio of blood lead to erythrocytes lead for 6 month- old child (1/2–2/5), infants (7/10–7/11), adult (5/12) irrespectively. Increased delta amino levulinic acid, haemolysis, anaemia, curvilinear relationship between plasma lead and whole blood is within the range (2.13–3.97 μg/dl), chelation is not recommended at >45 μg/dl	—	—	—	—	—	—
Reproductive	Low birth weight, premature birth, anomaly, abortion	—	—	Decreased libido	—	—	—
Renal	—	—	Renal insufficiency	—	—	—	—
Immunological	—	—	—	—	Humoral and cellular immunity is affected	—	—
Respiratory	All the toxic doses can affect respiration						

Note: All the reported threshold limits set for blood lead are wrong; — = System is affected by the dose.

Table 3.
Toxicological indices of lead poisoning in human.

injurious to haematological, neurological, cardiovascular, reproductive, renal, immunological and respiratory systems (**Table** 3). The calculated maximum tolerated dose of lead for 70 kg weighed man was 337.1 mg/kg. Bioavailability was 82.3%, whereas 62% of lead was cleared in the urine and 42% sequestrated in various tissues of 70 kg weighed man. Inhaled lead (525 μg/dl) would translate to 622 μg/dl over a period of 5 months with elimination rate of 1.2 h.

3.1 Effects of lead on intelligence quotient

Lead in the brain affects intelligence quotient (IQ) of school age child. IQ measured at 3.8 years is affected by 5 μg/dl of lead concentration in the brain [44]. The established Benchmark limit doses of 1% extra risk are for intelligence quotient (IQ- $BMDL_{01}$) (12 μg/dl), systolic blood pressure, SBP-$BMDL_{01}$ (36 μg/dl) and chronic kidney disease, CKD- $BMDL_{01}$ (15 μg/dl) respectively. Increased blood lead of 1–6.7 μg/dl is associated with mortality from ischaemic heart disease and cardiovascular disease [45] This may likely affect 600,000–900,000 population of Sweden that consume game meat [46].

4. Discussion

4.1 Median lethal effects of lead bullet in human

The reported LD_{50} (450 mg/kg) of lead in human indicates that lead is very dangerous to life. The concentration, 100 mgpb/m^3 is unsafe [33]. However, blood concentration of lead (525 μg/dl) after 5 months caused epilepsy and death, but 10–60 μg/dl for 21 days caused neurological signs [47], as 6.25 μg/dl (0.3 μM) damaged and reduced dopamine uptake [48] and up to 97.2 μg/dl can cause acute death [49]. The concentration of pb (>50 μg/dl) at 60-day increased D_1 receptors in the striatum, but decreased D_1 receptors in the nucleus accumbens [50]. Lead (5.2–20.8 μg/dl) reduced glutamine synthetase activity [51], as 38.2 μg/dl caused abnormal oligodendrocytes [52]. Where blood lead level is below 45 μg/dl, chelation is not recommended [53]. The calculated 1080 mg of lead poisoning antidote agrees with the report indicating that, 500–1000 mg of penicillamine can be used for treatment of plumbism in man [54]. Accumulation of lead in astrocytes altered neurotransmitter release, receptor density, impaired development and function of oligodendrocytes, caused abnormal myelin function, neurotrophic factor expression, abnormal dendritic branching patterns, disruption of blood brain barrier, thyroid hormone transportation to brain, lowered IQ, impaired neuropsychological function and impaired academic achievement [55]. Interspecies comparison of lead LD_{50} between rat and mouse using regression analysis, showed high correlation of 0.8 and 0.9, respectively. LD_{50} variability showed 90% probability; 54% in one category, and 44% in adjacent category suggesting the possibility of an alternative method to conventional in-vivo acute oral toxicity test [56]. Blood lead concentration was significantly higher among Australian consumers of meat contaminated with lead-based ammunition (≤18.1 μg/dl daily), as compared to non-consumers of lead-based ammunition meat (≤7.4 μg/dl rarely) [57].

4.2 Clinical implication of delayed lead bullet elimination

The lead clearance of 1.2 l/kg/h agrees with the reported value of 1.18 l/kg/h [58]. Our findings agree with the report indicating that, other methods can complement the application of LD50 for discovery of potential toxicants. Such methods could aim at encouraging replacement, refinement and reduction [23]. Many scaling factors are determined experimentally, as all scaling factors have uncertainty associated with them. Mathematics of translation from one species to another requires multiple experimentally estimated scaling factors [59]. The developmental effects of lead occur at the age (>2 years). Low level of lead (>10 μg/dl) is associated with adverse effect in the developing child [60] and inversely proportional to neuropsychological development in the first 7 years of life [61]. The reported average blood lead concentration in child aged 1 and 5 years are 0.03 mg/l (3 μg/dl) and 0.11 mg/l (11 μg/dl), respectively. The elimination half-life in adult is 1 and 10 months in children [62]. Circulation of lead after absorption is 30 days. It diffuses into soft tissues including brain, and after 2 min diffuses into bone with blood half-life of 30 days and bone half-life of 20–30 years [63]. Also, half-life of lead in blood is 1–1.5 months and 25–30 years in bone respectively. However, Center for Disease Control (CDC) has defined poisoning level of lead equals or greater than 5 μg/dl [64]. Blood lead concentration of 9.1 μg/dl causes bad mood, headache, memory loss, daylight drowsiness, trembling, tingling of limb among others. Hence there is no known level of lead exposure considered safe [65]. This confirms that lead can enter brain because, it has a molecular weight of 207.2 g [66]. The total elimination half-life of lead is greater than 18 months. The primary route of elimination is urine [67], suggesting that urine is the most important sample in forensic toxicology of lead poisoning. Therefore, governments at various levels and law enforcement agents should curtail the use of lead bullet, so as to avoid damage to physical and intellectual capacity of affected humans [68]. Blood lead concentration (391 μg/dl) requires the use of calcium EDTA, but lead (49 μg/dl) can be neutralized using 600 mg succimer, three times daily for 14 days [69].

4.3 Relationship between brain damage caused by lead, low intelligence quotient and renal dysfunction

Acute encephalopathy occurs in children of blood lead concentration of ≥80 g/dl [70], therefore low threshold of 30–70 g/dl has been suggested [71]. Every increase of 10 g/dl in blood lead caused a loss of 4—7IQ points, hence it is difficult to identify a threshold for decrement in IQ [72, 73]. Renal dysfunction was caused by lead concentration of blood at <40–70 g/dl, and 10 g/dl was associated with 9% reduction in creatinine clearance [74, 75]. Nevertheless, 85 g/dl blood lead caused increased susceptibility to cold and >50 g/dl caused significant immunological changes [76], such as increase in lymphocytes, abnormal T-cell subsets and cellular immune function [77, 78]. Lead concentration of >62 g/dl inhibited conversion of vitamin 2 into 1.25—dihydroxy vitamin 2 which was reduced in children with severe renal insufficiency, at blood lead concentration of 33–55 g/dl [79]. Nevertheless, blood lead concentration of 14 g/dl caused low birth weight, premature birth and increased risk of developmental abnormalities [80]. Threshold level for hypohaemoglobinaemia is 50 g/dl in adult and ≤40 g/dl in children, respectively [38]. Regulatory bodies such as Control of Lead at Work (CLAW) and Scientific Committee on Occupational Exposure Limit (SCOEL) have recommended 30 g/dl for female workers of child-bearing capacity and 60 g/dl for men and others. However, European Lead Association has recommended 30 g/dl for men and 10 g/dl for women with reproductive capacity, respectively [81, 82]. Mean blood lead concentration of pigs that fed on venison was 2.29 g/dl which is 3.6 times higher than that of pig that did not feed on venison (0.63 g/dl). The venison-fed pig eliminated lead within 6 days of last ingestion [45]. Blood concentration of lead >5 g/dl is associated with high risk of spontaneous abortion in woman and the concentration > 40 g/dl is associated with decreased libido, sperm count and abnormal morphology of sperm cells [83, 84].

4.4 Effects of lead bullet on human and wildlife, diagnosis and therapeutic benefit of plumbism

About 0.4 million water birds of 33 species die every year from lead shot in European Union wetlands, and it cost European Union 105 million euros to replace 0.7 million captive-bred birds for killed ones. Restriction of water birds hunting cost greater than 100 million euros [85–87]. The milk plasma concentration ratio for lead is 50–100:1 after 24 h in mice, indicating a higher efficient concentration of lead milk of lactating mice as compared to that of non-lactating mice [88]. Linear biokinetic model of prehistories/preindustrial children's blood of 0.06–0.12 g/dl was calculated for two lead intakes, which was lower than CDC threshold limit value of 10 g/dl. Toxicokinetics of bone lead that causes resorption with metabolic stimuli is of great concern for baby growth [89]. However, plumbism in birds cause death in 3 weeks [90]. The metabolizing enzymes that play very great role in the toxicokinetics of lead are d-amino-levulinate dehydratase d–ALA–d and porphobilinogen synthetase [91]. The activity of d-ALA-d, an allosteric enzyme with 28 thiol group is inhibited by lead [92], leading to accumulation of d-amino levulinic acid (d-ALA), whose concentration in urine of human and other animals is used to diagnose lead poisoning [93]. Sublethal dose of lead (0.2–0.5 ppm) has been reported with ≥0.5 ppm showing a significant decreased of d-ALA-d, causing brain damage which can be reversed by zinc. Haemosynthetase, ALA-dehyrotase and ferrochelatase have antidotal effects [94]. The latter enzyme binds iron to protoporphyrin, an indicator of blood lead, 40 ppm of the protoporphyrin is a clear proof of plumbism, over 500 pm affects neuromuscular activity with a consequent change in the motor functions [95–97]. Dimercaprol, a diethylene triamine pentaacetic acid, D-penicillamine, thiamine and calcium disodium ethylene diamine tetraacetate chelate lead for elimination. Highly hunted birds such as red grouse, mallard partridge, pheasant, woodpigeon, woodcock and deer could have lead fragments that exceeded threshold values of 100–10,000 ppb [98]. Many lead fragments in the carcasses of killed animals weighed >12–25 mg each, concentration of blood lead (5.9–18.1 g/dl) has been reported for consumers of game meats in Greenland and Switzerland and >4.1 millions shots have been reported against macropods, deer, red foxes, feral pigs, European rabbits and feral goats in Australia, annually [74], signifying that Australia may have high incidence of plumbism among wildlife. One million wild fowl estimated to have been killed by lead poisoning and ≥3 million sublethally poisoned [17], including Anseriformes, Falconiformes and Accipitriformes. They were severely poisoned with lead blood concentration of (>100 g/dl) [18]. Lethal lead concentration range (56–120 g/dl) has been reported for bearded vulture, Cape vulture and golden eagle [99–103] suggesting variation in susceptibility to lead poisoning among wild birds. However, concentration range of 10–47 g/dl was survived, and associated with different isotopes of lead

[100, 104, 105]. Clinical threshold limit values for lead toxicosis of blood (>0.5 mg/kg), liver and kidney (>6 mg/kg) have been reported. Fragment sample size of 0.5 to >5 mm radiate from the wound channel [2]. Concentration of lead in the liver (28.9 ppm) for bald eagles and 19.4 ppm for golden eagles are sources for concern [106]. However reduced circulatory erythrocyte volume reduce uptake of lead by blood [107].

4.5 Exposure to environment lead

Exposure to lead arises from air and surfaces, and absorption occurs via ingestion, inhalation, percutaneous and transdermal routes. The first two are relevant to firing ranges, 0.1–5 μm lead can be inhaled, absorbed through the lung and 50% gets distributed to various parts of biological system. Absorption of ingested lead is >8–10% [108]. However, 12.5 g/m^3 of airborne lead particles of ≤1 μm is of public health significance and the particles higher than >1 μm are deposited in the upper respiratory tract [109]. About 70% of workers exposed to lead (50 g/m^3) had blood lead of 405 g/dl and 6% had >505 g/dl respectively [110]. However, 94% of samples of deer killed with bullets contained fragments of lead, which portend very high risk for scavengers [111]. Blood lead levels increased with time after injury up to 3 months with fragments and increasing age, which is 30% higher in the patient whose torsos are affected. Hence, blood level could be higher (11.8%) at 3 months and 2.6% at 12 months, respectively. Therefore, there is need for continued surveillance after gunshot [112]. The uncertainty in predictive power of algometric scales remains a concern in plumbism caused by lead bullet. Hence, the scales can only apply for exploratory research [113]. The uncertainty and availability, both in terms of inter-subject and application associated can be significant [114]. Natural isotopes of lead; 204 pb, 206 pb, 207 pb, and 208 pb constitute manufactured lead in various percentages, and their measurements in human and wildlife could be compared with their potential sources for environment risk assessment [2].

4.6 Lead causes cognition impairment

Lead causes impairment of neurodevelopment, cognition and behavioural development in the foetus and young child. The source of plumbism from wild birds killed by ammunition is significant among 5 million people in European Union countries [45]. The half-life of lead in blood and bone is 30 days and decades, respectively [115]. Unfortunately, maximum level (ML) for lead in game animals has not been set in the Codex Alimentarius General Standard for contaminants and toxicants [116], and by European Union [117], leading to concentration of 690 μg of lead fragments in wild-shot moose carcasses in Finland, Norway and Sweden [45]. Daily blood lead (12 μg/l) and lead intake (0.5 μg/kg) can affect intelligence quotient (IQ) of a child [118]. Bullet position may preclude surgical removal in order to avoid exacerbation of neurologic damage. The complication of the removal may be due to immediate migration of the fragment [119]. Retention of lead fragments in joint space is associated with increased risk of lead poisoning, and joint disruption leading to synovial metaplasia [120]. Good radiography and clinical findings are highly essential, for identification and complete surgical removal of bullet fragments, that may have high potential of distribution to various parts of biological system [121]. Injuries from bullet are most severe in brain and liver, causing temporary cavitation far from the actual bullet track. Bone and subcutaneous fats are highly resistant to bullet injury [122, 123]. Toxic leads widely used to hunt game animals and varmints are a source of environmental pollution. Lead and bismuth are highly frangible [26] and about 90% of the total burden of lead is found in bone and 5% in plasma, which pass through the cell membrane and cause toxic effect in brain, red blood cells, liver among others. In view of this, the knowledge of lead kinetics is of prime importance to a greater and better understanding of lead toxicity, as the risk of its adverse effects is very high [124]. Substitution of toxic lead bullets for non-toxic bullets such as steel, bismuth and tungsten may be possible alternative of curtailing lead poisoning from firearms, and phasing-out period of lead bullets could reduce cognition impairment [125]. Rationales used to remove lead from paints, gasoline and household items should be applied to lead-base ammunition globally, an issue that regularizes international intervention [126]. About 45% of surveyed states and provinces in the USA and Canada have non-toxic short regulation above federal water fowl regulations [127].

4.7 Forensic implication of lead poisoning

Regulatory toxicology consists of collection, processing and evaluation of epidemiological and experimental toxicological data, that end up in a decision for protection of health against toxic substances [128]. Clinicians treating plumbism from gunshot must be aware of potential incompatibilities between drugs and lead [129]. Mathematical modelling is becoming increasingly relevant for drug development [130]. One in every five injuries caused by firearm is fatal [131]. Ballistic weapon can move with a velocity of 915 m/s, whereas bullet can move up to 610 m/s [132]. Hence there is need for anatomical mapping of the target organs. Neck injuries caused by bullet are described according to the anatomical zones (1–111). Zone I extends from clavicle to cricothyroid membrane, zone II from cricothyroid membrane to the mandibular angle and zone III from mandibular angle to base of the skull [133]. But advanced neurotrauma research can improve the quality of life of patients that suffer from traumatic brain injuries [134].

4.8 Relationship between lead poisoning and brain over claim syndrome

Brain over claim syndrome (BOS) is about the relationship between neuroscience and criminal responsibility, distinguishing between internal and external critiques based on neuroscience [135]. The brain holds the key to mind and behaviour, which is useful to the law [136]. Criminal behaviour and violence are worldwide public health problem, since criminal behaviour has neurobiological basis with judicial implication. The affected brain pathways are genetic (foetal neural development), hormones and neurotransmitters (cortisol and testosterone), psychophysiology (e.g., low resting heart rate, low electroencephalography), brain imaging and neurology (reduced frontal lobe function) with attendant legal context (punishment, prediction and prevention) [137], respectively. Morality is part of human judgment, behaviour and mind. Frontal, temporal and cingulate cortex mediate between emotion and reasoning, amygdala, hippocampus and basal ganglia play vital role in morality. Therefore, genetic polymorphism, endocrine and environmental factors could modify the psychology of morality. Hence, abnormal behaviour can arise from structural brain stimulation [138], especially the anterior cingulate which causes empathy, orbital prefrontal cortex (causes regret), ventromedial prefrontal cortex (PFC) (ethical discussion), ventrolateral PFC (inhibits behaviour) and dorsolateral PFC is for reasoning [139]. Relationship between lower intelligence, crime and custodial outcomes has been established [140]. Also established is a very strong association between preschool lead and subsequent crime rate trends over decades in USA, Britain, Canada, France, Australia, Finland, Italy, West Germany and New Zealand [141]. Nevertheless, removal of lead from petrol since 1975 has led to the decline of crimes in the USA [142], because inhalation of lead content of petrol from 2 g to 0.5 g per gallon between 1975 and 1980 was highly reduced [143]. Atmospheric exposure could cause aggressive crime in children [144].

4.9 Arsenic can mar litigation caused by lead bullet

Since lead decreases arsenic bioavailability [145], it can reduce the chance of arsenic poisoning and vice versa. Hence there is need for knowledge of toxicokinetic changes of lead for better evaluation and interpretation of preclinical safety and clinical hazard [146]. Also the dose of bullets can be used to deduce lead concentration in the body, and the area under curve (AUC) base line should be compared with lead AUC response to eliminate uncertainty and variability [147]. This may be highly beneficial in biopsy [148] and autopsy of living or dead person tissues, affected by lead bullets. Under this condition, statistical moment theory instead of the compartmental model may be used to calculate mean residence time [149]. Elimination and absorption rate constants and volume of distribution may vary with age, gender, weight, clinical status, genetic variability and co-administration of lead with another drug or toxicant. Hence therapeutic monitoring of plumbism is very important [150]. Therefore, Pharmacokinetic/Pharmacodynamic (PK/PD) relationship is very important guide for identifying susceptibility and treatment potential of poisoning from lead bullets [151]. Lead distribution and clearance were 2.5 and 4 times higher in lactating and non-lactating animals respectively [152], and 10 μg/dl limit issued by Centre for Disease Control (CDC) is relatively high [89]. Relationship between blood lead concentration and lead intake is non-linear, [153], but at low concentration the kinetic is linear and at 60 μg/dl in erythrocytes which corresponds to blood level of 25 μg/dl, the kinetic becomes non-linear [153], indicating that lead kinetics is Michaelis–Menten. Accessibility pool parameters (Vd, Clb, β, MRT) can be used compartmentally and non-compartmentally [154]. Gunshot residue and shooting distance could be used to determine contact and near contact wound in putrefied or charred bodies [155, 156]. In conventional rifles and gun bullet projection, the projectile requires high altitude and glides with subsonic speed and a good ratio lift/drag. This is applicable with bullets having projectiles of 2–5 times [157]. Threshold level (25 $\mu g/m^3$) in air is dangerous to health [158]. Velocity of 150–170 fps is required by bullet to penetrate skin [121]. But bones change the speed of bullets greatly, by changing their course and slowing them down [159]. Origin of bullet can be determined using the major/minor axis which determines the impact angle, although modern laser methods provide better results. Semi-automatic gun and bullet system (7.62 mm) is more effective [160]. Toxicosis from lead ammunition in predatory and scavenging birds have been reported in Argentina, Chile, Swiss Alps, Namibia, South Africa, Botswana, Israel, French Pyrenees, Spain, Iberian Peninsula, Sweden, USA, Granada, UK, Japan, Poland, Finland, Ireland, Portugal, Italy and Canada [17]. International suspension limit of blood lead is 10–70 μg/dl in females and 20–70 μg/dl in males, respectively. However, 5–80 μg/dl and above can cause hypertension, kidney dysfunction, neurocognitive deficits, colic, gout, sperm abnormalities, anaemia, peripheral neuropathy and encephalopathy (**Table** 3). Hence, there is narrow margin of safety between blood lead suspension and subclinical effects [161]. Therefore, the

1899 Hague Declaration is about abstinence from the use of bullets; an effective treaty applied for over 100 years, but may likely face modern challenges [162]. At short range of shooting bullets, the amount of energy absorbed is increased which is proportional to striking velocity [163]. Jauhari experimented on bullet crochet, defined as deflection of a bullet from its course by firing low velocity handgun cartridges on targets [164].

4.10 The importance of ban on the use of lead ammunition

Gun at 0.436° hit the centre of a target 1 m off the ground and 1 km away with an air temperature of 27.2°C. Hence hollow bullet has more drag and hit the centre of the target at a different angle [165]. Bullets from high velocity modern rifles produce lead fragments, and lead shot (6.1 μg/g) could kill birds, when the meats from such birds were consumed, blood concentration (15–128 mg/l) was detected in the blood of human consumers, as well as 24–50 and 9–180 μg/l were detected in mothers and newborns, respectively [166]. Low blood lead concentration (LBLC) is associated with decreased intelligent quotient (IQ) in children [167]. Hence the use of lead ammunition has been banned in the USA, Canada, Mexico, Oceania, Austria, Japan, South Africa, Bennin, Guinea-Bisau, Sudan, Denmark, Norway, Netherland, Finland and Sweden on some categories and species of birds [168]. But 3 mm lead pellet and 3.4 mm steel pellet each weighed 250 mg. Increasing diameter by 0.5 mm compensates for steel's lower density [169]. Over 90% of ammunitions manufactured in the world contain lead [170]. Pattern density is the primary factor that influences types of ammunition performance [171]. A high lead load (45–52 mg) per 100 g wet weight and the embedded pellet per body mass (1.21/100 g) in woodcock portend high health risk to consumers [172]. Exit wound caused by bullets are very rare at close range [173]. But sabot bullet made from lead alloy and plastic tends to be the most dangerous in soft and medium density materials. However, the effect of lead ammunition in non-quarry species of animals is unknown [174]. All these are very specific in forensic toxicology that can be relied upon in justice delivery, and provision of solution for criminal cases [175]. Hence forensic scientists play critical role in the determination of various risk factors in litigations related to the medical and legal cases [176], which are related to complete penetration of bullet into brain, that may cause death or incomplete penetration that may cause death or survival [177]. Hence, there is need to reduce level of lead exposure in overall population with a view to having healthy and safe environment [161], >0.1 mg/kg concentration has been reported for bovine, sheep, pigs and poultry, a dose that exceeds European Union Maximum level of 100 ppb [178], fulfilling the expectations of the community and justice [179], bearing in mind that wildlife could serve as source of potential lead bullet poisoning [3, 5, 173, 180–185]. Nevertheless renal damage could be confirmed legally by applying the reported investigation protocol [186]. European Chemical Agency (ECHA) has proposed a restriction on lead use in sports shooting, hunting and fishing. The restriction could reduce lead emissions by 630,000 tonnes over 20 years, representing 72% lead reduction [187].

5. Conclusion

Lethality of lead bullet is dependent on the body weight, median lethal time, doses of lead fragments released per unit time, concentration of lead in the brain, volume of distribution, elimination rate constant, mean residence time and elimination half-life of the lead fragments, which could be detected within 100 days after gunshots. Brain damage caused by lead fragments appears to be associated with low level of intelligence and brain over claim syndrome. Hence, forensic pathologists, police and the concerned judges should take note of prevailing conditions during gunshot attack.

Author details

Saganuwan Alhaji Saganuwan
Department of Veterinary Pharmacology and Toxicology, College of Veterinary Medicine, Federal University of Agriculture, Makurdi, Benue State, Nigeria

*Address all correspondence to: pharm_saga2006@yahoo.com

References

[1] Linden MA, Manton WI, Stewagt RM, Thal ER, Feirt H. Lead poisoning from retained bullets: Pathogenesis, diagnosis and management. Annals of Surgery. 1982;**195**(3):305-313

[2] Golden NH, Warner SE, Coffey MJ. A review and assessment of spent lead ammunition and its exposure and effects to scavenging birds in the United States. Reviews Contamination and Toxicology. 2016;**237**:123-191

[3] Pattee OH, Carpenter JW, Fritts SH, Rattner BA, Wiemeyer SN, Royle JA, et al. Lead poisoning in captive Andean condors (vulture gryphus). Journal of Wildlife Disease. 2006;**42**:772-779

[4] Carpenter JW, Pattee OH, Fritts SH, Rattner BA, Wiemeyor SN, Royle JA, et al. Experimental lead poisoning in Turkey vultures (*Cathartes aura*). Journal of Wildlife Disease. 2003;**39**: 96-104

[5] Pattee OH, Wiemeyer SN, Mulhern BM, Sileo L, Carpenter JW. Experimental lead-shot poisoning in bald eagles. Journal of Wildlife Management. 1981;**45**:806-810

[6] Peraza MA, Ayala-Fierro F, Barber DS, Caseren E, Rael LT. Effects of micronutrients on metal toxicity. Environmental Health Perspective. 1998; **106**(1):203-216

[7] Bressler JP, Goldstein GW. Mechanisms of lead neurotoxicity. Biochemical Pharmacology. 1991;**41**: 479-484

[8] Burger J, Gochfeld M. Effects of lead on birds (lavidae): A review of laboratory and field studies. Journal of Toxicology Environmental Health. 2000; **3**:59-78

[9] Garces G, Bernado J, Artuz M, Ignacio R. Secondary lead poisoning: A projectile housed in the human body. Columbia Medicine. 2012;**43**(3):230-234

[10] Anderson KE, Sassa S, Bishop DF, Desnick RJ. Disorders of heme biosynthesis: X-linked sideroblastic anemia and the porphyrias. In: Vale MD, editor. The Online Metabolic and Molecular Basis of Inherited Diseases. New York: McGraw Hill; 1996

[11] Silbergold EK, Hruska RE, Bradley D. Neurotoxic aspects of porphyry no parties: Lead and succinyl acetone. Environmental Research. 1982;**29**: 459-471

[12] Zawia NH, Henry GJ. Developmental exposure to lead interferes with glial and neuronal differential gene expression in the rat cerebellum. Toxicology Applied Pharmacology. 1996;**138**:43-47

[13] Wilson MA, Johnston MV, Goldstein GW, Blue ME. Neonatal lead exposure impairs development of rodent barrel field cortex. Proceeding National Academy Science USA. 2000;**97**(10): 5540-5545

[14] Bellinger DC. Very low lead exposures and children's neurodevelopment. Current Open Pediatrics. 2008;**20**:172-177

[15] Rehman MA, Umer N, Sepah TJ, Wajid MA. Bullet-induced synovitis as a cause of secondary osteoarthritis of the hip joint: A case report and review of literature. Journal of Medical Case Report. 2007;**1**:1-4

[16] Knott J, Gilbert J, Green RE, Hoccom DG. Comparison of the lethality of lead and copper bullets in deer control operations to reduce incidental lead poisoning: Field trials in England and Scotland. Conservation Evidence. 2009; **6**:71-78

[17] Pain DJ, Mateo R, Green RE. Effects of lead from ammunition on birds and other wildlife: A review and update. Ambio. 2019;**48**:935-953

[18] Franson JC, Pain D. Lead in birds. In: Beyer WN, Meador JP, editors. Environmental Contamination in Biota, Interpreting Tissue Concentrations. 2nd ed. Boca Ralon, FL: Taylor & Francis Group LLC; 2011. pp. 563-593

[19] Mazer-Amirshashi M, Stolbach A, Nelson LS. Correction to ACMT Position Statement: Addressing the Rising Cost of Prescription Anridotes 2018;**14**:174-176

[20] Cairns R, Buckley NA. The poisoning severity score: If it did not exist, we would have to invent it. Journal Medical Toxicology. 2017;**13**:131-134

[21] Saganuwan SA. Principles of Pharmacological Calculations. 1st ed. Nigeria: Ahmadu Bello University Press Zaria; 2012. p. 529

[22] Saganuwan SA. The new algorithm for calculation of median lethal dose (LD_{50}) and effective dose fifty (ED_{50}) of *Micranus fulvinus* venom and antivenom in mice. International Journal of Veterinary Science and Medicine. 2016; **4**(1):1-4

[23] Saganuwan SA. Toxicity studies of drugs and chemicals in animals: An overview. Bulgarian Journal of Veterinary Medicine. 2017;**20**(4): 291-318

[24] Bruce RD. An up-and-down procedure for acute toxicity testing. Fundal Applied Toxicology. 1985;**5**(1): 151-157

[25] van den Heuivel MJ, Clark DG, Eielder RJ, Koundakjian PP, Oliver GJ, Pelling D, et al. The international validation of a fixed dose procedure as an alternative to the classical LD_{50} test. Food Chemistry and Toxicology. 1990; **28**(7):469-482

[26] Stroud RK, Hunt WG, Gunshot wounds: A source of lead in the environment. In: Watson RT, Fuller M, Pokras M, Hunt WG (eds). Ingestion of Lead from Spent Ammunition: Implications for Wildlife and Humans. The Peregrine Fund, Borse, Idaho, USA DOI 10.4080/ilsa.2009.0109

[27] Ragsdale BD. Gunshot wounds: A historical perspective. Military Medicine. 1984;**149**:301-305

[28] Rhee PM, Moore EE, Joseph B, Tang A, Pandit V, Vercruysse G. Gunshot wounds: A review of bathistics, bullets, weapons and myths. Journal of Trauma and Acute Care Surgery. 2016;**80**(6): 853-867

[29] Dimaro VJ, Copeland AR, Besant-Matthews PE, Fletcher LA, Jones A. Minimal velocities necessary for perforation of skull by air gun pellets and bullets. Journal of Forensic Science. 1982; **27**(4):894-898

[30] Yoganandan N. Frontiers in Head and Neck Trauma: Clinical and Biomechanical. Amsterdam: IOS Press; 1998

[31] Versace J. A review of the seventy index. No 710881 SAE Technical paper 1971

[32] Cy J. Surface area and volume of a single red blood cell. Journal of Membrane Boil. 1971;**5**:200-214

[33] Bergdahl IA, Schutz A, Gerhardson L, Jensen A, Skerftving S. Lead concentrations in human plasma, urine and whole blood. Scandinavian Journal of Work and Environmental Health. 1997;**23**(5):359-363

[34] Sanganuwan SA. Comparative therapentic index, lethal time and safety margin of various toxicants and snake antivenoms using newly derived and old formulas. Philadelphia: Biomedical Central Research, Notes. 2020;**13**(292): 1-7

[35] Clark JN. Oxygen toxicity. In: Bennett PB, Elliott DH, editors. The Physiology and Medicine of Diving. 4th ed. Philadelphia: WB Saunders; 1983. pp. 121-169

[36] Lambertsen CJ. Extension of oxygen tolerance in man. Philosophy and significance. Experimental Lung Research. 1988;**14**:1035-1058

[37] Paxton JW, Kim SN, Whitfield LR. Pharmacokinetic and toxicity scaling of the antitumor agents amascarine and C1-921, a new analogue in mice, rats, rabbits, dogs and humans. Cancer Research. 1990;**50**:2692-2697

[38] Bide RW, Armour SJ, Tee E. Estimation of Human Toxicity from Animal Inhalation Toxicity Data: Minute Volume-Body Weight Relationships between Animals and Man. Canada: Defence Research Establishment Suffield (DRESS), National Defence; 1997

[39] Amantana A, Chen T, Tyavanagimatt SR, Jones KF, Jordan R, Chinsangaram J, et al. Pharmacokinetics and interspecies allometric scaling of ST-246, an oral antiviral therapeutic for treatment of orthopoxyvirus infection. PLOS One. 2013;**8**(4):1-10

[40] Vozmediano V, Ortega I, Lukas JC, Gungalo A, Rodriguez M, Lucero ML. Integration of preclinical and clinical knowledge to predict intravenous pk in humans: Bilastine case study. European Journal of Drug Metabolism and Pharmacokinetics. 2014;**39**(1):33-41. DOI: 10.1007/S13318-0131-3

[41] Knibbe CAJ, Zuideveld KP, Aarts LPHJ, Kuks PFM, Danhof M. Allometric relationships between the pharmacokinetics of propofol in rats, children and adults. British journal of Clinical Pharmacology. 2005;**59**(6): 705-711

[42] Mahmood I, Bahian JD. The pharmacokinetic principles behind sealing from preclinical results to phase I protocol. Clinical Pharmacokinetics. 1999;**36**(1):1-11

[43] Quijano-Mateos A, Castillo-Alanis LA, Bravo-Gomeg ME. Mathematical models employed to predict the time frame of intoxications as interpretation tool in forensic cases. Journal of Forensic Toxicology and Pharmacology. 2017; **6**(1):1-9

[44] Reuben A, Caspi A, Belsky DW, Broadbert J, Harrington H, Sugden K, et al. Association of childhood blood lead levels with cognitive function and socioeconomic status at age 38 years and with IQ change and socioeconomic mobility between childhood and adult. Journal of American Medicine Association. 2017;**317**:1244-1251

[45] Green RE, Pain DJ. Risks to human health from ammunition derived lead in Europe. Ambio. 2019;**48**:954-968

[46] Ankarberg EH, Bjerselius R, Kollander B, Sand S, Scherling K, Linne

C, et al. Lead in Game in Sweden. Sweden: National Food Agency; 2013. pp. 1-33

[47] Fox DA, Campbell ML, Blocker YS. Functional alterations and apoptotic cell death in the retina following developmental or adult lead exposure. Neurotoxicology. 1997;**18**:645-664

[48] Hanbauer SM. The effect of lead exposure and serum deprivation on mesencephalic primary cultures. Neurotoxicology. 1997;**18**:331-339

[49] Struzynska L, Dabrowska-Bouta B, Rafalowska U. Acute lead toxicity and energy metabolism in rat brain synaptosomes. Acta Neurobiology and Experiment. 1997;**57**:275-281

[50] Widzowski DV, Finkelstein JN, Pokora MJ, Cory-Schlecta DA. Time course of postnatal lead-induced changes in dopamine receptors and their relationship to changes in dopamine sensitivity. Neurotoxicology. 1994;**15**: 853-865

[51] Sierra EM, Tiffany-Castiglioni E. Reduction of glutamine synthetase activity in astroglial exposed in culture to low levels of inorganic lead. Toxicology. 1991;**65**:295-304

[52] Dabrowska-Bouta B, Sulkowski G, Bartosz G, Walski M, Rafalowska U. Chronic lead intoxication affects the myelin membrane status in the central nervous system of adult rats. Journal of Molecular Neuroscience. 1999;**13**:127-139

[53] Gracia RC, Snodgrass WR. Lead toxicity and chelation therapy. American Journal of Health System Pharmacy. 2007;**64**:45-53

[54] Gurer H, Ercal N. Can antioxidants be beneficial in the treatment of lead poisoning? Free Radical Biology and Medicine. 2000;**29**:927-945

[55] Lidsky TI, Schneider JS. Lead neurotoxicity in children : Basic mechanisms and clinical correlates. Brain. 2003;**126**(1):5-19

[56] Hoffmann S, Kinsner-Ovaskainen A, Prieto P, Mangelsdorf I, Bieler C, Cole T. Acute oral toxicity: Variability, reliability, relevance and interspecies comparison of rodents LD50 data from literature surveyed for the acutetox project. Regulatory Toxicology and Pharmacology. 2010;**58**:395-407

[57] Hampton JO, Laidlaw M, Buenz E, Arnemo JM. Heads in the sand: Public health and ecological risks of lead-based bullets for wildlife shouting in Australia. WildLife Research. 2018;**45**:287-306

[58] Mcintyre TA, Han C, Xiang H, Bambal R, Davis CB. Difference in the total body clearance of lead compounds in the rat and mouse: Impact of pharmacokinetic screening strategy. Xenobiotica. 2008;**38**(6):605-619

[59] Rogers JA, Wilbur J, Cole S, Bernhardt PW, Bupp JL, Lennon MJ, et al. Quantifying uncertainty in predictions of hepatic clearance. Statistical Biopharmaceutic Research. 2011;**3**(4):515-525

[60] Sanders T, Liu T, Buchner V, Tchounnon PB. Neurotoxic effects and biomarkers of lead exposure: A review. Reviews in Environmental Health. 2009; **24**(1):15-45

[61] Baghurst PA, McMichael AJ, Wigg NR, Vimpani GV, Robertson EF, Roberts RJ, et al. Environmental exposure to lead and children's intelligence at the age of seven years. The Port Pirie Cohort Study. New England Journal of Medicine. 1992; **327**:1279-1284

[62] Goldstein GW, Asbury AK, Diamond I. Pathogenesis of lead encephalopathy. Uptake of lead and reaction of brain capillaries. Archives of neurology. 1974;**31**(6):382-389

[63] Rehani B, Wissman R. Lead poisoning from a gunshot wound. South Medical Journal. 2011;**104**:57-58

[64] Paulson JA, Brown MJ. The CDC blood lead reference value for children: Time for change. Environment Health. 2019;**18**(16):1-3

[65] De Araujo GCS, Mourao NT, Pinheiro IN, Xavier AR, Gameiro VS. Lead toxicity risks in gunshort victims. PLoS One. 2015;**10**(10):1-10

[66] Winecker RE, Rofero-Miller JD, Broussard LA, Hammett-Stabler CA. The toxicology of heavy metals: Getting the lead out. Laboratory Medicine. 2018, 2002;**33**(12):934-947

[67] Ling LJ, Rosen CL. Harwood-Nuss' Clinical Practice of Emergency Medicine. Philadelphia: Wolters Klower, Lippincott, William and Wilkins; 2009

[68] Jones BL. Reducing Lead Contamination and Exposure on Military Firing Ranges Through the Practical Application of Ballistic Containment System, 4th ed. Fort Belvoir. 1999. p. 24

[69] McNutt TK, Chambers-Emmerson J, Dethlefsen M, Shah ZR. Bite the bullet: Lead poisoning after ingestion of 206 lead bullets. Veterinary and Human Toxicology. 2001;**43**(5):288-289

[70] National Poisons Information Service (NPIS) US. Lead TOXBASE. Birmingham: Health Protection Agency; 2010

[71] Davis JM, Svendsguard DJ. Nerve conduction velocity and lead: A critical review and meta-analysis. In: Johnson BL, Anger WK, Durao A, Xinteras C, editors. Advances in Neurobehavioural Toxicology: Applications in Environmental and Occupational Health. Chelsea, MI: Michingan Lawis Publishers; 1990. pp. 353-376

[72] Winneke G, Brockhaus A, Ewevs U, Kramer U, Nent M. Results from the European multicemter study on lead neurotoxicity in children: Implications for risk assessment. Neurotoxicology and Teratology. 1990;**12**:553-559

[73] Committee on Toxicity of Chemicals (COT) in Food Consumer Products and the Environment. COT Statement on the 2006 UK Total Diet Study of Metals and Other Elements. Vol. 2008. London: Food Standards Agency;

[74] Ehrlish R, Robins T, Jordaan E, et al. Lead absorption and renal dysfunction in a South African battery factory. Occupational Environmental Medicine. 1998;**55**:453-640

[75] Tsaih SW, Kornick S, Schwartz J, et al. Lead, diabetes, hypertension and renal function: The normative ageing study. Environmental Health Perspective. 2004;**112**:1178-1182

[76] Kimber J, Stonard ND, Gidlow DA, Niewola Z. Influence of chronic low-level exposure to lead on plasma immunoglobulin concentration and cellular immune function in man. International Archive of Occupational and Environmental Health. 1986;**57**: 117-125

[77] Coscia GC, Discalzi G, Ponzetti C. Immunological aspects of occupational lead exposure. Medical Lav. 1987;**78**: 360-364

[78] Wang L, Wang JT, Bailt LXF, Wan F. Impact of excessive blood- lead levels

on T cell subsets in lead exposed workers. Zhonzuo shi Tan Xue Xue Za Zhi. 2011;**19**:150-1511

[79] Koo WW, Succop PA, Bornschem RL, et al. Serum vitamin D metabolites and bone mineralization in young children with chronic low to moderate lead exposure. Pediatrics. 1991;**87**:680-687

[80] Health Protection Agency. Chemical Hazards and Poisons. Report from the Chemical Hazards and Poisons Division; 2009. p 1-75

[81] Recommendations from the Scientific Committee on Occupational Exposure Limits for Lead and Its Inorganic Compounds. SCOEL/SUM. European Commission; 2013. pp. 1-10

[82] The Agency for UK REACH Work Programme 2021/2022. Health and Safety Executives, June 2021. pp 1-37

[83] Agency for Toxic Substances and Disease Registry (ATSDR). Appendix G: Calculating Exposure Doses, Atlanta. 2005

[84] Borja-Aburto VH, Hertz-Picciotto I, Rojas Copez M, Farias P, Rios C, Blanco J. Blood lead levels measured prospectively and risk of spontaneous abortion. American Journal of Epidemic Lead. 1999;**150**:590-597

[85] ECHA. Annex XV Restriction Report on Lead in Shot and Appendix. Proposal for Restriction. Helsonki, Finland: ECHA; 2017

[86] True G, Drost W, Stock F. An elevation of the proposal to regulate lead in hunting ammunition through the European Union's REACH regulation. Environmental Science Turkey;**32**(68):1-18

[87] Andreoti A, Guberti V, Nardelli R, et al. Economic assessment of wild bird mortality induced by the use of lead gun shot in European coastlands. Science and Total Environment. 2018:610-611; 1505–1513

[88] Hallen P, Johnson S, Karlsson MO, Oskarsson A. Toxicokinetics of lead in lactating and non lactating mice. Toxicology and Applied Pharmacology. 1996;**136**(2):342-347

[89] Mushak P. New directions in the toxicokinetics of human lead exposure. Neurotoxicology. 1993;**14**(2–3):29-42

[90] Friend M. Lead poisoning. In: Friend M, editor. Field Guide to Wildlife Diseases. Vol. 1. Washington DC, USA: Department of the Interior, Fish and Wildlife Service; 1987. pp. 175-189

[91] Friend M. Interpretation criteria commonly used to determine lead poisoning problem areas. US Fish and Wildlife Service, Washington DC. Fish Wildlife Deseases. 1985;**2**:1-4

[92] Pain DJ. Lead poisoning in waterfowl. Proc an IWRB Workshop Brussels, Belgium 13-15 June 1991. In: IWRB Special Publication No. 16, Gloucester; 1992, pp. 95-97

[93] Humphreys DJ. Toxicolgia Veterinaria, Interamericana. Madrid, Espafia: McGraw Hill; 1990

[94] Pain DJ. Haematological parameters as predictors of blood lead and indicators of lead poisoning in the Black duck, *Anas rubripes*. Environmental Pollution. 1989; **60**:67-81

[95] Roscoe DE, Nielsen SW, Eaton HD, Rousseau JE. Chronic plumbism in rabbit: A comparison of three diagnostic tests. American Journal of Veterinary Research. 1975;**36**:1225-1229

[96] US Fish and Wildlife Service. Lead Poisoning in Water Fowl. Washington,

DC: US Fish and Wildlife Service; 1990. pp. 1-15

[97] Lumeij JT. Clinicopathologic aspects of lead poisoning in birds: A review. Veterinary Quarterly. 1985;7:133-138

[98] Pain DJ, Cronne RL, Newth J, Brown MJ, Crutcher E, Hardman P, et al. Potential hazard to human health from exposure to fragments of lead bullets and shot in the tissues of game animals. PLoS One. 2010;**5**(4):1-17

[99] Ganz K, Jenni L, Madry MM, Kraemer T, Jenny H, Jenny D. Acute and chromic lead exposure in four avian scavenger species in Switzerland. Archive of Environmental contaminants and Toxicology. 2018;**75**:566-575

[100] Naidoo V, Wolter K, Botha CJ. Lead ingestion as a potential contributing factor to the decline in vulture populations in south African. Environmental Research. 2017;**152**: 150-156

[101] Madry MM, Kraemer T, Kupper J, Naegeli H, Jenny H, Jenni L, et al. Excessive lead burden among golden eagles in the Swiss Alps. Environmentals Research Letters. 2015;**10**:034003

[102] Hovowitz IH, Tanco E, Nadler RV, Anglister N, Landau S, Elia R, et al. Acute lead poisoning in a griffon vulture (*Gyps fulvus*) in Israel. Israel Journal of Veterinary Medicine. 2014;**69**:163-168

[103] Langner HW, Domenech R, Slabe VA, Sulivan SP. Lead and mercury in fall migrant golden eagles from Western North America. Archive of Environmental Communication and Toxicology. 2015;**69**:54-61

[104] Garbett R, Maude G, Hancock P, Kenny D, Reading D, Amar A. Association between hunting and elevated blood lead levels in the critically endangered African white-backed vulture *Gyps africanus*. Science and Total Environment. 2018;**630**:1654-1665

[105] Mateo-Tomas P, Olea PP, Jimenez-Moreno M, Camarero PR, Sanchez-Barbudo IS, RCR M-D, et al. Maping the spatio-temporal risk of lead exposure in apex species for more effective mitigation. Proceedings of Royal Society of Biological Science. 2016;**283**:20160662

[106] Russell RE, Franson JC. Causes of mortality in eagles submitted to the National Wildlife Health Centre 1975-2013. Wildlife Society and Bulletin. 2014;**38**:697-704

[107] Kochen J, Greener Y. Levels of lead in blood and haematocrit: Implications for the evaluation of the newborn and arsenic patient. Pediatric Research. 1973; 7:937-944

[108] O'Flaherty EJ. Physiologically based models for bine seeking elements: Kinetic of lead disposition in humans. Toxicology and Applied Pharmacology. 1993;**118**(1):16-29

[109] Park DU, Paik NW. Effect on blood lead of airborne lead particles characterized by size. Annals of Occupation. 2002;**46**(2):237-243

[110] Snee RD. Models for the relationship between blood lead and air lead. International Archive of Occupational and Environmental Health. 1982;**50**(4):303-319

[111] Hunt G, Burnham W, Parish C, Burnharm K, Mutch B, Oaks JL. Bullet fragments in deer remains: Implications for lead exposure in scavengers. In: Watson RT, Fuller M, Pokras M, Hunt WG, editors. Ingestion of Lead from Spent Ammunition: Implications for

Wildlife and Humans. Boise Idaho, USA: The Peregrine Fund; 2009

[112] McQuirter JL, Rothenberg SJ, Dinkins GA, Kondrashov V, Mando M, Todd AC. Change in blood lead concentration up to 1 year after a gunshot with a retained bullet. American Journal of Epidemiology. 2004;**159**(7): 683-692

[113] Mahmood J. Prediction of drug clearance in children: A review of different methodologies. Expert Opinion on Drug Metabolism and Toxicology. 2015;**11**(4):573-587

[114] Riley R, Wilson CE. Cytochrome P450 time-dependent inhibition and induction: Advances in assays, risk analysis and modeling. Expert Opinion Drug Metabolism Toxicology. 2015; **11**(4):557-572

[115] United States Agency for Toxic Substances and Disease Registry (USATSAR). Toxialogical Profile for Lead. US. New York: Department of Health and Human Services; 2007. pp. 1-582

[116] Codex Alimentarius. Standard for contaminants and toxicants in food and feed LXb 1993–1995. Adopted in 1995. Raised and Amended 2018. Rome: Food and Agricultural Organization. 2018; **364**:5-24

[117] EC. European Commission Regulation EC 1881/2006. Setting maximum levels for certain contaminants in food stuffs. Official Journal of European Union. EC 1881/ 2006;**364**:5-24

[118] EFSA 2010. Scientific opinion on lead in food. EFSA panel on contaminants in the food chain (CONTAM). European Food and Safety Journal. 2010;**8**(4):1570

[119] Zaforte RD, Watanabe T, Mann NR. Moving bullet syndrome: A complication of penetrating head injury. Archive of Physics and Medical Rehabilitation. 1998;**79**:1469-1472

[120] Ragsdale BD, Lehmer LM. Soft tissue pseudocysts associated with retained bullets: A series of 4 cases. Journal of Ortho Trauma Research. 2017; **1**(1):003

[121] Wilson AJ. Gunshot injuries: What does a radiologist need to know? RadioGraphic. 1999;**19**:1358-1368

[122] Dimaio VJM. Gunshot Wounds: Practical Aspects of Firearms, Ballistics, and Forensic Techniques. Boca Raton, FL: CRC Press; 1985. pp. 163-265

[123] Swan RK, Hunt WG. Gunshot wounds: A source of lead in the environment. In: Watson RT, Fuller M, Pokras M, Hunt WG, editors. Ingestion of Lead from Spent Ammunition: Implications for Wildlife and Humans. Boise, Idaho: The Peregrine Fund, USDA; 10.4080/i/sa.2009.0109

[124] Moreira FR, Moreira JC. Lead kinetics in human body and its significance to health. Cienc Sande Colectiva. 2004;**9**(1):167-181

[125] Treu G, Drogt W, Slock F. An evaluation of the proposal to regulate lead in hunting ammunition through the European Union's REACH regulation. Environmental Science European. 2010; **32**(68):1-18

[126] Arnemo JM, Andersen O, Stokke S, Thomas VG, Krone O, Pain DJ, et al. Health and environmental risks from lead-based ammunition: Science versus socio-politics. EcoHealth. 2016;**13**: 618-622

[127] Tranel MA, Kimmel RO. Impacts of lead ammunition on wildlife, the environment and human health—A literature review and implications for Minnesota. In: Watson RT, Fuller M, Pokras M, Hunt WG, editors. Ingestion of Lead from Spent Ammunition: Implications for Wildlife and Humans. Boise, Idaho, USA.: The Peregrine Fund;

[128] Schwank M, Werner M, Younes M. Regulatory toxicology: Objectives and tasks defined by the working group of the German Society of Experimental and Clinical Pharmacology and toxicology. Toxicology Letters. 2002;**126**(31): 145-153

[129] Papich MG. Drug compounding for veterinary patients. American Association of Pharmaceutical Scientist Journal. 2005;**7**(2):281-287

[130] van der Graaf PH, Benson N, Peletier LA. Topics in mathematical pharmacology. Journal of Dynamics, Diffusion Equation. 2016;**28**:1337-1356

[131] Barlett C. Clinical update: Gunshot wound ballistics. Clinical Orthopaedics and Related Research. 2003;**408**:20-57

[132] Fackler N. Civilian gunshot wounds and ballistics: Dispelling the myths. Emerging Clinical North America. 1998; **16**:1-8

[133] Godhi S, Mittal GS, Kukreja P. Gunshot injury in the neck with an atypical bullet trajectory.Journal of Oral and Maxillofacial Surgery. 2011;**10**(1): 80-84

[134] Young L, Rule GT, Bocchieri RT, Waliko TJ, Burns JM, Ling G. When physics meets biology: Low and high-velocity penetration, blunt impact, and blast to the brain. Frontiers in Neurology. 2015;**6**:89

[135] Morse SJ. Brain over claim syndrome and criminal responsibility: A diagnostic note. In: Conference on the Mind of a Child, Moriz College of Law. Columbus: The Ohio State University; 2005. pp. 397-412

[136] The Royal Society. Brain waves module 4: Neuroscience and the law. RS Policy Document. 2011;**05**(11):1-135

[137] Glenn L, Raine A. Neurocriminology:Implications for the punishment, prediction and prevention of criminal behaviour. Natural Reviews of Neuroscience. 2014;**15**:54-63

[138] Fumagalli M, Priori A. Functional and neuroanatomy of morality. Brain. 2012;**135**:2006-2021

[139] Mobbs D, Lau HC, Jones OD, Frith CD. Law, responsibility and the brain. PLoS Biology. 2007;**5**(4):0693-0700

[140] Freeman J. The relationship between lower intelligence, crime and custodial outcomes: A brief literary review of a vulnerable group. Working Life Stress, Rehabilitation Counselling and Inclusion. 2012;**3**(1)S:1-15

[141] Nevin R. Understanding international crime trends: The legacy of preschool lead exposure. Environmental Research. 2007;**104**:315-336

[142] Hall W. Did elimination of lead from petrol reduce crime in the USA in the 1990s? F1000. Research. 2013;**2**(156):1-10

[143] Land K. National Child and Youth Well-being Index (CWI). Vol. 2. New York: Foundation for Child Development, F1000 Research; 2013. p. 156

[144] Taylor NP, Forbes MK, Opeskin B, Parr N, Lanphear BP. The relationship

between atmospheric lead emissions and aggressive crime: An ecological study. Environmental Health. 2016;**15**(23):1-10

[145] Diacomanolis V, Noller BN, Ng JC. Interaction effects of lead on bioavailability and pharmacokinetics of arsenic in rat. Environmental Geochemical Health. 2013;**35**:757-766

[146] Ploemen JPHT, Kramer H, Krajnc EI, Martin I. The use of toxicokinetic data in preclinical safety assessment: A toxicologic pathologist perspective. Toxicological Pathology. 2007;**28**(5): 1081-1089

[147] Scheff JD, Almon RR, DuBois DC, Jusko WJ, Androulakis IA. Assessment of pharmacologic area under curve, the curve when baselines are variable. Pharmaceutical Research. 2011;**28**(50):1081-1089

[148] Testa B, van de Waterbeemd H. Comprehensive Medicinal III, Vol 5: ADME-Tox Approaches. 1st ed. Amsterdam: Elsevier. 2006. pp. 1181

[149] Zhang A, Sun H, Jiao G, Wang X. Synergism effects of active ingredients from YCHT. Serum Pharmacochemistry of Traditional Chinese Medicine. 2017: 59-71

[150] Loftsson T. Essential Pharmacokinetics: A Primer for Pharmaceutical Scientists. 1st ed. Amsterdam: Elsevier; 2015. pp. 1-175.

[151] Sykes JE, Papich MG. Pharmacodynamics of antimicrobial drugs. In: Canine and Feline Infectious Diseases. Amsterdam: Elsevier; 2014. pp. 900

[152] Gulson BL, Jameson CW, Mahaffey KR, Mizon KJ, Patison N, Law AJ, et al. Relationships of lead in breast milk to lead in blood, urine, and diet of the infant and mother. Environment Health Perspect. 1998;**106**(10):667-674

[153] Leggett RW. An age-specific kinetic model of lead metabolism in humans. Environmental Health Perspectives. 1993;**101**(7):598-616

[154] Foster DM. Accessible pool parameters. In: Daniel CE, Markey SP (eds) Principles of Clinical Pharmacology, 2nd ed. Washington DC: Academic press; 2007. p. 545

[155] Gradascevic A, Resic E, Saralic N, Franjic B, Sallaic A, Ozuzdanoric-Pasalic A. Is it possible to determine firearm caliber and shooting range from the examination of gunshot residue in close range gunshot wounds? An experimental study. Journal of Health Science. 2013; **3**(3):b232-b237

[156] Bolonkin A. Long distance bullets and shells. International Journal of Aero Science. 2013;**2**(2):29-36

[157] Greenberg N, Frimer R, Meyer R, Derazane E, Chodick G. Lead exposure in military outdoor firing ranges. Military Medicine. 2016;**181**:1121-1126

[158] Ordog GJ, Wasserberger J, Balasubramamiam S. Shortgun wound batistes. Journal of Trauma. 1988;**28**: 624-631

[159] Wei Z, Wang F. Overall parameters design and optimization system for gun and bullet. International Journal of Military Medicine. 2008;**6**(1):1-7

[160] Coupland R, Loye D. The 1899 Hague declaration concerning expanding bullets. A treaty effective for more than 100years faces complex contemporary issues. IRRC. 2003;**85**(849):286-287

[161] Gidlow DA. Lead toxicity. Occupational Medicine. 2015;**65**:348-356

[162] Kent RH. The Theory of the Notion of a Bullet About Its Centre of Gravity. In Dense Media, With Applications to Bullet Design. Aberdeen Proving Ground, Maryland: Ballistic Research Laboratories, Report No. X-65; 1957

[163] Jauhari M. Mathematical model for bullet cachet. Journal of Criminal Law, Criminal Police Science. 1970;**61**(3): 469-473

[164] Wade A. Goth of ballistic: Bullet trajectories. Underground Journal of Mathematic Model: One of Two. 2013; **4**(1):1-9

[165] Johansen P, Asmund G, Riget F. High human exposure to lead through consumption of birds hunted with lead shot. Environment Pollut. 2004;**127**: 125–129

[166] Coburn HL, Snary EL, Kelly LA, Wooldridge M. Qualitative risk assessment of the hazards and risks from wild game. Veterinary Record. 2005;**157**: 321-322

[167] Mateo R, Kanstrup N. Regulations on lead ammunition adopted in Europe and evidence of compliance. Ambio. 2019;**48**(9):989-998

[168] Kanstrup N, Thomas VG. Transition to lead-free ammunition use in hunting: Socio-economic and regulatory considerations for the European Union and other jurisdiction. Environmental Sciences Europe. 2020; **32**(91):1-11

[169] Mammo. Ammunition Handbook. 6th ed. 2021. pp 1-189

[170] Pierce BL, Roster TA, Frisbic MC, Mason CD, Roberson JA. A comparison of lead and steel shot loads for harvesting and mourning doves. Wildlife Society Bulletin; 2015;**39**(1): 103-115

[171] Andreotti A, Borghesi F, Aradis A. Lead ammunition residues in the meat of hunted avodock: A potential health risk to consumers. Italian Journal of Animal Science. 2016;**15**(1):22-29

[172] Smith WDF. Air rifle ammunition and its influence on wounding potential. Archive Emergency Medicine. 1984;**2**: 25-29

[173] De Francisco N, Troya JDZ, Aguera E1. Lead and lead toxicity in domestic and free living birds. Avian Pathology. 2003;**32**:3-13

[174] Quy R. Review of Evidence Concerning the Contamination of Wildlife and the Environment Arising from the Use of Lead Ammunition. A Report to DEFRA. Sand Hutton: The Food and Environment Research Research Agency; 2010. pp. 2-56

[175] Yadav M, Tiwari A. Forensic toxicology and its relevance with criminal justice delivery system in India. Forensic Research and Criminology International Journal. 2017; **4**(4):121-127

[176] Ateriya N, Saraf A, Meshram V, Shekhawat RS, Satia P. Quadruple hanging: a rare scenario in flicide-suicide. Egyptian Journal of Forensic Science. 2019;**9**(56):1-5

[177] Webster JE, Gurdjian ES. Acute physiological effects of gunshot and other penetrating wounds of the brain. Journal of Neurophysiology. 1943;**6**(4): 255-262

[178] Pain DJ, Cromie RL, Newth J, Broan MJ, Crutcher E, Hardman P, et al. Potential hazard to human health from

exposure to fragments of lead bullets and shot in the tissues of game animals. Plors One. 2010;**5**(4):1-17

[179] Denton JS, Segovia A, Filkins JA, Segovia A, Filkins JA. Practical pathology of gunshot wounds. Archive of Pathology and laboratory Medicine. 2006;**130**:1283-1289

[180] Carneiro MA, Oliveira PA, Brandao R, Francisco ON, Velavde R, Lavin S, et al. Lead poisoning due to lead pellet injestion in griffon vultures (Gyps fulvus) from the Iberian Peninsula. Journal of Avian Medicine and Surgery. 2016;**30**:274-279

[181] Carpenter JW, Pattee OH, Fritts SH, Rattner BA, Wiemeyer SN, Royle JA, et al. Experimental lead poisoning in Turkey vultures (Cathartes cura). Journal of Wildlife Diseases. 2003;**39**:96-104

[182] Wiemeyer GM, Perez MA, Bianchini LT, Sampietro L, Bravo GF, Jacome NL, et al. Repeated conservation threats across the Americas: High level of blood and bone lead in the Andean condor widen the problem to a continental scale. Environmental Pollution. 2017;**220**:672-679

[183] Degerness LA, Redig PT, Freeman ML. Treatment of lead poisoning in trumpeter swans *Cygrums buccinators*. Wildlife Rehabilitation. 1990;**8**: 15-20

[184] Zin P, Zheng N, Tu T, Tu S, Sun W, McEachern D, et al. Preclinical pharmacokinetics of MI -219, a novel human double minute 2 (HDM_2) inhibitor and prediction of human pharmacokinetics. Journal of Pharmacology and Pharmaceutical Science. 2012;**15**(2):265-280

[185] Epps CW. Considering the switch transitional to non-hunting ammunition. The Condor: Ornithology Application. 2014;**116**:429-434

[186] Sagnuwan SA. The use of body surface area for determination of age, body weight, urine creatinime, serum creatinime , plasma creatinime, urine volume and creatinime clearance: the reliable canomical method of assessing renotoxicity in animals. Comparative Clinical Pathology. 2018;**27**:1531-1536

[187] European Chemical Agency (ECHA). Lead in Short Bullets and Fishing Weight. Helsinki, Finland; 2020. p. 3021 https://ECHA.Europa.EU

Section 3

Environmental Accumullation and Remediation of Pollutants

Chapter 8

Enzymatic Bioremediation of Dyes from Textile Industry Effluents

Ane Gabriele Vaz Souza, Tainá Carolini Maria, Luciana Maria Saran and Lucia Maria Carareto Alves

Abstract

The use of synthetic dyes began in 1865 with the discoveries of researcher William Henry Perkin. Its production and use only grew due to the high demand of several industrial sectors, mainly textiles. At the same time, concerns about environmental problems arose due to the disposal of wastewater with dyes, being the textile industry's effluents the most polluting in the world. According to their structure, dyes can be more or less harmful, whereby azo dyes are the most worrisome from an environmental point of view. Problems, such as carcinogenicity, mutagenicity, and genotoxicity, are related to dyes, as well as contamination of water, and soil, and damages to agricultural plantations. Some of the methods used in the treatment of textile industrial effluents are membrane filtration, coagulation, chemical oxidation, biodegradation, photocatalytic degradation, phytoremediation, and enzymatic remediation. Enzyme remediation is considered an efficient, ecological, and innovative technique, through which enzymes can be used in free or immobilized form. The main enzymes involved in the degradation of azo dyes are azoreductases, laccases, and peroxidases. In some cases, harmful by-products are formed during the reactions and require proper management. Thus, this chapter addresses the main aspects of enzymatic bioremediation of dyes present in effluents from the textile industry.

Keywords: azo dyes, azoreductases, dyes and colorants, emerging pollutants, enzymatic remediation, microbiological remediation, wastewater treatment

1. Introduction

The history of dyes began over 4000 years ago, and for many years, dyes were extracted from natural sources, such as flowers, vegetables, wood, insects, and roots, among others [1]. The synthetic dye industry began with the synthesis of mauveine, by researcher William Henry Perkin, in 1865. This dye, which until then was extracted from coal tar, was synthesized by Perkin while the researcher was looking for a new synthetic route for quinine, a drug used to treat malaria [2]. Perkin's discovery marked the creation of a new generation of dyes [3].

Synthetic dyes are organic compounds that are produced from raw materials of petrochemical origin. Such compounds may or may not be soluble in water, are generally easily absorbed, and quickly impart color to substrates [1]. Structurally, dyes contain three essential groups: the chromophore, which is the active site of dyes where atoms interacting with visible electromagnetic radiation are located [2]; auxochrome, which has functional groups that introduce the chromophore, increase the fiber's affinity to color, and decrease its solubility in water [4] and conjugated aromatic structures, such as benzene, anthracene and perylene rings [2]. Dyes are classified according to their chemical structure and application mode. Thus, according to the chemical structure of the dye, this is classified into azo, anthraquinone, sulfur, phthalocyanine, and triarylmethane [2]. Depending on its method of application, the dye is classified as reactive, direct, dispersed, basic, and by vat dyeing [5].

The chemical composition of the dye reflects in its pigmentation (formation of its color), being also responsible for the lighter or darker tone of each dye. The coloring is due to the absorption of light of a certain wavelength in the visible range of the electromagnetic spectrum, that is, the dye is a molecule capable of absorbing certain light radiations and then reflecting the complementary colors [6]. **Table 1** brings together the main classes of dyes used in the textile industry, the types of fiber or substrates to which the dyes of each class are applied, the types of interaction between dye and fiber or substrate, and the methods of application or dyeing.

Dyes are materials of great importance in different industrial sectors, such as fabric production, papermaking, plastics, cosmetics, as well as in medicine and biology [8]. Currently, the world production of dyes is about 800 tons a year and most of the dyes produced, about 70 million tons a year, are used in the textile industry [1].

With high world production, the textile industry occupies the second place among the industrial sectors that most pollute since during the dyeing stage a large amount

Classes	Fiber type	Interaction between dye and fiber	Method of application
Acid dye	nylon, wool, silk	Electrostatics; hydrogen bond	Neutral to acid dye baths.
Basic dye	modified nylon, polyester	Electrostatics	Acid baths.
Direct dye	cotton, rayon, leather, nylon	Intermolecular forces.	Neutral or slightly alkaline baths containing additional electrolytes.
Dispersed dye	polyester, polyamide, acetate, plastic, acrylic	Hydrophobic - solid-state mechanism	High or low-temperature pressure transport methods.
Reactive dye	cotton, nylon, silk, wool	Covalent bond	Under the influence of heat and pH of the medium, which must be alkaline, the dye reacts with the fiber functional group, with which it covalently bonds.
Sulfur dye	cotton, rayon	Covalent bond	Aromatic substrate covered with sodium sulfide and reoxidized to sulfur-containing products, insoluble in fiber.
Vat dye	cotton, rayon	Impregnation and oxidation	Water-insoluble dyes are solubilized by reduction with sodium hydrosulfite and then exhausted into the fiber and reoxidized.

Table 1.
Main classes of dyes used in the textile industry, types of fiber to which the dyes of each class are applied, types of interaction between dye and fiber, and methods of application or dyeing [7].

of dyes is released into the environment due to the nonadhesion of the dye to the substrate to be dyed [2]. Therefore, the search for economically viable and ecologically sustainable alternatives for the treatment of effluents containing textile dyes is of extreme importance and interest, whereupon bioremediation is a process that can help to solve this industrial problem.

This chapter brings together the main and most recent information reported in the scientific literature on the enzymatic bioremediation of dyes from textile industry effluents. In this context, the negative impacts of dyes used in this industrial segment on human and animal health are discussed, as well as methods conventionally used for the treatment of industrial effluents containing dyes, the principles of enzymatic bioremediation, the enzymes used in this process, and their by-products.

2. Negative impacts of textile dyes on human and animal health

Textile industry effluents are considered the most polluting compounds both by the volume generated and discarded and by their toxicity [9]. Wastewater from the textile industry is estimated to contain between 10 and 200 mg L^{-1} of dyes, as well as other organic chemicals, inorganic compounds, and additives. Even after the treatment of such effluents, about 90% of the dyes are still dumped in water bodies without undergoing chemical changes [1]. The biodegradation of such dyes is hampered by their xenobiotic nature, aromatic structure, high thermal resistance, and photostability [4].

In recent studies, Gita et al. [9] have observed that the toxicity of dyes is generally low for mammals and aquatic organisms, however, secondary products formed by biodegradation, especially aromatic amines from anaerobic dye reduction, can be harmful. In addition, these authors found that the concomitant presence of dyes and other pollutants in textile wastewater, such as heavy metals, can have a synergistic effect, causing considerable damage to the aquatic environment.

The main concern about the discharge of dyes is the presence of genotoxic, mutagenic, teratogenic, and carcinogenic effects, observed in animal studies [9]. Carcinogenicity is related to the formation of ions that bind to DNA and RNA, causing mutations and leading to the formation of tumors. In this sense, benzidine and 2-naphthylamine dyes are associated with a high incidence of bladder cancer [10]. Azure-B dye is capable of interspersing in the helical structure of the DNA and may have cytotoxic effects since it is an inhibitor of monoamine oxidase A (MAO-A), an enzyme that acts on the central nervous system and is important to human behavior [10]. Sudan 1 dye, widely used in the textile industry, although illegal in many European countries and the US, is also used in foods, such as paprika. Such dye, when present in the body of humans and animals, is transformed by the action of enzymes in carcinogenic aromatic amines [10]. Furthermore, human exposure to dyes can still generate skin and lung irritations, headaches, congenital malformation, and nausea [11].

Triphenylmethane dyes are phytotoxic to agricultural plantations, cytotoxic to mammals, and generate tumors in several fish species [10]. The violet crystal dye is also a powerful carcinogen, capable of inducing tumors in fish, such as hepatocellular carcinoma and reticular cell sarcoma in several organs [10].

Some of the main environmental problems related to the disposal of synthetic dyes are—*i*. contamination of surface water, which leads to decreased penetration of light, with damage to photosynthesis and consequent oxygen deficiency; *ii*. accumulation of nonbiodegradable organic dyes along with the food chain; *iii*. Soil and water contamination, and *iv*. inhibition of growth and development of various crops of agricultural interest [4].

In the literature, a correlation is described between the increase in the concentration of dyes and the decrease in the growth of microalgae, reaching the total suppression of their growth [9]. In that study, different concentrations of three dyes were used to evaluate the specific growth rate of green algae *Chlorella vulgaris* exposed to dyes. Such findings are important because the inhibition of microalgae growth causes disturbances in the trophic transfer of energy and nutrients in aquatic environments [4].

Aquatic macrophytes are used as natural ecological markers to quantify the phytotoxicity of textile dyes when exposed to effluents that contain those since there is a change in all their parameters [4]. In the presence of two textile dyes, *Lemna giba*, an aquatic macrophyte, had its growth rate and photosynthetic pigment content decreased. The authors of the study concluded that this species can be used as a bioindicator of polluting dyes [12]. High concentrations of dyes are reported to decrease vital elements, such as P, Mg, Ca, S, and Ca in plants of *Eichhornia crassipes* and *Salvinia natans*, which also presented damaged roots, chlorosis, and necrosis in leaves [13].

Among thousands of dyes studied, found in effluents, more than 100 have the potential to form carcinogenic amines. However, these potentially toxic dyes are still marketed and used, especially in small textile factories. In several places around the world, the demands of export and cheap labor sustain the existence of factories with a small-scale activity that clandestinely releases toxic dyes into water bodies [10].

2.1 Textile industry effluents: Composition and conventional methods of treatment

Textile industry effluents contain large quantities of biodegradable organic compounds and nonbiodegradable compounds [14]. According to the literature, there are more than 8000 substances, such as acids, surfactants, salts, metals, oxidizing agents, reducing agents, as well as dyes and their auxiliaries [15]. Wastewater from the textile industry contains characteristic color, resulting from the mixture of dyes, in addition to the presence of metals, organic carbon, ammonium salts, nitrate, and orthophosphate [5].

Due to the environmental impact of this type of effluent, pretreatment is necessary before such compounds are released into natural water bodies, and the textile industry shows interest in controlling this problem [14]. However, even after treatment, effluents are still discarded in rivers with up to 90% of dyes that have not undergone chemical changes [1]. **Table 2** shows information related to the studied treatment processes for the removal of textile dyes from industrial effluents and the main results obtained, as reported in the literature.

The composition, as well as the standards allowed for each substance present in the composition of effluents from textile factories, aiming at its release in surface water bodies, vary according to the standards of each country. In China, the chemical oxygen demand (COD) and chrominance of wastewater from dyeing and finishing processes cannot exceed 80 mg L^{-1} and 60, respectively, so that such effluents can be

Name of dyes	Treatment Method	Main Results	Reference
Reactive Yellow 138, Reactive Red 231, and Navy HEXL® Procion	Electrolysis, carried out in a filter-press cell, under galvanostatic conditions.	Complete discoloration (99%) was observed in all cases.	[14]
Reactive Red 120	Biodegradation and dye biosorption by *Pseudomonas guariconensis.*	The immobilized VITSAJ5 bacterium exhibited maximum adsorption of 87%. There was only 37% of removal without immobilization of the microorganism.	[15]
Malachite Green, Reactive Red 198, and Direct Yellow 31	Chitosan adsorption.	The amount of dye adsorbed depends on the mass of the adsorbent and decreased with its increase.	[16]
Basic Blue 9 (MB), Basic Green 4 (MG), and Acid Orange 52 (MO)	Adsorption using synthesized materials	Fast adsorption of MB, MG, and MO in the initial 60 min. After 240 min, adsorption equilibrium is reached.	[17]
Basic Blue 26 (BB26), Basic Green 1 (BG1), Basic Yellow 2 (BY2), and Basic Red 1 (BR1)	Adsorption on carbonaceous materials (acai seeds and Brazil nut shells), activated in the following ways: chemical activation with H_3PO_4, heat treatment, and oxidation with HNO_3.	The adsorbents activated by heat treatment showed good performance for the removal of BB26 (87 and 85%) and BG1 (100 and 99%) but were not efficient for the removal of BY2 and BR1. Chemical activation was the most efficient for all dyes tested. Oxidation with HNO_3 showed the worst results.	[18]
Diamine Green B (DG-B), Acid Black 24 (AB-24), and Congo Red (CR)	Cellulose adsorption on cationized rice husk (CRHC).	Maximum adsorption capacities of DG-B, AB-24, and CR: 207.15, 268.88, and 580.09 mg g^{-1} at pH = 8, respectively, following the order CR > DG-B > AB-24.	[19]
Methylene Blue (MB)	Photocatalytic degradation of organic dyes with nanocomposites	Synthesized nanocompounds showed high catalytic activity for the reduction of methylene blue under solar irradiation, efficiency of up to 90.1%, simple and low-cost method.	[20]
Basic Yellow 28 (BY28), Acid Brown 75 (AB75)	Adsorption of cationic and anionic dyes by natural clays rich in smectite.	BY28: removal efficiency increased (97%) with increasing pH. AB75 anionic dye: adsorption was high in acidic medium (86%).	[21]
Reactive Violet 5 (RV5)	Decolorization of azo-reactive dyes using sequential chemical treatment and activated sludge.	Almost complete decolorization was obtained for dye concentrations up to 300 mg L^{-1}. Fenton's reagent was unable to decolorize at concentration $\geq$ 500 mg L^{-1} (87.4% dechlorination).	[22]

Name of dyes	Treatment Method	Main Results	Reference
Procion Red HE-3B (RR120)	Photoelectrocatalysis	Treatment proved to be efficient, with up to 100% of decolorization in 30 min, concentration 10 mg L^{-1} of the dye RR120. The efficiency is only effective at low concentrations, with increasing concentration the decolorization occurs to a certain extent, then stabilizes.	[23]
Reactive Red 120	Simultaneous adsorption, filtration, and photoelectrocatalytic oxidation processes	The simultaneous performance of the treatments demonstrated that the dye was completely removed in solution. No pretreatment of intermediate by-products was necessary.	[24]
Acid Blue 25	Adsorption	The absorbent material was shown to reach an equilibrium constant in 270 min, as was observed to reduce absorption with alkaline solutions. The mortality rate of *Daphnia similis* reduced from 50–10% using 30 mg of quaternary chitosan granules when compared to the control.	[25]
Acid Blue 25	Adsorption Chitosan beads (CB) and chitosan beads with immobilized *Saccharomyces cerevisiae* by zeta potential (CBY)	The adsorbent with immobilized *S. cerevisiae* reached equilibrium faster than the chitosan polymer alone. The adsorption capacity increased in both treatments with acidification, and also varied with temperature. There was a significant decrease in toxicity with the CBY treatment.	[26]

Table 2.
Examples of treatment processes used to remove textile dyes.

released into the environment. In the United States, according to the Environmental Protection Agency (EPA), the limit value for COD is 163 kg per ton of fabric, however, in practice, cod effluents are up to 15 times higher than the legal standard [27]. Therefore, it is essential to apply efficient treatment strategies that ensure the complete removal of pollutants or that ensure the sustainability of the environment for future generations through physical, chemical, and biological technologies or a combination of them [10].

Physical methods, such as membrane filtration (nanofiltration, reverse osmosis, electrodialysis), sorption techniques, or chemical methods, such as coagulation or flocculation combined with flotation and filtration, flocculation by precipitation, electroflotation, and electrokinetic coagulation, considered for the removal of various dyes, do not degrade them. Such methods simply promote the reduction of the concentration of dyes, converting them from one chemical way to another, thus creating secondary pollution [6]. Among the several processes used for the removal of wastewater dyes, such as chemical oxidation, biodegradation, electrochemical treatment, adsorption, and photocatalytic degradation, the use of photocatalyst provides good results with high efficiency, low cost, speed, and better performance in environmental conditions when sunlight is used in the process [28].

Several natural materials, such as chitosan, are used in physical dye adsorption processes. Chitosan is a modified natural biopolymer, derived from the deacetylation of chitin, which is the most abundant polymer on the planet, derived from important biomass produced by inferior plants and animals, such as arthropods, shells of crustaceans, lobsters, shrimps, crabs, and squid [16]. Adsorption is one of the most efficient methods for removing dyes, however, there is a need for further treatment of the residue resulting from the process.

In addition to the physical and chemical processes aimed at the removal of dyes from wastewater, biological processes also play an important role. Among the biological methods that can be used to remove dyes from industrial wastewater, phytoremediation is a process that has advantages compared to chemical and physical methods of removal. The removal of textile dyes by plants occurs by adsorption, accumulation, and subsequent degradation, mediated by enzymes [29].

In situations where the application of chemical products must be continuous, the use of microorganisms may be considered a simpler and low-cost process, since microorganisms can be added only once in the effluent to be treated, as they have the potential to multiply [30]. Within this context, the activated sludge is commonly used in bioreactors for effluent treatment, which is one of the most used processes by the textile industry [10]. Another possible biological method for the treatment of effluents is the use of bacterial cultures. The isolation of pure cultures from textile wastewater is usually not performed, as it can be a slow and laborious process. Thus, mixed bacterial cultures are commonly used, which, due to cooperation to achieve a potentiated effect, provide better results in discoloration and mineralization of toxic aromatic amines [1].

3. Principles of enzymatic bioremediation

Bioremediation techniques have been gaining increasing prominence worldwide due to high public acceptance, low cost compared to conventional remediation methods, high availability of enzymes, and minimal impact on the environment [31]. The exploration of enzymes for bioremediation has been of great interest due to their ability to function in wider ranges of pH and temperature, in the presence of contaminants and saline concentrations [32]. Enzymatic bioremediation is an ecological, economical, promising, and innovative technique. The process consists of exploring the typical characteristics of microorganisms or genetically modified organisms capable of producing specific enzymes to catalyze or metabolize the pollutant, transforming the toxic form into a nontoxic form and sometimes into new products [33].

Among the enzymes involved in bioremediation processes are laccases, dehalogenases, and hydrolases. Laccases are enzymes capable of catalyzing the oxidation of phenolic compounds, aromatic amines, and their compounds. Dehalogenases degrade a wide range of halogenated compounds by cleaving C – X bonds (X = halogen atom, such as Cl). Hydrolases break chemical bonds using water and convert larger molecules into smaller molecules, decreasing their toxicity. These enzymes facilitate the cleavage of C – C, C – O, C – N, S – S, S – N, S – P, C – P bonds [33].

Enzymes can be used in free or immobilized form, the latter having the following advantages—long-term operational stability, easy recovery, and reuse in industrial applications, which improve process performance and lower overall cost [34].

Immobilization consists of coupling the enzyme with an insoluble support matrix to maintain an adequate geometry, which guarantees greater stability to the enzyme [32]. The bioremediation process using microbial enzymes can be slow and so far, only a few bacterial species have been able to produce enzymes with potent biodegradation capacity. Thus, the use of genetically modified organisms is more common due to their ability to produce large amounts of enzymes under optimized conditions [33].

Enzymes from aerobic bacteria, such as *Pseudomonas*, *Alcaligenes*, *Sphingomonas*, *Rhodococcus,* and *Mycobacterium*, are often used in the bioremediation of pesticides and hydrocarbons, while those produced by anaerobic bacteria are more used in bioremediation of polychlorinated biphenyls (PCBs), trichloroethylene (TCE) decolorization, and chloroform. The main enzymes used in bioremediation processes include those of the cytochrome P450 family, laccases, hydrolases, dehalogenases, dehydrogenases, proteases, and lipases [33]. Fungi can also biodegrade, generally mediated by enzymes, such as azoreductases, lignin peroxidases, manganese peroxidases, and laccases. White rot fungi, for example, are capable of degrading textile dyes through peroxidases and laccases [10].

In the treatment of effluents from the textile industry, enzymes act on the dyes, generating precipitates that can be easily removed or chemically transformed into easy-to-treat compounds [35]. The rate of dye degradation by enzymes will depend on the chemical structure of the dye, salt content, the concentration of metal ions, pH, and temperature of the wastewater [36]. The enzymatic degradation of pollutants in textile effluents has several advantages, such as specificity and selectivity to the substrate, in addition to being an accessible, efficient method that meets the principles of green chemistry [37]. The requirement of large amounts of enzyme, high cost, thermal instability, inhibition of enzymatic activity, attack of certain enzymes by proteases, and the formation of undesirable by-products are the main difficulties or challenges related to the use of enzymatic degradation for wastewater treatment [30].

Some of the problems listed can be solved, at least partially, by immobilizing effective enzymes in low-cost matrices, leading to their separation and reuse, in addition to application in continuous bioreactors [30]. To control the reactions in the biodegradation process, the use of enzymes is often more advantageous than the use of cells [37]. As for the high cost of the enzymes themselves due to the fact of trying to obtain an enzymatic solution as pure as possible, the tendency is that it will decrease as technologies and techniques advance and the exploration of cheaper growth substrates for the reproduction of microorganisms increases.

3.1 Main enzymes used in the bioremediation of textile dyes and toxicity of degradation by-products

Enzyme-mediated bioremediation has gained notoriety due to its versatility and efficiency in the degradation of persistent organic pollutants, thus being applied in industrial, biotechnological, and environmental processes [38]. These enzymes can be obtained from the extraction of intracellular and extracellular metabolites from cultures of certain species of bacteria, fungi, algae, and plants [39].

Table 3 shows some studies related to the degradation of dyes by enzymes produced by microorganisms. As it is shown, many of the tested can decolorize the dyes, as well as provide a decrease in their toxicity, as in the case, for example, of horseradish peroxidase, which promotes the decrease in the toxicity of the methyl orange dye.

Study objective(s)	Results and by-products of degradation	Reference
Use of ionic liquids (ILs) with surfactant characteristics in the degradation of Indigo Carmine (IC) dye by laccase.	Rapid and significantly higher discoloration of the IC dye in 0.5 h. Color removal percentage: 82% (against 6% obtained without ionic liquids). By-products from IC oxidation induced by laccase: indole-2,3-dione, which is decomposed into aminobenzoic acid. Both are less toxic than the IC.	[38]
Use of the isolate of *Oudemansiella canarii* to produce laccase and evaluation of its potential in the degradation of Congo Red (CR).	The *O. canarii* laccase was efficient in decolorizing the red of the dye. Accumulation of various intermediates during degradation as naphthalene derivatives, for example. These products are less toxic than CR.	[40]
Validation of a novel bioinformatics amalgamation and bacterial remediation approach using non-native strains for decolorization and degradation of azo dyes: Drimaren Red CL-5B (Reactive Red 195).	The gas chromatography–mass spectrometry (GC–MS) analysis of the degradation products indicated the formation of low molecular weight metabolites, confirming the dye degradation. Need to carry out microbial toxicity, cytotoxicity, and phytotoxicity tests before large-scale bioremediation.	[41]
Development of an airlift bioreactor for the use of copper alginate laccase in the degradation of dyes: Indigo Carmine (IC), Remazol Brilliant Blue R (RBBR), Bromophenol Blue (BB), Crystal Violet (CV), Malachite Green (MG), Congo Red (CR), Direct Blue 15 (DB) and Direct Red 23 (DR).	100% decolorization of IC and RBBR, quickly. Discoloration percentages of MG, BB, and CV: 82; 64.4, and 48.5%; respectively. Percentages of discoloration of azo dyes CR, BD, and DR: 64, 54, and 22%, respectively. Isatin sulfonic acid was confirmed as the main degradation product.	[36]
Development of a hydrogel blended with an agarose-chitosan polymer for plant-based horseradish peroxidase (HRP) immobilization and its use in the degradation of synthetic textile dye RB-19.	During the degradation process, the chromophore was fragmented into respective smaller fractions, leading to discoloration. The RB-19 has degraded into its possible daughter compounds. There is no result of toxicity studies of these compounds.	[42]
Use of a packed bed reactor equipped with polyacrylamide gel-immobilized horseradish peroxidase (PAG-HRP) for the purpose of sequentially degrading the Methyl Orange (MO) dye.	PAG-HRP biocatalytic system: efficient in biologically based degradation. The MO degradation efficiency was 93.5% at pH 6. Significant reduction in the toxicity of azo textile dyes according to the results of acute toxicity bioassays together with phytotoxicity.	[43]
Study the potential of *Aspergillus niger* for detoxification and discoloration of Congo Red (CR) dye.	High CR removal (85%). 97% of discoloration results from the combination of two processes: adsorption and enzymatic biodegradation. Detoxification by *A. niger* indicates degradation of amines in solution. According to phytotoxicity and microtoxicity analysis results, the metabolites generated after the CR biodegradation are less toxic than the crude dye.	[44]

Study objective(s)	Results and by-products of degradation	Reference
Evaluate the performance of a new *Meyerozyma guilliermondii*, *Yarrowia* sp. and *Sterigmatomyces halophilus* (MG-Y-SH) oleaginous yeast consortium in the decolorization and detoxification of textile dyes Reactive Black 5 (RB5), Reactive Red 120 (RR120), Reactive Blue 19 (RB19), Reactive Green 19 (RG19), Blue Remazol R (RBBR), Bromophenol Blue (BPB), Azure B (AB), Methylene Blue (MB), Methyl Red (MR), Malachite Green (MG), Congo Red (CR) and Scarlet GR (SGR).	Maximum decolorization efficiency: ranged between 55.81 (blend III) and 80.56% (blend VI) in 24 h of treatment with MG-Y-SH at 18°C and static conditions. Maximum decolorization efficiency by MG-Y-SH reached 100% for 100 mg L^{-1} of RR120 in 3 h. Phytotoxicity results indicate the ability of MG-Y-SH to convert the toxic azo dye RR120 into non-toxic metabolites.	[45]
Test a new consortium of oleaginous yeasts that produce lipase and xylanase in the removal of Sigma-Aldrich, Reactive Black 5 (RBB), Reactive Green 19 (G19R), Reactive Red 120 (HE3B), Reactive Blue 19 (B19R), Reactive Violet 5 (V5R) and Reactive Orange 16 (O3R) textile dyes.	Discoloration rate obtained by the *Yarrowia* sp., *Barnettozyma californica*, and *S. halophilus* (Y-BC-SH) consortium: higher than that of pure yeast cultures. Phytotoxicity assay results: metabolites generated after biodegradation of RBB are less toxic when compared to the original dye.	[46]
Examine Methylene Blue (MB) dye removal performance by an immobilized enzyme.	The immobilized enzyme showed the highest removal efficiency (99%) compared to the pure nanocarrier and the free enzyme (81 and 36% removal, respectively). No result of toxicity analysis of by-products was presented.	[47]
Evaluation of a new strain of white-rot fungus, *Ceriporia lacerata*, of its ability to discolor Congo Red (CR) in a statically open system and the effect of toxicity of degradation products.	The discoloration occurred by the absorption of mycelia and by degradation by manganese peroxidase (MnP) and laccase enzymes. By-products or intermediates identified: naphthylamine and benzidine (very toxic to an organism). At 48 h the by-products were more toxic than the original dye, demonstrating the dye can take a long time to become harmless.	[48]
Immobilization of lignin peroxidase (LiP) on Ca-alginate granules, its application in the degradation of dyes, and its potential for reducing the cytotoxicity of Reactive Red 195a (VR), Reactive Blue 21 (AR21), Reactive Blue 19 (AR19); Reactive Yellow 154a (AR154); Sandal-Fix Black CKF.	Discoloration efficiencies: 66, 59, 52, 40, and 48% were observed for VR, AR21, AR19, sandal-fix black CKF, and AR154, respectively with free LiP, which increased to 93, 83, 89, 70, and 80% with immobilized LiP. It was an efficient catalyst for the decolorization and detoxification of synthetic dye solutions. Results of the hemolytic and brine shrimp lethality tests—they showed that Ca-alginate beads entrapped LiP may be an effective biocatalyst for bioremediation of dye-based textile industry effluents.	[49]
Biochemical characterization of stable azoreductase enzyme from *Chromobacterium violaceum* and its application in the degradation of Methyl Red, Methyl Orange, and Amaranth dyes present in industrial effluent.	The lower value of the Michaelis–Menten constant (K_M) indicates a very high affinity of the three dyes with the azoreductase enzyme. Azo dye metabolites resulted from the action of enzyme: they had reduced toxicity on fibroblast cell lines (L929) as compared to raw and intact dye.	[50]

Table 3.
Main results of studies on dye bioremediation by enzymes and degradation by-products.

As reported in the literature, dye-decolorizing microorganisms produce a variety of enzymes, including azoreductase, riboflavin reductase, laccase, peroxidases, NADH-DCIP reductase, tyrosinase, reductase, and aminopyrine N-demethylase, lignin peroxidase, and veratryl alcohol oxidase [39]. Among those enzymes, the main ones responsible for the discoloration of azo dyes are azoreductases, laccases, and peroxidases [35].

Azoreductases are considered the main degradation enzymes produced by bacteria [30]. Such enzymes can be of two types—*i*. membrane-bound or *ii*. intracellular, which are thermostable, hydrophilic, and, in general, capable of degrading azo dyes more efficiently [51]. Laccases are copper-dependent and use oxygen to degrade lignin and other aromatic compounds, including textile dyes [32]. Because of their higher redox potential, fungal laccases, when compared to plant or bacterial laccases, are used to treat various xenobiotics, including textile dyes, present in water and soils [40].

Peroxidases also play a role in the degradation of the azo dye and are oxidoreductases, which contain heme. Peroxidases are present in plants, microorganisms, and animals. The mechanism of action of such enzymes is similar to that of laccases, providing the degradation of the dye without the production of toxic by-products [30]. Peroxidases act especially on synthetic dyes, degrading their respective constituents through the oxidative polymerization of phenolic compounds to form insoluble polymers [52]. An association between oxide-reducing enzymes can significantly reduce the toxicity of dyes [39].

Enzymes are proteins easily affected by changes in pH, and small variations in the medium's pH can result in changes in the ionization phase of the active site and the distribution of charge in the protein structure, possibly affecting its affinity for the substrate [52]. Thus, one of the main challenges of enzymatic treatment is the deactivation of the biocatalyst caused, mainly, by the denaturation of the enzyme, due to the pH of the medium or extreme temperatures, which can alter the conformation of the enzyme's active site [53]. Despite the many advances in enzymatic engineering, enzymes are still expensive and/or labile and, as a result, the industrial application of enzymes often requires their immobilization in a matrix (support) [54].

It is essential to evaluate the toxicity of effluents containing dyes after they have undergone enzymatic biodegradation, as some degradation products are mutagenic and carcinogenic, which represents a threat to human and animal health [30]. Thus, phytotoxicity tests are widely used and, according to the literature, among the bioindicators considered suitable for the detection of environmental toxicity, *Artemia salina and Daphnia magna* are cited [43].

Ali et al. [55] performed phytotoxicity studies, whose results indicate that MG-Y-SH can convert the toxic azo dye RR120 into nontoxic metabolites. However, many studies reported in the literature lack further tests to evaluate the by-products of enzymatic dye degradation, as well as the effects of these by-products on the environment.

4. Conclusions

Much of the textile dyes are still discharged into rivers without undergoing chemical changes, even with conventional effluent treatments. Pollution generated by dyes from textile industry effluents is harmful to human and animal health, presenting carcinogenic, genotoxic, mutagenic effects, in addition to having direct effects on the survival of aquatic species, as such dyes can accumulate in the food chain, conferring toxicity to water and soil and interfere with the development of crops of agricultural interest.

A more rigorous inspection of the release of dyes is important given its potential toxicity, as well as the factories that may be clandestinely dumping effluents containing toxic dyes in water bodies, without any treatment. Studies must be carried out to optimize effluent treatment methods, which must be ecological and efficient, making use of new technologies provided by modern science.

Among the methods currently used, photocatalytic degradation presents good results, is cheap, and uses sunlight, a clean source of energy. In addition to this method, there is phytoremediation, considered an ecologically correct process, and enzymatic remediation. The enzymes used in the enzymatic bioremediation of textile industry effluents are mainly azoreductases, laccases, and peroxidases.

Enzymatic bioremediation or even conventional treatment can generate by-products that are equally toxic to the starting compounds. But in some cases, less toxic intermediate compounds are generated, such as those presented in this chapter. Therefore, due importance must be given to these secondary products or by-products, identifying them, quantifying them, and subjecting them to proper handling and treatment.

The key point for the treatment of dyes is to have greater investment by companies to put the results of scientific research into practice. An alternative would be to carry out tests in simulation stations, as if on an industrial scale. In addition, genetic engineering has significantly revolutionized the field of bioremediation, with the possibility of modifying organisms or their metabolites so that they are more efficient in degrading pollutants.

Acknowledgements

This study was financed in part by the Coordenação de Aperfeiçoamento de Pessoal de Nível Superior – Brazil (CAPES) – Finance Code 001. We are grateful to this research funding agency and the Agricultural and Livestock Graduation Program, São Paulo State University (UNESP), School of Agricultural and Veterinarian Sciences (FCAV).

Conflict of interest

The authors declare no conflict of interest.

Author details

Ane Gabriele Vaz Souza, Tainá Carolini Maria, Luciana Maria Saran*
and Lucia Maria Carareto Alves
São Paulo State University (Unesp), School of Agricultural and Veterinarian Sciences (FCAV), Department of Agricultural, Livestock and Environmental Biotechnology, Jaboticabal, São Paulo, Brazil

*Address all correspondence to: lm.saran@unesp.br

References

[1] Jamee R, Siddique R. Biodegradation of synthetic dyes of textile effluent by microorganisms: an environmentally and economically sustainable approach. European Journal of Microbiology and Immunology. 2019;**9**:114-118. DOI: 10.1556/1886.2019.00018

[2] Benkhaya S, M'rabet S, Harfi AE. A review on classifications, recent synthesis, and applications of textile dyes. Inorganic Chemistry Communications. 2020;**115**:107891. DOI: 10.1016/j.inoche.2020.107891

[3] Holme I, Perkin SWH. A review of his life, work and legacy. Coloration Technology. 2006;**122**:235-251. DOI: 10.1111/j.1478-4408.2006.00041.x

[4] Sharma J, Sharma S, Soni V. Classification, and impact of synthetic textile dyes on Aquatic Flora: A review. Regional Studies in Marine Science. 2021;**45**:101802. DOI: 10.1016/j.rsma.2021.101802

[5] Yaseen DA, Scholz M. Textile dye wastewater characteristics and constituents of synthetic effluents: A critical review. International Journal of Environmental Science and Technology. 2019;**16**:1193-1226. DOI: 10.1007/s13762-018-2130-z

[6] Natarajan S, Bajaj HC, Tayade RJ. Recent advances based on the synergetic effect of adsorption for removal of dyes from wastewater using photocatalytic process. Journal of Environmental Sciences. 2018;**65**:201-222. DOI: 10.1016/j.jes.2017.03.011

[7] Verma AK, Dash RR, Bhunia P. A review on chemical coagulation/flocculation technologies for removal of colour from textile wastewaters. Journal of Environmental Management. 2012;**93**:154-168. DOI: 10.1016/j.jenvman.2011.09.012

[8] Fleischmann C, Lievenbrück M, Ritter H. Polymers and Dyes: Developments and Applications. Polymers. 2015;**7**:717-746. DOI: 10.3390/polym7040717

[9] Gita S, Shukla SP, Saharan N, Prakash P, Deshmukhe G. Toxic effects of selected textile dyes on elemental composition, photosynthetic pigments, protein content and growth of a freshwater chlorophycean alga *Chlorella vulgaris*. Bulletin of Environmental Contamination and Toxicology. 2019;**102**:795-801. DOI: 10.1007/s00128-019-02599-w

[10] Lellis B, Fávaro-Polonio CZ, Pamphile JÁ, Polonio JC. Effects of textile dyes on health and the environment and bioremediation potential of living organisms. Biotechnology Research and Innovation. 2019;**3**:275-290. DOI: 10.1016/j.biori.2019.09.001

[11] Madhav S, Ahamad A, Singh P, Mishra PK. A review of textile industry: Wet processing, environmental impacts, and effluent treatment methods. Environmental Quality Management. 2018;**27**:31-41. DOI: 10.1002/tqem.21538

[12] Hocini I, Benabbas K, Khellaf N, Djelal H, Amrane A. Can duckweed be used for the biomonitoring of textile effluents? Euro-Mediterranean Journal for Environmental Integration. 2019;**4**:34. DOI: 10.1007/s41207-019-0126-9

[13] Rápó E, Aradi LE, Szabó Á, Posta K, Szép R, Tonk S. Adsorption of Remazol Brilliant Violet-5R Textile

Dye from Aqueous Solutions by Using Eggshell Waste Biosorbent. Scientific Reports. 2020;**10**:8385. DOI: 10.1038/s41598-020-65334-0

[14] Orts F, Río AI, Molina J, Bonastre J, Cases F. Electrochemical treatment of real textile wastewater: Trichromy Procion HEXL®. Journal of Electroanalytical Chemistry. 2018;**808**:387-394. DOI: 10.1016/j.jelechem.2017.06.051

[15] Reddy S, Osborne JW. Heavy metal determination and aquatic toxicity evaluation of textile dyes and effluents using *Artemia salina*. Biocatalysis and Agricultural Biotechnology. 2020;**25**:101574. DOI: 10.1016/j.bcab.2020.101574

[16] Subramani SE, Thinakaran N. Isotherm, kinetic and thermodynamic studies on the adsorption behaviour of textile dyes onto chitosan. Process Safety and Environmental Protection. 2017;**106**:1-10. DOI: 10.1016/j.psep.2016.11.024

[17] Elmoubarkia R, Mahjoubia FZ, Elhalila A, Tounsadia H, Abdennouria M, Sadiqa M, et al. Ni/Fe and Mg/Fe layered double hydroxides and their calcined derivatives: preparation, characterization, and application on textile dyes removal. Journal of Materials Research and Technology. 2017;**6**:271-283. DOI: 10.1016/j.jmrt.2016.09.007

[18] Souza TNV, Carvalho SML, Vieira MGA, Silva MGC, Brasil DSB. Adsorption of basic dyes onto activated carbon: Experimental and theoretical investigation of chemical reactivity of basic dyes using DFT-based descriptors. Applied Surface Science. 2018;**448**:662-670. DOI: 10.1016/j.apsusc.2018.04.087

[19] Jiang Z, Hu D. Molecular mechanism of anionic dyes adsorption on cationized rice husk cellulose from agricultural wastes. Journal of Molecular Liquids. 2019;**276**:105-114. DOI: 10.1016/j.molliq.2018.11.153

[20] Ayyob M, Ahmad I, Hussain F, Bangash MK, Awan JÁ, Jaubert JN. A new technique for the synthesis of lanthanum substituted nickel cobaltite nanocomposites for the photo catalytic degradation of organic dyes in wastewater. Arabian Journal of Chemistry. 2020;**13**:6341-6347. DOI: 10.1016/j.arabjc.2020.05.036

[21] Chaari I, Fakhfakh E, Medhioub M, Jamoussi F. Comparative study on adsorption of cationic and anionic dyes by smectite rich natural clays. Journal of Molecular Structure. 2019;**1179**:672-677. DOI: 10.1016/j.molstruc.2018.11.039

[22] Meerbergen K, Crauwels S, Willems KA, Dewil R, Impe JV, Appels L, et al. Decolorization of reactive azo dyes using a sequential chemical and activated sludge treatment. Journal of Bioscience and Bioengineering. 2017;**124**:668-673. DOI: 10.1016/j.jbiosc.2017.07.005

[23] Khan SU, Perini JAL, Hussain S, Khan H, Khan S, Zanoni MVB. Electrochemical preparation of Nb_2O_5 nanochannel photoelectrodes for enhanced photoelectrocatalytic performance in removal of RR120 dye. Chemosphere. 2020;**257**:127164. DOI: 10.1016/j.chemosphere.2020.127164

[24] Martins AS, Lachgar A, Zanoni MVB. Sandwich Nylon/stainless-steel/WO3 membrane for the photoelectrocatalytic removal of Reactive Red 120 dye applied in a flow reactor. Separation and Purification Technology. 2020;**237**:116338. DOI: 10.1016/j.seppur.2019.116338

[25] Mendes CR, Dilarri G, Stradioto MR, Faria AU, Bidoia ED, Montagnolli RN.

The addition of a quaternary group in biopolymeric material increases the adsorptive capacity of Acid Blue 25 textile dye. Environmental Science and Pollution Research. 2019;**26**:24235-24246. DOI: 10.1007/s11356-019-05652-7

[26] Mendes CR, Dilarri G, Stradioto MR, Lopes PRM, Bidoia ED, Montagnolli RN. Zeta Potential Mechanisms Applied to Cellular Immobilization: A Study with *Saccharomyces cerevisiae* on Dye Adsorption. Journal of Polymers and the Environment. 2021;**29**:2214-2226. DOI: 10.1007/s10924-020-02030-0

[27] Li W, Um B, Yang Y. Feasibility of industrial-scale treatment of dye wastewater via bio-adsorption technology. Bioresource Technology. 2019;**277**:157-170. DOI: 10.1016/j.biortech.2019.01.002

[28] Attia EF, Zaki AH, El-Dek SI, Farhali AA. Synthesis, physicochemical properties and photocatalytic activity of nanosized Mg doped Mn ferrite. Journal of Molecular Liquids. 2017;**231**:589-596. DOI: 10.1016/j.molliq.2017.01.108

[29] Khandare RV, Govindwar SP. Phytoremediation of textile dyes and effluents: Current scenario and future prospects. Biotechnology Advances. 2015;**33**:1697-1714. DOI: 10.1016/j.biotechadv.2015.09.003

[30] Imran M, Crowley DE, Khalid A, Hussain S, Mumtaz MW. Arshad m. Microbial biotechnology for decolorization of textile wastewaters. Reviews in Environmental Science and Bio/Technology. 2015;**14**:73-92. DOI: 10.1007/s11157-014-9344-4

[31] Zhang X, Iqbal HMN. Immobilized ligninolytic enzymes: An innovative and environmental responsive technology to tackle dye-based industrial pollutants – A review. Science of The Total Environment. 2017;**576**:646-659. DOI: 10.1016/j.scitotenv.2016.10.137

[32] Bilal M, Asgher M, Parra-Saldivar R, Hu H, Wang W, Bilal M, et al. Immobilized ligninolytic enzymes: An innovative and environmental responsive technology to tackle dye-based industrial pollutants – A review. Science of The Total Environment. 2017;**576**:646-659. DOI: 10.1016/j.scitotenv.2016.10.137

[33] Bhandari S, Poudel DK, Marahatha R, Dawadi S, Khadayat K, Phuyal S, et al. Microbial Enzymes Used in Bioremediation. Journal of Chemistry. 2021;**2021**:1-17. DOI: 10.1155/2021/8849512

[34] Darwesh OM, Matter IA, Eida MF. Development of peroxidase enzyme immobilized magnetic nanoparticles for bioremediation of textile wastewater dye. Journal of Environmental Chemical Engineering. 2019;**7**:102805. DOI: 10.1016/j.jece.2018.11.049

[35] Routoula E, Patwardhan SV. Degradation of Anthraquinone Dyes from Effluents: A Review Focusing on Enzymatic Dye Degradation with Industrial Potential. Environmental Science Technology. 2020;**54**:647-664. DOI: 10.1021/acs.est.9b03737

[36] Teerapatsakul C, Parra R, Keshavarz T, Chitradon L. Repeated batch for dye degradation in an airlift bioreactor by laccase entrapped in copper alginate. International Biodeterioration & Biodegradation. 2017;**120**:52-57. DOI: 10.1016/j.ibiod.2017.02.001

[37] Ihsanullah I, Jamal A, Ilyas M, Zubair M, Khan G, Atieh MA. Bioremediation of dyes: Current status and prospects. Journal of Water Process Engineering. 2020;**38**:101680. DOI: 10.1016/j.jwpe.2020.101680Get rights and content

[38] Bento RMF, Almeida MR, Bharmoria P, Freire MG, Tavares APM. Improvements in the enzymatic degradation of textile dyes using ionic-liquid-based surfactants. Separation and Purification Technology. 2020;**235**:116191. DOI: 10.1016/j.seppur.2019.116191

[39] Mishra S, Maiti A. Applicability of enzymes produced from different biotic species for biodegradation of textile dyes. Clean Technologies and Environmental Policy. 2019;**21**:763-781. DOI: 10.1007/s10098-019-01681-5

[40] Iark D, Buzzo AJR, Garcia JAA, Côrrea VG, Helm CV, Corrêa RCG, et al. Enzymatic degradation and detoxification of azo dye Congo red by a new laccase from *Oudemansiella canarii*. Bioresource Technology. 2019;**289**:121655. DOI: 10.1016/j.biortech.2019.121655

[41] Srinivasan S, Sadasivam SK. Exploring docking and aerobic-microaerophilic biodegradation of textile azo dye by bacterial systems. Journal of Water Process Engineering. 2018;**22**:180-191. DOI: 10.1016/j.jwpe.2018.02.004

[42] Bilal M, Rasheed T, Zhao Y, Iqbal HMN. Agarose-chitosan hydrogel-immobilized horseradish peroxidase with sustainable bio-catalytic and dye degradation properties. International Journal of Biological Macromolecules. 2019;**124**:742-749. DOI: 10.1016/j.ijbiomac.2018.11.220

[43] Bilal M, Rasheed T, Iqbal HMN, Hu H, Wang W, Zhang X. Horseradish peroxidase immobilization by copolymerization into cross-linked polyacrylamide gel and its dye degradation and detoxification potential. International Journal of Biological Macromolecules. 2018;**113**:983-990. DOI: 10.1016/j.ijbiomac.2018.02.062

[44] Asses N, Ayed L, Hkiri N, Hamdi M. Congo Red Decolorization and Detoxification by *Aspergillus niger*: Removal Mechanisms and Dye Degradation Pathway. BioMed Research International. 2018;**2018**:1-9. DOI: 10.1155/2018/3049686

[45] Ali SS, Sun J, Koutra E, El-Zawawy N, Elsamahy T, El-Shetehy M. Construction of a novel cold-adapted oleaginous yeast consortium valued for textile azo dye wastewater processing and biorefinery. Fuel. 2021;**285**:119050. DOI: 10.1016/j.fuel.2020.119050

[46] Ali SS, Al-Tohamy R, Xie R, El-Sheekh MM, Suna J. Construction of a new lipase- and xylanase-producing oleaginous yeast consortium capable of reactive azo dye degradation and detoxification. Bioresource Technology. 2020;**313**:123631. DOI: 10.1016/j.biortech.2020.123631

[47] Ariaeenejad S, Motamedi E, Salekdeh GH. Application of the immobilized enzyme on magnetic graphene oxide nano-carrier as a versatile bi-functional tool for efficient removal of dye from water. Bioresource Technology. 2021;**319**:124228. DOI: 10.1016/j.biortech.2020.124228

[48] Wang N, Chu Y, Wu F, Zhao Z, Xu X. Decolorization and degradation of Congo red by a newly isolated white rot fungus, *Ceriporia lacerata*, from decayed mulberry branches. International Biodeterioration & Biodegradation. 2017;**117**:236-244. DOI: 10.1016/j.ibiod.2016.12.015

[49] Shaheen R, Asgher M, Hussain F, Bhatti HN. Immobilized lignin peroxidase from *Ganoderma lucidum* IBL-05 with improved dye decolorization and cytotoxicity reduction properties. International Journal of Biological

Macromolecules. 2017;**103**:57-64. DOI: 10.1016/j.ijbiomac.2017.04.040

[50] Verma K, Saha G, Kundu LM, Dubey VK. Biochemical characterization of a stable azoreductase enzyme from *Chromobacterium violaceum*: Application in industrial effluent dye degradation. International Journal of Biological Macromolecules. 2019;**121**:1011-1018. DOI: 10.1016/j.ijbiomac.2018.10.133

[51] Sarkar S, Banerjee A, Chakraborty N, Soren K, Chakraborty P, Bandopadhyay R. Structural-functional analyses of textile dye degrading azoreductase, laccase and peroxidase: A comparative in silico study. Electronic Journal of Biotechnology. 2020;**43**:48-54. DOI: 10.1016/j.ejbt.2019.12.004

[52] Wong JKH, Tan HK, Lau SY, Yap PS, Danquah MK. Potential and challenges of enzyme incorporated nanotechnology in dye wastewater treatment: A review. Journal of Environmental Chemical Engineering. 2019;**7**:103261. DOI: 10.1016/j.jece.2019.103261

[53] Jun LY, Yon LS, Mubarak NM, Bing CH, Pan S, Danquah MK, et al. An overview of immobilized enzyme technologies for dye and phenolic removal from wastewater. Journal of Environmental Chemical Engineering. 2019;**7**:102961. DOI: 10.1016/j.jece.2019.102961

[54] Gkaniatsou E, Sicard C, Ricoux R, Benahmed L, Bourdreux F, Zhang Q, et al. Enzyme Encapsulation in Mesoporous Metal–Organic Frameworks for Selective Biodegradation of Harmful Dye Molecules. Angewandte Chemie International Edition. 2018;**57**:16141-16146. DOI: 10.1002/anie.201811327

[55] Ali SS, Al-Tohamy R, Koutra E, Kornaros M, Khalil M, Elsamahy T, et al. Coupling azo dye degradation and biodiesel production by manganese-dependent peroxidase producing oleaginous yeasts isolated from wood-feeding termite gut symbionts. Biotechnology for Biofuels. 2021;**14**:61. DOI: 10.1186/s13068-021-01906-0

Chapter 9

Nonbiodegradable Hospital Waste Burden and Implications

Deepak S. Khobragade

Abstract

Hospitals and other healthcare facilities are very essential for the cure and care of persons suffering from health issues and also to promote health in society. As the health care services are improving and increasing their reach even in underdeveloped countries, so is the problem of health care waste (HCW) as hospitals generate a relatively huge amount of HCW, which consists of general as well as hazardous waste. The persons handling HCW are at immediate risk, followed by persons residing near HCW dumping/processing areas and the general public. Infectious HCW is a major threat to the health of humans and animals as it has the potential to spread various infectious diseases to the human and animal population. Due to the uncontrolled use of disposable nonbiodegradable materials by healthcare systems and their processing or lack of it, the HCW has emerged as one of the major sources of environmental pollution including the emission of the significant amount of greenhouse gases, which stands from 3 to 10% of total emissions of nations. HCW also leads to leaching chemicals, heavy metals like Pb, Cd, Cr, radioactive substances, and even generating carcinogens like dioxin in the environment contaminating air, soil, and water in general and especially in areas surrounding HCW dumping or processing affecting health and quality of life of not only of humans but cohabiting flora and fauna in those areas. Thus, the HCW is becoming one of the major sources of environmental pollution and collectively contributing to the problem of global warming. The HCW needs to be given the desired attention and priority in actions and policy. The chapter focuses on sources, types, and various environmental and health hazards related to HCW, its global environmental impact and management strategies for minimum effects with an eco-friendly and sustainable approach.

Keywords: health care waste, biodegradable, infectious waste, sharp, cytotoxic waste, radioactive waste, environment, carbon emission

1. Introduction

A biodegradable material can be decomposed by natural microorganisms, while nonbiodegradable material cannot be decomposed by natural microorganisms. The former will not be adding to pollution as it will be slowly broken down, but the latter acts as a source of pollution as it will remain as such in the environment for a very long time.

S. no.	Biodegradable waste	Nonbiodegradable waste
1	Decomposed and degraded by microbes.	Not decomposed and degraded by microbes.
2	Degradation process waste is rapid.	Degradation process is extremely slow.
3	Do not accumulated in environment but are cleaned up in a short time.	Accumulated in environment and are not easily cleaned up.
4	Becomes part of biogeochemical cycles, and are rapidly turned over in nature into useful components.	Never enter into biogeochemical cycles, and are therefore toxic and hazardous for nature.
5	Produce energy manure, compost, and biogas.	Can be separated and recycled and reused.
6	Decomposition process is natural and very affordable.	The process of treatment of waste is very expensive.

Table 1.
Difference between biodegradable and nonbiodegradable waste.

Biodegradable waste typically originates from some kind of organic materials from plant or animal sources and is commonly found as green waste, food waste, paper waste, and other biodegradable materials, like human waste, manure, sewage, slaughterhouse waste, etc.

Nonbiodegradable wastes are not decomposed or dissolved by natural biological processes. Most of the inorganic waste is nonbiodegradable. The major drawback of technological advancements in the creation of materials that nature cannot decompose, i.e. nonbiodegradable. Prominent examples of nonbiodegradable wastes are polyethylene and plastics, which are commonly used materials in almost every field, including the healthcare system. Now a day's improved, temperature resistant and more durable plastics are being produced making them even more long-lasting pollutants. Cans, metals, and chemicals form other chunks of nonbiodegradable waste.

It remains on earth for thousands of years unchanged and the threat caused is more significant. It not only causes air, water, and soil pollution but also act as a measure health hazard causing diseases like cancer (**Table 1**).

2. Health care waste (HCW)

The hospitals are considered as noble places, which treat sick persons and work for the health of society. The various adverse effects like high waste generation by them, their unplanned disposal, and their impact on the health of humans, animals, and the environment were generally neglected. A well-established and well-accepted fact is that Health care waste (HCW) or hospital waste is a potential challenge not only for the health care employees but for the general public and animals and plants of the surrounding environment.

HCW is anything that is produced by health care centers either of biological or nonbiological origin that needs to be discarded and is not intended for further use. It can be generated during the diagnosis, treatment, immunization, healthcare-related research activities, any such activity in healthcare centers, or hospitals. HCW may be composed of bio-waste like bodily parts and fluids, used medical materials, and also nonmedical general waste material which may be nonbiodegradable. Various sources of HCW are enlisted in **Table 2**.

Major sources	Minor sources
Hospitals/clinics/nursing homes • Teaching University hospital • General and District hospital • Primary healthcare center • Medical emergency services • Other health-care establishments • Obstetric and maternity hospitals • Dialysis centers • Dispensaries	• Physicians' offices • Specialized health-care establishments • Door to door health services
Medical and biomedical laboratories • Diagnostic centers • Autopsy centers	• Dental clinics
• Medical research & training centers	• Psychiatric hospitals
• Biotechnology research centers/institution/production units	• Disabled persons' institutions
• Animal houses	• Acupuncturists • Chiropractors
• Blood banks and blood collection services	• Ambulance services
• Home where health care is being provided	• Home treatment
• Mortuaries	• Funeral services
	• Cosmetic ear-piercing and tattoo parlors
	• Illicit drug users

Table 2.
Sources of biomedical waste.

3. Classification of biomedical waste

The medical waste generated is a multi-component waste and varies from regular nonhazardous waste. It consists of general items, biological materials to chemicals

S. no.	The EPA USA	The EU	The UK government	World Health Organization (WHO)
1	**General waste:** the major portion of medical waste consists of typical domestic and office waste.	Infectious waste including sharps.	**Infectious waste**: any waste generated by the treatment of patients or containing any infectious body fluids or material.	**Infectious waste:** any thing that's infectious or contaminated.
2	**Infectious waste:** any waste having potential to cause an infection e.g. blood, human tissue, or anything contaminated with bodily fluids, etc.	Pathological waste	**Cytotoxic/cytostatic waste**: drugs and materials that are cytotoxic and/or cytostatic and the items that are in contact with toxic or carcinogenic agents etc.	**Sharps**: waste like needles, scalpels, broken glass, razors, etc.

S. no.	The EPA USA	The EU	The UK government	World Health Organization (WHO)
3	**Hazardous waste:** waste that is potentially dangerous but non-infectious e.g. sharps, discarded surgical equipment, some chemical waste, etc.	Chemicals & pharmaceutics	**Medicinal waste**: All types of noncytotoxic medicine, pills,creams, etc.	**Pathological waste:** Human or animal tissue, body parts, blood, fluids, etc.
4	**Radioactive waste:** waste generated during radioactive treatments, like in cancer and due to the use of medical equipment, which use radioactive substances.	Cytotoxic & radioactive waste	**Anatomical waste**: waste from a human or animals including body parts, blood bags, etc.	**Pharmaceutical waste:** discarded, unused or expired medicines like tablets, capsules, syrups, creams, etc.
5		Nonrisk general waste	**Offensive waste**: non-infectious waste that includes sanitary,nappy waste, etc.	**Genotoxic waste:** hazardous waste containing drugs that are cytotoxic and carcinogenic, mutagenic, or teratogenic.
6			**Domestic or municipal waste**: all other general, nonclinical waste.	**Radioactive waste**: waste contaminated with radioactive materials
7				**Chemical waste**: hazardous waste congaing chemicals, disinfectants, liquid waste from machines, batteries, etc
8				**General/other waste**: nonhazardous waste containing stationary or other general daily use items.

Table 3.
Classification of medical waste.

including radioactive substances. The classification of medical waste, as per EPA (USA), EU, the government of UK, and WHO is depicted in **Table 3**.

All these classifications have commonly focused on Infectious waste, hazardous waste, chemical waste, and general waste. WHO's classification is most elaborate and very specific and generally followed irrespective of country and continent.

4. The problem of hospital waste

The healthcare sector can be a great nuisance, if HCW is not given due importance and handled properly and become the worrisome source that emits different greenhouse gases and is home to different pathogens that can cause damage to human and animal health and affect the environment. HCW also is the source of particulate matter and the area close to HCW dumping or processing site has a relatively very high level of the same [1].

Considering the segregation of HCW, the nonhazardous waste usually constitutes 80–85% of the total HCW and hazardous waste is about 15–20% based on rough estimations provided by WHO [2]. HCW is a worldwide issue as the AAMC found that globally approximately 4.4% of all greenhouse gas emissions and over 5 million tons of waste come from hospitals [3].

This estimation needs to be further investigated with respect to the degradation potential of total health care waste as the nonhazardous waste may not be biodegradable. **Table 4** gives the classification of overall HCW based on biodegradation. The list indicates that though the waste may not be hazardous but it may also not be biodegradable thus aggravating the problem of long-term environmental pollution and subsequent effects.

Various studies reported an increased incidence of health issues among employees and the resident population living nearby of waste processing facilities especially living near landfill sites, incinerators, composting facilities, and nuclear installations. Studies also reported that pathogens originating at HCW treatment plants pose a high risk of gastrointestinal infections [4].

Biodegradable waste	Partially biodegradable waste	Nonbiodegradable waste
Human anatomical waste: •Human tissues •Organs •Body parts	Liquid waste generated from laboratory and washing, cleaning, house keeping	**Sharps:** Needles, syringes, ampoules, scalpels, blades, glass, etc.
Animal waste: •Animal body parts, tissues, and organs •Carcasses •Animal blood •Waste generated by veterinary hospitals and research centers, colleges, and animal houses	Ash from the incineration of any Biomedical/HC waste	**Solid waste:** Tubings, catheters, intravenous sets, oxygen sets, dialysis sets, PPE gowns, gloves, masks, empty bottles and plastic containers, and polybags Disposable items Materials used during test for diagnostics
Microbiological & biotechnology waste •Laboratory cultures •Microorganisms specimens or stocks •Unused or partially used vaccines (live or attenuated) •Cell culture (human and animal) •Infectious agents (from research and industry) •Production of Biologicals •Toxins		**Chemical waste** Chemicals used in the production of drugs and biologicals Unused drugs and medicines Chemical Materials used during surgery Chemicals used in disinfection and cleaning Radioactive waste Insecticides, etc.)

Table 4.
Biodegradable and nonbiodegradable medical waste.

Rapid and uncontrolled growth of medical care facilities are resulting in an increase in waste generation because of the marked increase in the use of disposable items and their illegal recycling. Illegal recycling affects the local community, especially health workers, hospital employees, waste processing staff, and rag pickers [5]. A study in Iranian some selected hospitals indicate that the average of total medical waste generated was about 3.48 kg/bed of which approximately 1.039 kg/bed was hazardous-infectious waste, and 2.439 kg/bed-day was general waste [6]. Some studies reported the concern that large quantity of nonbiodegradable HCW such as disposable syringes, infusion bags, IV fluid bottles and administration sets, oxygen masks, etc. Are dumped in-properly by health care facilities and picked up by rag pickers and returned back into the market without any processing, posing a dangerous threat to the health of patients [7]. Exposure to HCW may spread communicable diseases through skin contact, injection, inhalation, and improper sterilization of containers and plastic materials before recycling [8].

HCW directly impacts on the health of the community, healthcare workers, animals, and surrounding environment. The HCW is saturated with infectious and hazardous waste. Impromptu, haphazard, and nonscientific disposal of HCW results in exposing the public in general and healthcare workers in specific to pathogenic waste which can cause different diseases. This also leads to contamination of all components of the surrounding environment by various hazardous content of HCW especially nonbiodegradable. Hence, HCW requires due attention and specific treatment and management prior to its final disposal.

Most of the times, the HCW gets mixed with domestic waste before disposal creating different types of problems in the long run. In economically developing or underdeveloped countries, the public, health workers, and waste processing personnel in particular, are not aware of the hazards of HCW or trained in management of HCW leading to the escalation of dangers of HCW. Also, in these countries, the lack of sufficient funds and proper information and awareness is a barrier for HCW management [9, 10].

One of the problems with HCW is that due to well-developed, superior, and well spread medical facilities available, the quantum of the pollution by HCW is much more than that of developing or poor countries, which have relatively underdeveloped and scarcely available health care systems [11, 12]. However, the global increment of the HCW production worldwide is increasing at an alarming rate, The middle and low-income countries contributing to this as HCW production is sharply increasing due to improved healthcare services and in the wealthy nations, the rapidly aging population

S. No.	national income level	Type of waste	Annual waste generation (kg/person)
1	High-income countries	All of the HCW	1.1–12.0
		Hazardous HCW	0.4–5.5
2	Middle-income countries	All of the HCW	0.8–6.0
		Hazardous HCW	0.3–0.4
3	Low-income countries	All of the HCW	0.5–3.0
		Hazardous HCW	Negligible (0.02–0.1aprox)

Table 5.
HCW generation and economic status of country.

Continent	Mean(kg/bed/day)	Sample size
Africa	0.8	8
America	4.41	6
Asia	2–44	18
Europe	3.10	10
Combined	2.57	42

Table 6.
Healthcare waste generation rates in different continents.

that need frequent usage of health care systems is increasing HCW generation rate (HCWGR) [13]. **Table 5** illustrate the average rate of HCW generation with respect to the economic status of the country and **Table 6** indicates that of continents [14].

As per WHO report of 2018, in general, hazardous medical waste generation per hospital bed per day in high-income countries is on an average up to 0.5 kg [3].

5. HCW and carbon emissions

It is estimated that in the USA alone, 8–9% of the total annual carbon dioxide emissions (33.34 MT) is contributed by the healthcare industry (HCI) [15, 16]. Just to understand the contribution of HCI in CO_2 emission, if we consider that the average value of 5% of total carbon dioxide emission is by HCI the amount of carbon dioxide emission by the top 10 carbon dioxide emitting countries in the year 2020 can be of large quantum as is given in the following **Table 7** [17].

The research shows that three groups of countries i.e. North America (29%), East Asia/Pacific (30%), and Europe/Central Asia regions (19%) contribute about 78% of health care emissions. The remaining 22% of global health care emissions is shared by Latin America (6%), South Asia (2%), and the remaining 14% is shared by

S. no.	Country	Total CO_2 Emission (Mt)	CO_2 Emission by HCI (Mt)
1	China	11680.42	584.02
2	United States	4535.30	226.77
3	India	2411.73	120.59
4	Russia	1674.23	83.71
5	Japan	1061.77	53.09
6	Iran	690.24	34.51
7	Germany	636.88	31.84
8	South Korea	621.47	31.07
9	Saudi Arabia	588.81	29.44
10	Indonesia	568.27	28.41
Total			1223.45

Table 7.
Top ten countries with CO_2 emission rates and contribution of HCS

S. no.	Primary factor	Secondary factor	Impact
1	Increased CO_2 level	Air pollution	Asthma, cardiovascular disorders, effect are generally more prominent in persons having lung and heart diseases.
		Increased allergens	Respiratory allergies, asthma, skin disorders, tiredness with minimum physical activity.
2	Rising temperature	Extreme hot conditions	Disorders related to heat and illness and may be deaths, cardiac disorders including cardiovascular failure.
		Severe weather conditions	Migration and social effects, injuries, mental health impacts, and fatalities.
3	Rising sea level	Impact on water quality	Infections like cholera, leptospirosis, cryptosporidiosis, campylobacter, and algal growth.
		Food and water supply impact	Food and drinking water problems, malnutrition, diarrheal, and other infective diseases.
4	Extreme weather conditions	Environmental degradation	Disturbed weather cycles, food and water supply problems, increased diseases, migration, civil conflict, and mental health impacts.
		Changes in ecology (especially vector)	Changed life cycles and growth in previously unfavorable areas leading to the spread of diseases like malaria, dengue, chikungunya, encephalitis, hantavirus, Rift Valley Fever, Lyme disease, West Nile virus, etc.
5	Acid rain	Decreased pH of water bodies	Decreased portability and utility e.g. not good for swimming, digestive, and skin problems.
		Increased particulate matter	Asthma or chronic bronchitis, make it hard for people to breathe, lungs infections.

Table 8.
Impact of environmental pollution on human health [21].

the combined health sectors of Sub-Saharan Africa, Middle East, and North African countries [18].

If we consider HCI a country, it would be at least the fifth-largest emitter of greenhouse gases on the planet. The HCI's carbon footprint can be the same as the emissions of 514 coal-fired power plants [19].

Studies have reported that greenhouse gas emissions from the health sector in various countries range from 3 to 10% of the national emissions. The energy consumption and other waste generation make it a significant factor in changing climatic conditions due to various pollutions. US Environmental agency has reported that HCW is the third major cause of dioxin pollution and 10% of overall mercury emission. The burning of medical waste such as plastic materials, which are generated from polyvinyl chloride (PVC) products is the major producer of dioxin [20]. The effect of climate change has a multifaceted effect on human health which is summarized in **Table 8**.

6. Health hazards of carbon emissions

Exposure and inhalation of CO/CO2 lead to a variety of health issues which include difficulty in breathing, increased heart rate, profound sweating, tiredness, restlessness, dizziness, headaches, a tingling sensation, hypertension, coma, asphyxia, and convulsions. Continuous exposure to CO in the closed area may even lead to death.

Higher average temperatures and changes in weather disturb rain and snow patterns which leads to the migration of invasive species to new areas. Pathogens and even their hosts which were not able to survive low temperatures will spread to new areas as the average temperature rise due to global warming. Insect pest infestations of plants and crops will increase as pests will be able to take advantage of weakened plants due to atmospheric and weather conditions (**Table 9**).

Marine animals are severely affected by the increase in carbon dioxide in the atmosphere. This is because the ocean absorbs CO_2 in the atmosphere and becomes more acidic. Though the increase of CO_2 in the ocean may have little impact on big marine animals, marine phytoplankton multiplies rapidly with more CO_2, and more phytoplankton support larger aquatic animal populations.

The major impact of a more acidic ocean is on animals like corals, sea urchins, and mollusks that produce calcium carbonate shells. Acidification not only causes difficulty for these animals to produce shells but cause the shells to actually dissolve due to the change in the chemical balance of ocean water. Decreased number of shelled animals can impact the ocean ecosystem and trigger a chain reaction in wide range of organisms that depend on these animals for their food (**Table 10**).

CO_2 level	Conditions
400 ppm	Normal level of outdoor air.
400–1000 ppm	Typical level is found in normally populated spaces having good air circulation.
1000–2000 ppm	Poor air quality is prominently indicated by complaints of drowsiness.
2000–5000 ppm	Health issues like increased heart rate, respiratory disorders, slight nausea, poor concentration, loss of attention, headaches, sleepiness, and stagnant, stale, and stuffy air.
5000 ppm	This is the maximum permissible exposure limit. Toxicity and oxygen deprivation occur. High levels of other gases may be present leading to more severe effects.
40,000 ppm	Very dangerous due to deprivation of oxygen.

Table 9.
Potential health problems with increased levels of CO_2 in the air [22].

City/country	Population (Million)	HCW generated	Additional HCW generated due to COVID	% Increase due to COVID
Manila	14	47	280	496
Jakarta	11	35	212	506
Kuala Lampur	10.5	35	210	500
Bangkok	8	27	160	493
Ha Noi	7.8	26	154	492

Table 10.
Increase in waste generation by COVID-19 in some cities.

According to Practice Green-health, an organization working for more sustainable hospitals, about 25% of the waste generated by hospitals is plastic. The National Health Service (NHS), UK creates.

133,000 tons of plastic annually with only 5% of it being recyclable [23] and hospitals in the USA produce more than 5 million tons of waste each year, 1.25 million tons of which is plastic. About 16 billion injections are utilized worldwide every year, but not all of them are properly disposed of afterward generating a huge amount of nonbiodegradable waste [24].

HCW that contains chemicals like pharmaceuticals, laboratory and diagnostic reagents, disinfectants, cleaners, solvents, and waste containing metals and heavy metals is considered chemical healthcare waste. Chemical waste accounts for about 3% of waste originating from health care activities [25].

The literature reveals even in small and economically not so sound countries like Pakistan hospitals produce 2.0 kg of waste, per bed per day, of which at least 0.5 kg can be categorized as hazardous HCW and the average daily HCWG from both public & private sector hospitals is approx 0.8 million tons [26].

7. COVID and HCWG

In 2019, an unprecedented medical emergency in the form of the COVID-19 pandemic was experienced by the whole world. The infection spread to the majority of areas and more than 370 million confirmed cases and over 5.6 million deaths have been reported globally. Tens of thousands of tons of extra HCW have been produced due to the medical efforts to treat and deal with COVID-19. The WHO Global analysis of HCW in the context of COVID-19 states that approximately 87,000 tons of personal protective equipment (PPE) were distributed to various countries from March 2020 to November 2021. It also points out that over 140 million test kits, generating 2,600 tons of plastic non-infectious waste and 731,000 liters of chemical waste have been shipped to support countries. Globally more than 8 bn vaccine doses have been administered generating 144,000 tons of added HCW in the form of nonbiodegradable syringes, needles, and safety boxes. Approximately 129 bn masks and 65 bn gloves were utilized per month globally during the COVID-19 epidemic increasing the burden of HCW immensely [27]. Wuhan in China, which is considered as the starting point of the COVID-19 outbreak has to manage a rise of HCWG of 600% during that period. **Table 8** shows an increase in HCW during COVID-19 outbreak in some cities. In Taiwan, it is reported that HCW generation has increased to 40,407 Mt. in 2019from 35,747 Mt. in 2016, an increase of 4.17% in three years span [28].

In a highly populous country India, about 420,461 kg/day of HCW is generated out of which only 240,682 kg/day of waste is treated [29]. India generated 550.9 tons/day of HCW in 2020 as per the estimation of ASSOCHAM (Associated Chambers of Commerce and Industry of India).

8. Effect of HCW on Environment

The HCW affects all components of the environment. The effect on water, soil, and air is discussed below.

8.1 Impact of biomedical waste on water

HCW is a multi-component waste; improper disposal of HCW causes leaching out of pollutants from the waste dumping sites into the surrounding water bodies including groundwater affecting water quality. The water near landfills and dumping sites contain a relatively higher amount of pollutants including heavy metals [30–32] found that incinerated biomedical waste contains the elevated percentage of heavy metals and polycyclic aromatic hydrocarbons (PAHs), and may pollute surface and groundwater by percolation of toxic substances. The analysis of water near HCW ash showed increased hardness at the levels of 1320 mg/L and chloride at 8500 mg/L. The levels of Al, V, Cr, Mn, Co, Ni, Ba, Fe, and especially Pb content in leachate were above the acceptable levels as per drinking water guidelines of WHO and EPA. Hence, it is also important to detoxify ash before disposal into landfills or reutilization [33, 34]. They cause indirect health hazards by conversion into other materials, breakdown, and decomposition. Consumption of contaminated drinking water and the resulting health issues may include cardiovascular disorders, neuronal damage, renal injuries, and risk of cancer and diabetes. Fabián Fernández-Luqueño et al. has comprehensively revived the health hazards of various metal contaminants on human health [35] Water is considered as the blood of the ecosystem. Heavy metals are extremely toxic to aquatic animals and cause histopathological changes, especially in fish even at low concentrations. They get accumulated in aquatic organisms as well as in vegetables and fruits grown using contaminated water and thus enter the food chain and propagate into other animals who feed on them thus increasing toxic effects to many folds [36].

8.2 Impact of biomedical waste on soil

Soil quality near waste dumping sites is greatly affected by improper and unscientific disposal of HCW, resulting in alteration of physical and chemical soil properties. The chemistry and biology of the soil ecosystem may change due to different pollutants getting mixed with the soil. The soil samples near the HCW incinerator and dumping sites were found to have very high concentrations of heavy metals like Fe, Cu, Zn, Cr, Cd, Pb, and Ni [37–40]. Soils at these sites showed high pH, TDS, and EC regime in comparison to control sites resulting in deteriorating soil quality and a decrease in vegetation [41]. The study in china indicated that the HW ashes contained large amounts of metal salts of various common metals with a concentration range of 1.8–315 g /kg. Abundant precautions and measures are needed to further prevent and reduce soil damage due to HCW with increased waste development due to increased establishment and utilization of healthcare facilities [42].

8.3 Biomedical waste and its impact on air quality

Greenhouse gas and particulate emissions are challenging issues for HCW dumping sites. Hospitals produce a huge quantity of waste mostly disposed of by incineration. Incineration is the conventional and most common method of choice for the treatment of HCW. The burning of HCW pollutes the environment by discharging fly ash and toxic metals in the incinerated ash. Burning HCW results in higher incidences of cancer, respiratory disorders, innate abnormalities, and hormonal disorders other issues related to the burning of HCW are contribution to global warming, acidification, ozone or smog formation, and eutrophication. This also releases various gases and particulate materials into the air contaminating the environmental air. Dust, particulate matter, black carbon, metals, acid gases, ammonia, sulfate, and nitrate are the major contaminants released in the air. Burning of HCW emits harmful organic compounds like acetone, octane, decane, dodecane, methenamine, cyclo-butane, diethyl phthalate, nonane, carbon disulfide, and diperoxide [43]. The incineration of plastic-rich hospital waste results in emissions of HCl, CO, C_2H_4, C_2H_6, C_3H_8,C_3H_6 in the concentrations of 3.3–5.3, 1.4–1.8, <0.002, <0.010, <0.012, and < 0.011 g/kg, respectively [44]. A high concentration of dioxin and furan in the atmosphere near medical waste incinerators was reported [45]. The high prevalence of self-reported

S. no.	Heavy metal contaminant	Toxicity
1	Mercury (Hg)	CNS injuries
		Renal dysfunction
		Gastrointestinal ulceration
		Hepatotoxicity
2	Lead (Pb)	CNS injury
		Lungs dysfunction
		Hematological disorders like anemia
		gastrointestinal colic
		Liver damage
		Reduced pulmonary function
		Cardiovascular dysfunction
3	Chromium (Cr)	Kidney dysfunction
		Gastro intestinal disorders
		Dermal diseases
		Increasing the incidence of cancers including lungs, larynx, bladder, kidneys, testicular, bone, and thyroid
		Genomic instability
4	Cadmium (Cd)	Degenerative bone disease
		Renal dysfunction
		Liver disorder
		GI disorders
		Lungs injuries
		Disorders in the metabolism of metals like Zn and Cu
		Cancer
5	Arsenic (As)	Cardiovascular dysfunction
		Skin and hair changes
		CNS injury
		Gastrointestinal discomfort
		Liver damage

Table 11.
Health hazards of heavy metal contaminants in HCW [52].

health symptoms such as fatigue, sleepiness, and headaches among residents near waste sites was reported in most of the studies [46–48]. The process of incineration may convert solid and liquid toxic waste into gaseous emissions, particulate matters, oxides of nitrogen, and oxides of sulfur causing acute effects such as eyes and respiratory irritation. It also increases the toxic effects of heavy metals and contributes to acid rain. The plastic waste made up of chlorine releases dioxins that are known as human carcinogens [46].

The increased level of these pollutants is dangerous to human health causing various types of health issues especially respiratory problems [49]. Studies have also reported the prevalence of adverse health effects other than respiratory problems like birth defects with low birth weight, cancers, etc. in individuals residing near HCW processing and dumping sites [50]. The study findings suggest a relatively higher prevalence of various health issues among people living in proximity to waste dumping and processing sites than those living far from these sites particularly respiratory illness (23% v 10%), eye irritation (20% v 9.5%) and stomach problem (27% v 20%) [51–53].

Heavy metals generate reactive oxygenic species (ROS) and induce oxidative stress which is responsible for various diseases and health conditions. Acting as metabolic poisons they react and inhibit sulfhydryl (SH) enzyme systems which are involved in cellular energy production. Heavy metals have been reported to be carcinogenic, mutagenic, and teratogenic [54]. The harmful effects of heavy metals which are the main pollutants from HCW are depicted in **Table 11**.

9. Management of nonbiodegradable wastes

Management of waste involves steps right from the generation to disposal of the treated waste. For nonbiodegradable waste, special care has to be taken during collection, storage, transport, and disposal. All are separated from general biodegradable and nonhazardous waste.

As nonbiodegradable wastes cannot be broken down by decomposers, their disposal poses a grave problem. Nonbiodegradable wastes can be managed by practicing the principle of **4RDs** i.e. Reduce, Reuse, Recycle, Recover, and Dispose. The fifth R i.e. Refuse is also very important in controlling HCW.

9.1 Reduce

The best mode to control pollution is reducing the release of pollutants in the environment, which can be achieved by reducing the usage of polluting materials. Without giving a thought, often more things are utilized than are actually needed resulting in the generation of more quantum of waste. The generation of waste needs to be reduced by reducing the usage of nonbiodegradable waste generating materials. Consume maximum and throw away minimum should be the guiding principle in the selection and utilization of materials in general and nonbiodegradable materials in specific. Thoughtful planning for use of nonbiodegradable materials for minimum waste generation should be the priority of all healthcare activities.

9.2 Reuse

Increased use of the single-use materials leads to increased generation of waste. Hospitals should try to make it a practice to utilize reusable materials wherever possible. Certain things can be used for more than one purpose and if we reuse them for the same or other purposes, we can reduce the waste generation. This can be employed not only for nonclinical use like eatery and other nonclinical purposes use but also for clinical uses wherever possible. Use glass or metal containers and trays which can be cleaned and even sterilized after every use. Also use cloth gowns and masks instead of plastic protective units in areas where they can be used.

9.3 Recycle

The process by which waste materials are utilized in the production/creation of new products is called recycling. The materials used/reused in recycling are substitutes for raw materials obtained from natural resources thus reducing the exploitation of natural recourses to some extent and also reducing contamination of the environment by waste disposal. It also prevents wasting potentially useful materials and reduces demand for new raw materials. Generally, materials like glass, metal, plastic, wood and paper are collected, separated, and recycled to make new things. The energy generation from waste treatment is also a part of the recycling process. Recycling can be internal (in-house) or external.

Following steps can be undertaken for nonbiodegradable waste management.

- Setting up nonbiodegradable waste collection centers in specific wards or divisions where the waste is temporarily stored before further processing.
- Segregation of waste into BW and NBW.
- NBW is taken for a separate treatment process.
- Transport with care to avoid spillage.

9.4 Recycling of nonbiodegradable waste

In the case of nonbiodegradable wastes, in addition to the 3 Rs of managing waste, a 4th R of Refuse should be considered. So, Refuse, Reduce, Reuse and Recycle, and Dispose is the best policy for reducing nonbiodegradable waste.

The nonbiodegradable waste goes for processing and treatment at specific waste treatment plants where they are recycled. Usually, the treatment of nonbiodegradable waste is done on the basis of the nature of the material it is made up of. Different procedures employed according to the major types of recycled waste are.

Iron metal materials: Iron is the most recycled metal. Recycled by separating by magnetic methods, melting in a furnace, and used for the production of other iron materials or steel.

Non-iron metal materials: Other metals like aluminum, copper, and alloys like brass are ground into fine pieces and molten to be recast in new materials.

Glass: Glass is crushed, decolorized, and put into the furnace for melting. This can be remolded into other articles of required shape and size. Molten glass is also used for layering on roads as glassphalt.

Plastic: Plastics are of various types and grades that all cannot be mixed together for treatment and need to be sorted. The plastics can be further processed remolded and used for making new materials.

9.5 Recover

Every material requires and intakes a lot of energy during its manufacture and the energy in waste materials cannot be wasted. It is cost-saving and eco-friendly to recover energy from waste materials.

Energy from biodegradable waste can be extracted relatively easily and efficiently by biomass energy conversion, composting, biogas plants, etc. This process converts biological energy into a usable form of energy like gas and electricity [55].

Energy retrieval from nonbiodegradable is somewhat difficult and requires a complex process. NBW is subjected to a process of thermal decomposition or pyrolysis, which involves the breaking of intermolecular bonds to release energy in the form of heat. The residue obtained is in the form of ash or degraded product which can be safely dumped or discarded.

9.6 Dispose

9.6.1 Ways to dispose of nonbiodegradable waste

Not all waste fits into the criteria of reuse or recycle. These waste needs to be disposed off in a way to have minimal impact on the environment. Disposal of biodegradable waste is very simple and can be done employing easy methods like landfilling, composting, etc.

The NBW cannot be decomposed naturally and need special disposal techniques for minimizing hazardous effects on environments and people handling it. Let us look at some nonbiodegradable waste management methods commonly used.

9.6.2 Incineration

Usually used for nonrecyclable nonbiodegradable waste and bio-hazardous waste from hospitals, etc. Incineration involves decomposition by combustion of waste using high heat, i.e. above 500°C. It is also referred to as the thermal treatment of waste. Incineration of waste converts it primarily into ash, flue gas, and heat. Heat can be used for various heat-based processes. The gases and fumes must be treated properly to prevent or at least reduce environmental pollution. Air filters are nowadays employed for the same. Modern methods of incineration such as gasification, pyrolysis, and anaerobic digestion can be utilized for energy recovery. Useful content from the residual ash contains metals that can be recovered using separate treatments. **Table 10** depicts some methods of incineration for waste disposal (**Table 12**).

Incinerators reduce the mass of the waste by 80–85% and the volume by 95–96%, depending on the composition and degree of recovery of materials such as metals from the ash for recycling [53].

9.6.3 Landfills

Solid waste landfill is a separate area of land or excavation where waste is collected. It provides long-term storage for nonbiodegradable waste. Ideally, landfills should be carefully situated and designed to prevent waste contamination from entering the neighboring environment. They are designed to reduce odor and pests to the maximum possible extent.

S. no.	Type of Incineration	Features	Concerns
1	Burn pile	Carried out in the open ground. A mound of combustible waste materials is piled on and set on fire.	Cause pollution. Spread uncontrolled fires. Incomplete combustion of waste produces particulate pollution.
2	Burn barrel	It holds the burning waste material inside a metal barrel having a metal grating over the exhaust. The spread of burning material is prevented by the barrel and residue after processing settles down in the barrel.	Cause pollution. Do not result in full combustion of waste and therefore produce particulate pollution.
3	Fixed grate	Simplest and most common form. It has a brick-lined chamber and a fixed metal grate over a lower ash pit. There are two openings, one either at the top or side for loading waste and another on the side for removing residue.	Cause pollution. The combustion is partial. Do not result in full combustion of waste and therefore produce particulate pollution.
4	Moving grate	Consists of an opening called "throat" for feeding waste at one end of the grate. The waste burns and moves through the descending grate to the ash pit present at the other end and is removed through a water lock.	Complete combustion. Advanced designs cause reduced pollution and can be utilized for energy generation.
5	Rotary-kiln	Contains a primary chamber and secondary chamber. The primary chamber has an inclined refractory lined cylindrical tube where volatilization, destructive distillation, and partial combustion reactions convert waste into gases that are completely burned in the secondary chamber.	Complete combustion Cause pollution. Prone to the production of gas and particulate pollution though can burn in afterburner.
6	Fluidized bed	It consists of a waste processing chamber where a strong airflow is forced through a sand bed until a fluidized bed is created. At this point the fuel and waste are introduced, mixing and churning occurs, and waste is incinerated. As the bed is mixed and agitated with force, content forms a fluid-like state making all of the mass of waste, fuel, and sand fully circulating through the furnace for efficient incineration.	Complete combustion Highly efficient process Can cause pollution if generated gases and ash not properly managed
7	Specialized incinerator	These are designed for incineration of special waste content lime chemicals, resin powder, and flammable substances. The process has higher control and prevents burn back.	Complete and controlled combustion Can handle critical waste components. Generated gases and ash need to be properly managed.
8	Liquid injection incinerator	It has a waste burner feed system, a supporting fuel system, and an air supply system attached to the combustion chamber for maximum incineration.	Used for waste in liquid form. Complete combustion. Cause pollution. Can be used to recover metals and energy.
9	Multiple hearth incinerator	Consist of a number of circular hearths or kilns superimposed over each other. Waste is introduced from the top and moved by rotating "rabble arms", which move over the surface of each hearth to continuously shift the content.	Complete combustion. High flexibility and efficiency. Precise control of the temperature profile. Less pollution.

S. no.	Type of Incineration	Features	Concerns
10	Catalytic combustion	It is a chemical process in which a catalyst is used to speed up desired oxidation reactions and reduce the formation of undesired products.	Complete combustion. High flexibility and efficiency. Precise control of the temperature profile. Less pollution especially nitrogen oxide gases (NOx).

Table 12.
Methods of incineration for waste disposal.

Sanitary landfills are similar to normal landfills but are built in a planned and methodical way. Normal landfills cannot completely prevent the leaching or leakage of waste and toxic substances along with water into the ground. Sanitary landfills are closed areas built with concrete and with facilities to collect the leachate and gases released. These also are superior in preventing pest breeding and pathogen spread.

Large area requirements, cost and chances of leakage, and pollution are some disadvantages.

9.6.4 Plasma arc furnaces

They are referred to as "plasma recycling," and "plasma gasification. In this process, the waste is heated to super-high temperatures where it melts and then vaporizes producing gas that can be used for energy and rocky solid residue that can be used for various purposes like a building material. Unlike inclinators which convert waste to ash and gases, plasma arc furnaces first directly convert waste to plasma, the fourth state of matter, and then produce gasification. Thus, it's a cleaner, greener form of waste treatment.

9.6.5 Encapsulation

Encapsulation is covering of material with some kind of material uniformly resulting in a product called the capsule. In waste disposal by encapsulation method, the waste is crammed very compactly in an inert cover just like a capsule which does not allow any exchange of materials including gases. These capsules of waste are buried deep down into the ground resulting in safe and long-lasting waste disposal without any leakage, leaching, and contamination of the environment.

At the COP26, world leaders discussed strategies directly affecting climate change. The Centre for Sustainable Healthcare has requested world leaders to take initiatives to make sure that healthcare systems are Net Zero by 2040. They further stated to fund existing healthcare facilities to transfer them to environmentally sustainable healthcare systems. This includes collaboration with all players in the supply chain to de-carbonize medical devices. Reducing plastic medical waste is an essential strategy.

9.7 Refuse

It is the fifth "R" of waste management. Refuse should be the first choice which involves refusing a certain amount of waste production. Refuse means not using or

REFUSE	The concept is about refusing the use of materials that add on to the nonbiodegradable waste burden. If we refuse to use them and stop buying these materials in the first place, then automatically we will not have to deal with them as waste.
RETHINK	Thinking about any material we use and try to adopt a Zero Waste practice thus rethinking the way we carry out hospital services so as to minimize waste generation.
REDUCE	Reducing unnecessary waste generation by using fewer materials should be a priority and adopted policy from the start. Also reducing energy consumption can indirectly help in reducing environmental pollution.
REUSE	Reusing any material, which can otherwise be a waste results in reduced waste generation. Applying some creative thinking and processing can result in the consumption of new materials and waste generation.
RECYCLE	Recycling all the waste to create new materials or products can reduce environmental hazards to a great extent. Using recycled products wherever available and possible can also serve the purpose to great extent.
RECOVER	The recovery of waste is of two types processed and without any pre-processing. Waste oils can be burnt for energy or energy can be recovered by processing waste with novel techniques to generate energy and thus reducing dependence on nonrenewable energy sources to some extent.
REPAIR	Repairing means fixing or restoring supposed to be waste material for use or reuse. This should be applied wherever possible instead of just discarding damaged materials /items as waste.
REPURPOSE	Repurposing comprises of using items for a different purpose than they were meant for. This is also termed as up-cycling Utilizing waste material for another use instead of disposing of it ending in hazardous waste. Some products can be repurposed using creativity and the possibilities are endless.
DISPOSE	The process of getting rid of HCW by one or other way like landfilling or incineration when all of the above means are exhausted. This should also be done scientifically and very carefully to have minimum effect on the environment and health.

Table 13.
Strategies for HCW management.

discontinuing use of waste-generating things, especially nonbiodegradable and hazardous things. Refuse can act as the most prominent measure in reducing waste generation. By refusing the usage of certain materials, one can avert the HCW generation thus not requiring any treatment or processing and saving a lot of financial resources, and preventing health and environmental hazards waste. For example, the refusal to single-use plastic in HCI will not only decrease the amount of plastic in HCW but will also prevent the related effects of plastic waste. It can look impractical and difficult, but there are some better and less waste generating options that can be opted for. It's the most effective way to reduce the amount of waste HCI is producing.

The measures are summarized in **Table 13** with enlisting more R's.

10. Causes for failure of waste management efforts

10.1 Lack of awareness about the hazards related to healthcare waste

Not only the general public but even highly educated people including healthcare professionals are not fully aware of the hazardous effects of HCW on health and the environment. Due to this, the HCWM does not gather the importance needed resulting in a casual and careless approach. Not all the hospital staffs have knowledge of standard protocol for collection, segregation, and disposal of HCW. In most of the cases, health care staff does not receive occupational safety education and has no knowledge of the safe handling of hazardous substances. They also are not properly trained for using personal protective equipment. A large number of waste handlers and cleaners are casual labors and are illiterate or relatively very less educated unvaccinated and untrained personnel. They generally never use proper personal protective equipment and do not understand the threats of HCW thus putting their and other's health in danger. HCW is transported by hand in regular waste risking spilling of toxic or infectious materials, or injuries to handlers from sharps like needles or other substances. Either, they are unaware or have very little knowledge and a careless approach towards safety measures like spillages and accidents. As the cleaners and waste handlers are in close contact with HCW, they are the worst sufferers of the effects of poor and improper safety procedures [56]. These factors lead to escalation of HCW which could be reduced if given needed importance and attention.

10.2 The low priority is given to the waste management

The HCW management requires the highest consideration and assiduousness to avoid the significant health challenges related with poor HCWM practices like exposure to infectious HCW and toxic material therein. It is one of the most prominent results of failure of HCWM. Sometimes even though the importance of safe management of HCW is sometimes known and understood but the efforts required are not undertaken.

It is generally regarded especially by the general public that waste management is the sole duty and responsibility of government and local administration and that the public is not supposed to contribute [57]. Waste management's success depends upon the active participation of all, the government through local administration, hospital management, and workers and patients. The guidelines related to waste management should be made mandatory to be followed by the hospital staff and regular monitoring of the same can lead to improved compliance. Hospital management is focused on earning more profit from the services without any regard for the environment and HCWM resulting in illegal and uncontrolled disposal of untreated waste increasing the severity of the problem.

The vital issue is the clear ascription of responsibility and accountability of apt handling and processing of HCW. According to the concept of "you pollute you clean or you pay", the responsibility of HCW management lies with the waste producer, the healthcare provider, or the establishment involved in related activities being the one. This needs to be made known to the healthcare system and fixing accountability with them can only bring some seriousness in their attitude.

10.3 Lack of legal framework and absence of waste management and disposal systems

Many countries either do not have proper regulations, have very nominal regulations, or do not enforce them strictly. Research indicates that having adequate legal framework results positively in the development of a waste management system [58] while the dearth of adequate policies [59] and not so strong regulations [60, 61] are disadvantageous to it. Lack of pollution and environmental control systems and systems for evaluation of the real impacts of pollution is a major concern, especially in middle and lower middle-income countries. The developed countries have strong legislative frameworks and control systems which is lacking in developing and underdeveloped countries. In these countries/societies, the condition is relatively better in urban areas but practically missing in remote village areas [62]. Thus, there is no system of waste management and disposal and most of the waste including HCW remains dumped anywhere without treatment. If we consider a ban on disposable plastics it is somewhat functional in urban areas but completely nonexistent in rural areas where nonbiodegradable plastic enters but is never returned. The HCW is also treated as general waste most of the time and disposed off without due care and precautions.

10.4 Insufficient financial and human resources

The developing and underdeveloped countries are facing the problem of a dearth of financial resources to address the rising quantity of HCW resulting due to rapid urbanization and healthcare facilities. Lack of the proper utilization of available finances has hampered the delivery of proper waste management services [63]. The available resources are primarily allocated to the high-income urban areas with higher tax yields habituating residents with more political influence. This leads to vast area which is poor and suburban housing major population that is relatively economically weaker unnerved. Huge expenditure is needed to provide the service [64] inadequate and insufficient funds and resources local government cannot finance adequate levels of service required for waste management in general and HCWM in particular. In the absence of proper financial support, limited resources with reservations, and unwillingness of the users to pay for the waste management [65] contribute to the problem more.

10.5 Utilization of traditional ways instead of modern techniques

The technical issues hinder efficient and broader health care management. In most of places the conventional approach to deal with waste treatment especially health care waste is in practice. The modern techniques of collection, segregation, and processing are very expensive and adopted mostly only by developed and highly industrialized countries. These techniques are expensive to purchase and maintain, sophisticated, and difficult to operate, thereby often inadequate for the socioeconomic conditions of developing and underdeveloped countries to be used extensively. Even though if systems are procured and utilized after a short period of usage, usually only very few systems remain in operation for want of trained staff and maintenance cost. Other technical factors apart from insufficient technologies are lack of trained and technically skilled personnel within [66], poor infrastructure and roads, and old vehicles [67, 68]. There is a lack of validated and authenticated data systems making it unreliable to know the exact level of HCW generation, processing, and its effects [59].

Some key elements for improving healthcare waste management are

- Having a strong legal framework and guidelines.

- Spreading awareness towards risks associated with HCW and safe practices of its treatment and processing.

- Addressing responsibilities.
- Proper and sufficient resource allocation.
- Opting for safe and sound, environment-friendly HCW management options.
- Building a comprehensive system for handling, processing, and disposal.
- Protecting people from hazards when collecting, handling, storing, transporting, treating, or disposing of waste.
- Long-term planning for gradual and sustained improvements.
- Government commitment and support to local bodies and both public and private players involved in waste management.
- Incentives for best practices and performance.
- Universal cooperation and sharing of knowledge and technology.

11. Conclusions

The problem of HCW management in general and hazardous and nonbiodegradable portion thereof is too big to be ignored or else it will boomerang into something, which will be very difficult to manage. Though, at first sight, it does not look that severe a close analysis reveals that it is one of the major sources of greenhouse gas emission and comprehensively affects all the components of the environment and contributes to global warming. One of the serious aspects of HCW is its threat to the health of humans and animals as a good part of HCW contains infectious waste. The HCW contaminate the air, water, and soil of the surrounding environment releasing toxic substance like chemicals including heavy metals and radioactive substances, carcinogenic toxic gases like dioxin and furan, and causing many health issues not only in humans but also in animal species. The surrounding areas in dumping and processing sites are affected by these pollutants making them inhabitable. There is an urgent need for comprehensive research on the health hazards of HCW and measures to prevent them, processing of HCW and development of biomarkers for risk assessment of HCW, and a standard protocol for its processing that can be made mandatory to be followed by HCI. Unless there are universal consensus and framework for dealing with HCW the problem will not be solved. The healthcare industry needs to adopt eco-friendly approaches and operations and initiate whatever it takes to really become a health care provider and not itself become a threat to the health of living and nonliving environment by indiscriminate toxic HCW generation. Measures like extensive awareness and training programs, setting up environment-friendly hospitals, and avoiding single-use materials should be undertaken. Refuse, reduce, reuse, recycle, recover, and dispose should be the governing principles of HCW management. With collective responsibility, sincerity and honest efforts the menace of HCW in general and nonbiodegradable in specific can be not only controlled but contained for good of the environment in general and human health in specific.

Author details

Deepak S. Khobragade
Datta Meghe College of Pharmacy, Datta Meghe Institute of Medical Sciences, Wardha, India

*Address all correspondence to: ksdeepak31@gmail.com

References

[1] McMichael AJ, Woodruff RE, Hales S. Climate change and human health: Present and future risks. Lancet. 2006;**367**(9513):859-869. DOI: 10.1016/S0140-6736(06)68079-3

[2] Available from: https://www.aamc.org/news-insights/hospitals-race-save-patients-and-planet. [Accessed: February 21, 2022]

[3] Available from: https://www.who.int/news-room/fact-sheets/detail/health-care-waste. [Accessed: February 21, 2022]

[4] Giusti L. A review of waste management practices and their impact on human health. Waste Management. 2009;**29**(8):2227-2239. DOI: 10.1016/j.wasman.2009.03.028

[5] Srinivasa Chary, V,(2001), "Medical Waste Management Practices in urban India and Strategies for safe disposal, Proceedings of Southern Regional Conference on Biomedical Waste Management" Chennai, Tamilnadu

[6] Taghipour H, Mosaferi M. Characterization of medical waste from hospitals in Tabriz, Iran. The Science of the Total Environment. 2009;**407**(5):1527-1535. DOI: 10.1016/j.scitotenv.2008.11.032

[7] Lekwot VE, Nunyi BV, Ifeanyi E, Adamu OCI, B. Public health implication of improper hospital waste disposal in Zonkwa district of Zangon-kataf Local Government Area, Kaduna State. Journal of Research in Environmental Science and Toxicology. 2012;**1**(2):023-028

[8] Santappa M, Kumar VR. Hospital Waste Management Committee and Salient features of biomedical wastes, Proceedings of Southern Regional Conference on Biomedical Waste Management Chennai, India. 2002

[9] Ansari M, Ehrampoush MH, Farzadkia M, Ahmadi E. Dynamic assessment of economic and environmental performance index and generation, composition, environmental and human health risks of hospital solid waste in developing countries; A state of the art of review. Environment International. 2019;**2019**:132

[10] Patwary MA, O'Hare WT, Street G, Elahi KM, Hossain SS, Sarker MH. Quantitative assessment of medical waste generation in the capital city of Bangladesh. Waste Management. 2009;**29**:2392-2397. DOI: 10.1016/j.wasman.2009.03.021

[11] Pruss A, Giroult E, Rushbrook P. Safe Management of Wastes from Health-Care Activities. Geneva, Switzerland: World Health Organization; 1999

[12] Mbongwe B, Mmereki BT, Magashula A. Healthcare waste management: Current practices in selected healthcare facilities, Botswana. Waste Management. 2008;**28**:226-233

[13] Canadian Senate Committee. Part VII: Financing reform. In: The Health of Canadians. Ottawa, ON, Canada: Parliament of Canada; 2002

[14] Minoglou M, Gerassimidou S, Komilis D. Healthcare waste generation worldwide and its dependence on socio-economic and environmental factors. Sustainability. 2017;**9**:220

[15] Available from: https://news.yale.edu/2019/08/02/healthcare-industry-major-source-harmful-emissions

[16] Chung JW, Meltzer DO. Estimate of the Carbon Footprint of the US Health Care Sector. JAMA. 2009;**302**(18):1970-1972. DOI: 10.1001/jama.2009.1610

[17] Available from: https://worldpopulationreview.com/country-rankings/carbon-footprint-by-country

[18] Karliner J, Slotterback S. Health care's climate footprint, How The Health Sector Contributes To The Global Climate Crisis And Opportunities For Action Produced in collaboration with Arup . 2019. Available from: https://noharm-global.org/sites/default/files/documents-files/5961/HealthCaresClimateFootprint_092319.pdf

[19] Available from: https://echalliance.com/hospitals-produce-tonnes-of-plastic-waste-annually-how-can-they-reduce-this/

[20] Mercer C. How health care contributes to climate change. CMAJ. 2019;**191**(14):E403-E404. DOI: 10.1503/cmaj.109-5722

[21] Available from: https://www.cdc.gov/climateandhealth/effects/default.htm

[22] Available from: https://www.dhs.wisconsin.gov/chemical/carbondioxide.htm#:~:text=Exposure%20to%20CO2%20can%20produce,coma%2C%20asphyxia%2C%20and%20convulsions

[23] World Health Organization. WHO Guideline on the Use of Safety-Engineered Syringes for Intramuscular, Intradermal and Subcutaneous Injections in Health Care Settings. Geneva: World Health Organization; 2016

[24] Available from: https://www.who.int/medical_devices/Sun_pm_SAF_2_ALLEGRANZI.pdf

[25] Ilyas S, Srivastav RR, Kim H. Disinfection technology and strategies for COVID-19 hospital and bio-medical waste management. Total Environment. 2020;**2020**:749

[26] Kumar R, Khan EA, et al. Healthcare Waste Management (Hcwm) in Pakistan: Current Situation And Training Options. JAMC. 2010;**22**(4):101-105

[27] Joana C, Ana LP, Silva P, Walker TR, Duarte AC, Teresa RS. COVID-19 pandemic repercussions on the use and management of plastics. Environmental Science & Technology. 2020;**54**(13):7760-7765. DOI: 10.1021/acs.est.0c02178

[28] Tsai WT. Analysis of medical waste management and impact analysis of COVID-19 on its generation in Taiwan. Waste Management Research. 2021;**39**(1_suppl):27-33

[29] Subrammani T, Anitha P, Sekar S. Health-care waste management system. International Journal of Engineering Research and Applications. 2014;**4**(6):255-258

[30] Al Raisi SAH, Sulaiman H, Suliman FE, Abdallah O. Assessment of heavy metals in leachate of an unlined landfill in the sultanate of Oman. International Journal of Environmental Science and Development;**5**(1):60-63

[31] Oluseyi T, Adetunde O, Amadi E. Impact assessment of dumpsites on quality of near-by soil and underground water: A case study of an abandoned and a functional dumpsite in Lagos, Nigeria. International Journal of Science, Environment and Technology. 2014;**3**(3):1004-1015

[32] Kanmani S, Gandhimathi R. Assessment of heavy metal contamination in soil due to leachate migration from an open dumping site.

Applied Water. Science. 2013;**3**(1): 193-205

[33] Heera S, Rajor A. Bacterial treatment and metal characterization of biomedical waste ash. Journal of Waste Management. 2014;**2014**:1-7

[34] Gautam A, Pathak G, SahniA. Assessment of ground water quality at municipal solid waste dumping site-Sewapura, Jaipur. Current World Environment. 2006;**6**(2):279-282. DOI: 10.12944/CWE.6.2.12

[35] Fernández-Luqueño F. Heavy metal pollution in drinking water - a global risk for human health: A review. African Journal of Environmental Science and Technology. 2013;**7**(7):567-584. DOI: 10.5897/AJEST12.197

[36] Ali H, Khan E, Ilahi I. Environmental chemistry and ecotoxicology of hazardous heavy metals: Environmental persistence, toxicity, and bioaccumulation. Journal of Chemistry. 2019. Article ID: 6730305. DOI: 10.1155/2019/6730305

[37] Auta, T and. Morenikeji O. A . Heavy metal concentrations around a hospital incinerator and a municipal dumpsite in Ibadan City, South-West Nigeria. Journal of Applied Sciences and Environmental Management. 2013;**17**(3):419-422. DOI 10.4314/jasem.v17i3.11

[38] Adama M, Esena R, Mensah BF, Tawiah DY. Heavy metal contamination of soils around a hospital waste incinerator bottom ash dumps site. Journal of Environmental and Public Health. 2016, 2016:1-6. DOI: 10.1155/2016/8926453

[39] Agamuthu, P and. Fauziah S. H. Heavy metal pollution in landfill environment: A Malaysian case study; Bioinformatics and Biomedical Engineering (iCBBE); 4th International Conference; 2010; p. 1-4

[40] Abidemi O, Theresa OC. Environmental fate of heavy metals in soil of Ido-Osun waste dump site, Osogbo, Osun, Nigeria. American Journal of Environmental Protection. 2015;**3**(1):1-4. DOI: 10.12691/env-3-1-1

[41] Ali SM, Pervaiz A, Afzal B, Hamid N, Yasmin A. Open dumping of municipal solid waste and its hazardous impacts on soil and vegetation diversity at waste dumping sites of Islamabad city. Journal of King Saud University-Science. 2014;**26**(1):59-65. DOI: 10.1016/ j.jksus. 2013.08.003

[42] Amfo-Otu R, Kyerewaa SG, Ofori EA, andSadick. A. Comparative study of heavy metals in bottom ash from incinerators and open pit from healthcare facilities in Ghana. Octa Journal of Environmental Research. 2015;**3**(1):50-56

[43] Sabiha J, Tufail M, Khalid S. Heavy metal pollution from medical waste incineration at Islamabad and Rawalpindi, Pakistan. Microchemical Journal. 2008;**90**:77-81. DOI: 10.1016/j. microc.2008.03.010

[44] Allen RJ, Brenniman GR, Darling C. Air pollution emissions from the incineration of hospital waste. Journal of the Air Pollution Control Association. 1986;**36**:829-831. DOI: 10.5897/AJEST

[45] Coutinho M, Pereira M, Rodrigues R, Borrego C. Impact of medical waste incineration in the atmospheric PCDD/F levels of Porto, Portugal. Science of the Total Environment. 2006;**362**(1-3):157-165. DOI: 10.1016/j.scitotenv.2005.06.012

[46] Manzoor J, Sharma M. Impact of biomedical waste on environment and human health. Environmental Claims Journal. 2019;**31**(4):311-334. DOI: 10.1080/10406026.2019.1619265

[47] Vrijheid M. Health effects of residence near hazardous waste landfill sites: A review of epidemiologic literature. Environmental Health Perspectives. 2000;**108**(l):101-112. DOI: 10.2307/3454635

[48] Joshi HD. Health care waste management practice in Nepal. Journal of Nepal Health Research Council. 2013;**11**(23):102-108

[49] Ulutaş demir, N. et.al. The impacts of occupational risks and their effects on work stress levels of health professional (The sample from the Southeast region of Turkey). Environmental Health and Preventive Medicine. 2015;20(6):410-421. DOI: 10.1007/s12199-015-0481-3

[50] Karthikeyan S, Balasubramanian R, Iouri K. Particulate air pollution from bushfires: Human exposure and possible health effects. Journal of Toxicology and Environmental Health, Part. 2006;**A69**(21):1895

[51] Singh SK et al. Open dumping site and health risks to proximate communities in Mumbai, India: A cross-sectional case-comparison study. Clinical Epidemiology and Global Health. 2021;**9**:34-40. DOI: 10.1016/j.cegh.2020.06.008

[52] Adama M et al. Heavy metal contamination of soils around a hospital waste incinerator bottom ash dumps site. Journal of Environmental and Public Health. 2016;**2016**:6

[53] Njoku PO et al. Health and environmental risks of residents living close to a landfill: A Case Study of Thohoyandou Landfill, Limpopo Province, South Africa. International Journal of Environmental Research and Public Health. 2019;**16**:2125. DOI: 10.3390/ijerph16122125

[54] Balali-Mood M et al. Toxic mechanisms of five heavy metals: Mercury, lead, chromium, cadmium, and arsenic. Frontier in Pharmacology. 2021;**12**:643972. DOI: 10.3389/fphar.2021.643972

[55] Available from: https://silo.tips/download/waste-to-energy-in-denmark-christian-riber-ramboll-waste-to-energy

[56] Franka, E, El-Zoka H, Hussein A.H, Elbakosh M. M, Arafa, A. K and. Ghenghesh K. S. Hepatitis B virus and hepatitis C virus in medical waste handlers in Tripoli, Libya. Journal of Hospital Infection . 2009;72(3):258-261. DOI: 10.1016/j.jhin.2009.03.019

[57] Samuel CV, Yuen TS, Pilapitiya S. Municipal solid waste management in the Southern Province of Sri Lanka: Problems, issues and challenges. Waste Management. 2006;**26**(8):920-930

[58] Asase M, Yanful E, Mensah MM, Amponsah SK, Amponsah S. Comparison of municipal solid waste management systems in Canada and Ghana: A Case Study of the Cities of London. Ghana Waste Management. 2009;**29**(10):2779-2786. DOI: 10.1016/j.wasman.2009.06.019

[59] Mrayyan B, Hamdi MR. Management approaches to integrated solid waste in industrialized zones in Jordan: A Case of Zarqa City. Waste Management. 2006;**26**:195-205

[60] Seng B, Kaneko H, Hirayama K, Katayama-Hirayama K. Municipal solid waste management in Phnom Penh, capital city of Cambodia. Waste Management & Research. 2011;**29**(5):491-500

[61] Guerrero LA, Maas G, Hogland W. Solid waste management challenges for cities in developing countries. Waste Management. 2013;**33**(1):220-232. DOI: 10.1016/j.wasman.2012.09.008

[62] Zohoori M, Ghani A. Municipal solid waste management challenges and problems for cities in low-income and developing countries. International Journal of Science and Engineering Applications. 2017;**6**:39-48. DOI: 10.7753/IJSEA0602.1002

[63] Sharholy M, Ahmad K, Mahmood G, Trivedi RC. Municipal solid waste management in Indian cities – A review. Waste Management. 2008;**28**:459-467

[64] Kafeel MS, Vaishya RC, Gupta RD. Municipal solid waste characteristics and management in Allahabad, India. Waste Management. 2007;**27**(4):490-496

[65] Sujauddin MH, Hoque AT. Household solid waste characteristics and management in Chittagong, Bangladesh. Waste Managemnt. 2008;**28**(9):1688-1695. DOI: 10.1016/j.wasman.2007.06.013

[66] Hazra T, Goel S. Solid waste management in Kolkata, India: Practices and challenges. Waste Management. 2009;**29**:470-478. DOI: 10.1016/j.wasman.2008.01.023

[67] Moghadam M, Mokhtarani NR, Mokhtarani B. Municipal solid waste management in Rasht City, Iran. Waste Management. 2009;**29**:485-489. DOI: 10.1016/j.wasman.2008.02.029

[68] Henry RK et al. Municipal solid waste management challenges in developing Countries-Kenyan Case Study. Waste Management. 2006;**26**:92-100. DOI: 10.1016/j.wasman.2005.03.007

Section 4

Hormones Disturbance

Chapter 10

Endocrine Disruptors and Infertility

Selma Yazar

Abstract

Endocrine-disrupting chemicals (EDC) are known to interfere the body's endocrine system. EDCs can also be considered as industrial chemicals namely pesticides, cleaning materials, plastics, heavy metals, and cosmetics. Most of these compounds particularly at low doses, occurring in complex mixtures, have been reported as emerging contaminants. EDCs are currently present in environment (water, diet, food contact materials, personal care products, etc). The adverse effects of exposure to EDCs have already been extensively described such as infertility, cancers, disrupted thyroid function, neurological disorders, obesity, metabolic syndrome. EDCs may be blamed for increasing the human reproductive disorders especially infertility. This is a serious public health problem that should not be ignored. This chapter aims to summarize the major scientific advances in human infertility associated with exposure to EDCs with epidemiological and experimental evidence. The chemicals covered in this chapter are heavy metals (lead), pesticides (pyrethroids), and cosmetics (UV filters).

Keywords: endocrine disruptors, infertility, pesticides, heavy metal, cosmetics

1. Introduction

Industrialization and the development of technology make our lives easier, but they also bring negative effects on our health. Particularly, the reproductive health is the system most affected by these modern living conditions and environmental factors. In recent years, many environmental polluting chemicals have been shown to have the ability to interfere with the functioning of the body's hormone, which have been classified as endocrine-disrupting chemicals (EDCs). An EDC is defined by the United States Environmental Protection Agency (EPA) as, "an exogenous chemical substance or mixture that alters the structure or function(s) of the endocrine system and causes adverse effects at the level of the organism, its progeny, and populations or (sub)populations" [1–4].

These EDCs are extremely heterogeneous and can be divided into three groups;

1. Pharmaceuticals—(e.g., diethylstilbestrol, ethinyl oestradiol, naproxen, acetaminophen),

2. Natural and synthetics hormones—(e.g., phytoestrogens, 3-omegafatty acids; synthetic such as oral contraceptives).

3. Environmental EDCs—(e.g., polycyclic aromatic hydrocarbons, polybrominated diphenyl ethers heavy metals, pesticides, detergents, plasticizers, solvents, dioxin and cosmetics) [5, 6].

EDCs have been by far the biggest focus due to their widespread use and wide exposure. The major route of human exposure to these chemicals is through ingestion of contaminated water and food (e.g., meat, fish, dairy products, and vegetables), *via* inhalation, and through the skin. These chemicals are easily released into the environment for example through leaching into the soil and water. Some EDCs (such as some organochlorine pesticides, polychlorinated biphenyl, biphenol-A, phthalates, heavy metals) are known as persistent organic pollutants due to their high lipophilicity. These substances pass into the systemic circulation, can be metabolized to compounds that are more toxic than the parent chemicals, and are potentially eliminated through pathways such as urine, semen, and breast milk [6–9].

EDCs include different groups of chemicals such as persistent organic pollutants, industrial compounds, children's products (containing lead, phthalates, cadmium), food contact materials (e.g., bisphenol A, phthalates, linings of cans, or plastic bottles containing phenol), pesticides, chemical substances that are widely used in cosmetics such as phthalates, ultraviolet (UV) filter constituents, and parabens, as well as several heavy metals, polybrominated diphenyl ethers that are flame retardants used in agriculture, and many household and industrial products [2, 8].

Most EDCs have the potential to markedly affect the development of the steroid hormone dependent human reproductive system. EDCs can interfere with the normal secretion, synthesis, production, metabolism, transport, or effect of hormones. EDCs can alter cellular processes by different mechanisms, by binding to steroid hormone nuclear receptors and activating genomic and non-genomic pathways, activating ion channels, inducing proinflammatory cytokines and chemokines, promoting oxidative stress, and altering cell proliferation and differentiation [7, 8]. EDCs may contain a large number of molecules capable of inducing estrogenic or antiandrogenic effects. They may mimic the sex hormones estrogen or androgen or they may block the activities of estrogen or androgen. (i.e., be antiestrogens or antiandrogens) [4, 5, 10]. EDCs can indirectly produce an estrogenic response by a number of different mechanisms, such as increasing estrogen synthesis (e.g., peroxisome proliferators inducing aromatase activity, thus increasing circulating estradiol levels), facilitating estrogen receptor binding, or altering the estrogen ratio. Estrogens are a group of chemicals of similar structure primarily responsible for female reproduction but the existence of estrogen in men has been known for over 90 years. However, our knowledge of the general role of estrogens in the male reproductive and non-reproductive organs is clearly far behind that in females. In addition, exposure to exogenous estrogens, especially developmentally, has recently been shown to have deleterious effects on the male reproductive system in men [11, 12].

Estrogens are mainly produced by the ovaries, but also by the adrenal glands and adipose tissue. Estradiol is most potent member of the class of steroid hormones produced primarily by the ovaries [11, 13]. For instance, in either sex, androgens give rise to estrogens, through aromatase, so together they play a vital role in homoeostasis. In addition, EDCs can exert an antiestrogenic effect by preventing endogenous estrogens from interacting with their receptors and thus inhibiting their action. In general, estrogenic compounds promote the development of female sexual characteristics; antiestrogens inhibit the development of female characteristics, but not necessarily male characteristics [7, 13].

It is well known that chemicals interfering with hormonal pathways can seriously affect human reproductive disorders such as infertility, endometriosis, breast cancer, testicular cancer, poor sperm quality, and/or function [5, 6, 9, 14]. A growing body of scientific evidence indicates that reproductive health, and ultimately reproductive capacity, is under pressure globally. Unfortunately, relatively few studies have addressed the impact of environmental exposures on human reproductive function. It has been reported that the number of families applying to infertility clinics to have a child with the assisted reproductive techniques has increased significantly in recent years [4, 8, 15]. Infertility is defined as "a disease characterized by the failure to establish a clinical pregnancy after 12 months of regular and unprotected sexual intercourse." It affects 10–15% of all couples and varies between countries and geographic regions. Idiopathic infertility accounts for approximately 44% of male infertility cases and is the most common individual diagnosis [3, 16, 17].

The current chapter discusses the detrimental effects of EDCs exposure on male/female infertility, by providing an overview of experimental studies on humans and by reporting epidemiological studies in humans. The present section will focus on the relationship between hormone disruptors and female infertility. Specifically, pesticides pyrethroids, heavy metal such as lead as well as commonly used cosmetics like UV filters will be discussed.

2. Male infertility

The psychological, social, and economic consequences of reduced male capacity to have children are often severe and extend beyond individuals to entire families and society at large. The previously discussed subject of decline in male fertility is no longer controversial because many studies over the past 10 years have shown a decrease in semen quality [4, 17–19]. EDCs affect the maturation, function, and viability of sperm by acting directly on the sperm or altering the function of the epididymis as well as the sperm's ability to fertilize an egg. In normal human males, the number of sperm is close to what is normally required for fertility. While acute exposure can cause significant changes in spermatogenesis, it appears to occur with low-dose, chronic exposures to EDCs that impair spermatogenesis [5, 17, 20]. Therefore, even a small decrease in daily sperm production can cause infertility. Semen parameters are used to measure sperm quality and they are very important because they can be used to predict male infertility [5, 20]. However, for many reason, semen may be the least understood body fluid in terms of the distribution of its normal values in the general population. Since it is difficult to obtain semen fluid, men are not included in the study, therefore not many studies can be conducted to reveal the relationship between semen quality and chemical substances [21].

About 15% of couples worldwide are infertile and half is the male factor. Male infertility is considered as primary cause of infertility in 20% of couples and a contributing factor in 30–40% of cases. Infertility is caused by changes in the hypothalamic-pituitary-gonadal (HPG) axis or by direct effects on sperm and other semen parameters [4, 17]. Men with sperm parameters below the values specified in WHO are considered to have male factor infertility. The most important of these are low sperm concentration (oligospermia), poor sperm motility (asthenospermia), and abnormal sperm morphology (teratospermia). Other factors less correlated with infertility include semen volume and other seminal markers [15].

In a large review of international studies conducted by authors, it is reported that the average sperm count in men decreased from 113 million/mL to 66 million/mL and significant anomalies in sperm morphology/motility in 50 years (1940–1990) in the world [7, 22].

Sperm function is affected by reactive oxygen species (ROS) produced during the metabolism of these chemicals, which is another possible effect of infertility including EDCs. Oxidative stress plays an important role in the mechanism of male infertility. Oxidative stress is a balance between the production of ROS and the natural antioxidant defense of semen. Increased ROS levels can be due to many factors such as environmental pollutants and lifestyle factors [23, 24].

The effect of EDCs in testicles is mediated mainly by the nuclear estrogen receptors (ESR1 and ESR2) expressed by Sertoli and germ cells. These cells secrete masculinizing hormones that regulate sperm production, [6, 10, 25]. Because hormones tightly control the male reproductive system, anti-androgens or EDCs that mimic estrogens can interfere with spermatogenesis and have a profound effect on healthy sperm production [16]. Men exposed to estrogenic EDCs may reduce fertility and develop female secondary sex characteristics such as gynecomastia [13].

Different mechanisms of action related to the hormone-disrupting effects of pesticides are discussed, but the most common mention is the interaction with the recognition and binding of reproductive hormone receptors. Most EDCs are substances with estrogenic/anti-androgenic activity that act by interfering with the estrogen receptors (ER) or the androgen receptor (AR), which are commonly found in male reproductive tissues [26, 27]. For the last been, it has focused on the estrogenic effect of EDCs and it has been determined that many substances are "environmental estrogens." It is though that increased exposure to estrogens not only causes prenatal testicular damage, but may also contributes to postpartum inhibition of testicular function and spermatogenesis. Environmental estrogens affect fetal development by inhibiting the development of Sertoli cells, which determine the lifetime capacity of sperm production. These estrogens can also inhibit enzymes in testosterone synthesis and directly affect testosterone production [28–30].

2.1 Heavy metal (LEAD-Pb)

Rapid industrialization and over-growing urbanization and the toxic effects of heavy metals on the male reproductive system have become an important public health all over the world. Reproductive problems in males due to metal exposure are one of the most important areas of concern in toxicology [31]. In epidemiological and clinical studies, it has been found to be associated with impaired semen quality as a result of the direct effect of heavy metals on testicular function or hormonal changes. One of the heavy metals of greatest concern is lead (Pb). Lead exposure can cause toxicity to both the male and female reproductive systems. Pb is a natural compound and is regularly used in mining, smelting, refining, leaded gasoline (petrol), lead-acid batteries, paints, jewelry, children's products, and many other products. The general population is exposed to Pb through contaminated food and water and inhalation of airborne Pb. Lead in seminal plasma may increase with environmental pollutions, and industrial and dietary exposure [6, 32, 33].

In toxicology studies, it is argued that the determination of heavy metal levels in the seminal fluid may better indicate exposure, due to the accumulation of these substances in the male reproductive organs, rather than the determination of heavy metal levels in the blood [31, 32]. At low levels of occupational exposure in smelting industry workers, lead has been associated with reduced semen concentration, motility, and viability. Heavy metals cause toxicity by affecting the HPG axis, testicular function, spermatogenesis, and steroidogenic processes either directly or through the endocrine system [17, 31, 34].

Strong evidences confirm that male infertility in metal-exposed humans is mediated *via* various mechanisms such as production of reactive oxygen species (ROS). It is known that smoking causes oxidative stress by increasing oxidant levels or decreasing antioxidant levels in seminal plasma [34, 35]. Kiziler et al. [35] investigated Pb levels in blood and seminal plasma of the infertile and fertile groups. Pb levels in seminal plasma and blood were significantly higher in infertile men than those in fertile groups. It was revealed that sperm count, motility, and morphology were significantly decreased in infertile smokers than in non-smoker infertile and fertile men. He et al. [36] investigated whether oxidative stress is an intermediate mediator in regulating the associations between heavy metal exposure and impaired semen quality. A significant inverse relationship was found between Pb exposure and the percentage of normal sperm morphology [36], and a negative correlation was detected with the sperm count and motility [37]. Lead levels of non-occupational lead exposure in 341 infertile men were investigated by Wu et al. [32]. The research results showed a significant inverse correlation between the lead concentration in seminal plasma and the sperm count. These results showed a negatively correlation with standard semen parameters and biomarkers of sperm function. Therefore, the authors postulate that unexplained male infertility may be due to increased Pb levels [38].

It is known that semen quality has an effect on sperm motility, which is one of the most important factors in infertility [39]. Sperm motility depends on the synchronized movements proteins, sugars, ions, and small organic molecules. It is one of the main factors that facilitate the journey of sperm toward the egg and the subsequent fertilization process. Defects in sperm motility are a common reason for infertility in humans [34]. Li et al. [40] examined the positively relationship between increased blood Pb levels and low semen quality. Li et al. [41] also found a negative correlation between Pb concentrations and sperm motility. Therefore, authors suggest that among the semen parameters, sperm motility can be a sensitive indicator of semen quality.

It has been reported that 90% of male infertility problems are related to sperm count, and there is also a positive relationship between sperm count and semen parameters [15]. Famurewa and Ugwuja [42] found that seminal plasma Pb was significantly ($p < 0.05$) higher in oligospermic and normospernic men than in azospermic men. Significant inverse associations ($p < 0.01$) were found between blood lead and sperm count.

In conclusion, lead shows its effect on reproductive hormones by changing the reproductive hormone axis and hormonal control over spermatogenesis rather than having a direct toxic effect on the seminiferous tubules of testicles [43]. The overall results of these studies indicate that even considerably low levels of blood and seminal plasma Pb might reduce the human semen quality, it potentially reduces male fertility; however, more infertility studies are needed to show that lead has a direct effect on male infertility [42].

2.2 Pyrethroids

The most widely used group among pesticides is the group of synthetic pyrethroids. General population exposure to pyrethroids can occur primarily through dietary residues and inhalation or ingestion of contaminated house dust after indoor application. Because of high performance and low toxicity of pyrethroids, these chemicals are widely used both in agriculture and at home as a substitute for organochlorine insecticides [44, 45]. In recent years, hormone disruptors such as pyrethroids have been discussed with studies showing the male infertility relationship [28, 29]. It is suggested that pyrethroids can cross the blood testicular barrier, reach the nucleus of spermatogenetic cells, and affect sperm function, due to their hydrophobic and small molecular structure. Although associations between occupational exposure to pyrethroids and altered semen quality are generally reported, there are limited epidemiological data on the potential effects of non-occupational exposure to pyrethroids on male reproductive function [44]. In recent years, studies have reported that pyrethroid pesticides can reduce sperm count and motility, change sperm morphology, increase abnormal sperm count, cause sperm DNA damage, and also affect sex hormone levels [46–49]. It is emphasized that these findings may be of particular concern for male infertility due to increased use of pyrethroids and widespread human exposure. As a result, it is reported that these substances play an important role in reproductive toxicity [45].

The number of environmental pollutants such as pyrethroids determined to have anti-androgenic effects is increasing day by day. However, recently the relationship between androgenic/antiandrogenic effects of these substances and male infertility has been discussed [28, 29, 50, 51]. Androgens, like testosterone, are steroid hormones essential for normal male reproductive development and function and play a very important role in spermatogenesis, in adulthood [52]. Androgenes belong to the steroid superfamily and are mainly involved in gonadal development. Androgens are present in different levels in both men and women [27]. The differentiation of the male reproductive system depends on fetal testicular androgen production. In addition, disruption estrogen exposure in the fetal period may cause reproductive abnormalities by disrupting the sensitive androgen-estrogen balance [7, 27]. Anti-androgenic pyrethroids interfere with the androgen receptor signaling pathway by interacting with androgen receptors [51]. In recent years, cypermethrin, deltamethrin, fenvalarate, bifenthrin, permethrin, lambda cyholothrin, cyfluthrin are the most used pyrethroids in many countries, and the anti-androgenic effect of these substances has been reported [53–59]. Therefore, the identification of these chemicals is very important in many fields, including food production, reproductive toxicology, and risk assessment [57]. Although it has been suggested that some pyrethroids act as androgen receptor antagonists, more studies are needed to determine the mechanisms underlying the antagonism [50].

As a result of exposure to pyrethroids in different ways, it has been shown that these substances are rapidly metabolized in human by hydrolytic cleavage of the ester bond followed by oxidation [60]. Because of the rapid metabolism of pyrethroids, determination of their urinary metabolities is preferred for the estimation of pyrethroid exposures. 3-phenoxybenzoic acid (3-PBA) is a general metabolite of many pyrehroids (cypermethrin deltamethrin, permethrin, and others) and is a metabolite with the highest rate in non-occupational exposure. Therefore, determination of this metabolite in urine may indicate environmental exposure to different pyrethroids [44, 60]. In the literature, there are not many studies on the infertility relationship of anti-androgenic pyrethroids/metabolites [28, 29, 44, 46, 61]. In infertility studies, exposure to non-persistent pyrethroid metabolities has been associated with changes in reproductive hormones in men [62], as well as decreased semen quality and increased sperm DNA damage due to urinary metabolities of pyrethroid insecticides [29, 44, 63]. Han et al. [60] found an association between serum hormone levels and urinary 3PBA levels (between 3-BPA and LH and E2 hormones), in infertile men, as result of their investigation. The detrimental effect of pesticides such as pyrethroids on sperm concentration, motility, and morphology may result from impaired spermatogenesis due to various hormonal changes [64]. The information provided by examining sperm morphology in a complete semen analysis is becoming increasingly important clinically for infertility and fertility [65]. Abnormal sperm morphology due to secretory dysfunction of Leydig and Sertoli cells impairs sperm fertilization capacity. Sperm parameters such as sperm concentration, sperm motility, and sperm morphology are related to each other. The factors that cause deterioration in any of these parameters generally affect the others. It is reported that the best indicator of infertility is sperm concentration after sperm motility [64, 66]. More studies are needed to better elucidate the effects of exposure to potential endocrine-disrupting pyrethroid pesticides on semen parameters.

2.3 Cosmetics (UV filters)

Cosmetics include all non-pharmaceutical substances consumed or applied to improve personal health, hygiene, or appearance. These products contain many components such as phthalates, parabens, UV filters, polycylic musks, antimicrobials, formaldehyde, which are used different purposes. In addition, many cosmetic products contain heavy metals such as lead, cadmium, antimony, chromium, arsenic, mercury, nickel as ingredient or impurities [18, 67]. The main route of exposure is through the skin and through inhalation. The main endpoint of exposure is endocrine disruption. This is because of the many substances in cosmetics and UV filters that have endocrine active properties that affect directly damaging the testicular tissue. Recently, Peterson et al. [18] investigated the cosmetic exposure and associations with measures of semen quality in young Danish men. Despite the widespread use of multiple products, they found little an association with semen quality.

UV filters are used not only in cosmetic products such as skin lotion, beauty creams, lipsticks, and hair sprays, but also as additives in plastics, printing inks, shampoos, perfumes, and other products. Although UV filters are applied to the body surface, there is information that they are absorbed, metabolized, bio accumulated, and/or excreted from the skin. There is not much information about the metabolism of the UV filter in humans in the literature [68–70].

UV filters are new environmental pollutants that could potentially affect a large proportion of the population [71]. Men's exposure to these substances is likely due to contact with products containing these chemicals [72]. In fact, *in vitro* and *in vivo* studies in different species of mammals showed that some of these UV filters exhibit hormonal activity and are able to interact with estrogen, androgen, and thyroid signaling [68]. However, epidemiological studies on the relationship between hormone-disrupting effects of organic UV filters and infertility are very limited. Therefore, more research is needed to determine the health risks of these substances [73]. Frederiksen et al. [72] investigated the degree of exposure of human spermatozoa to UV filters in Danish men. They found that almost half of the men had measurable concentrations in their seminal fluid of at least one of the selected UV filters.

In recent studies, the mechanism of action of UV filters on sperm has been evaluated. Some processes in sperm depend on calcium ion channels opened in the cell membrane. CatSper ion channel, which is specifically expressed in spermatozoa, controls intracellular Ca2+ concentration and sperm motility. CatSper activation mediates an increase in intracellular Ca2+ levels in the sperm tail. The presence of an inactive CatSper protein in male mice has been reported to cause infertility [74, 75]. Schiffer et al. [74] investigated the effect of 96 different EDCs including UV filters (4-MBC, BP3, 3-BC, HMS, OD-PABA) on human sperm. Researchers reported that structurally diverse EDCs activate the sperm-specific CatSper channel, thereby inducing intracellular Ca2+ increase, motility response, and acrosomal exocytosis. Rehfeld et al. [76] also revealed that organic UV filters have been shown to induce a Ca2+ influx through CatSper. As a result, authors argue that EDCs (selected UV filters) interfere with various sperm functions and thus may impair human fertility. Sperm cell dysfunction is a common cause of infertility. Progesterone is a known inducer of acrosomal reaction in sperm cells, and suboptimal induction of acrosomal reaction in response to progesterone is correlated with fertility. Rehfeld et al. [77] examined the effects of organic UV filters on the human sperm cell function acrosomal reaction, sperm penetration into a viscous medium and hyperactivation, as well as on sperm viability. The result of these study showed that selected UV filters mimic the effects of progesterone on the activation of the CatSper Ca2+ channel in human spermatozoa.

Adoamnei et al. [78] investigated whether there are associations between urinary concentrations of BP-type UV filters and semen quality and reproductive hormone levels in young men. They found a significant positive association between urinary BP-type (BP1 and BP3) concentrations and some reproductive hormones (FSH, T/E2). They suggest that further research is needed in other male populations. When the relationship between semen parameters and reproductive hormones is evaluated in other studies with BP-type UV filters, it is reported that there is a significant relationship [79] and found no association between urinary concentrations of BP3 and idiopathic male infertility [80]. As a result, human exposure to these organic UV filters can interfere with sperm and impair fertility.

3. Female infertility

EDCs are thought to affect women's menstrual cycle, estrogen deficiency, infertility, and are also associated with diseases such as polycystic ovary syndrome (PCOS) and endometriosis, spontaneous abortions, birth defects, endometriosis, breast cancer, premature ovarian failure [23, 25]. Female are at a greater risk than men, especially with the rise in environmental estrogens. However, since research on these exposures often tends to focus on male fertility, it is unlikely that EDCs will answer questions about female fertility [25, 81]. Because females are relatively sensitive to estrogens and are heavily exposed to environmental estrogens, women will also be most affected by EDCs. The origin of endocrine disruption hypothesis was related to exposure to estrogens. Literature data also show that long-term and combined exposure to environmental estrogens will have an impact on female fertility. Although it has long been known that female fertility is impaired by estrogen exposure, there are limited data on whether long-term low-dose exposure to environmental pollutants with weak estrogenic effect causes problems such as infertility in women [81].

There is little epidemiological information about trends in female infertility. Data on the effects of EDCs on the female reproductive system and fertility are insufficient. However, it has been suggested that there is a relationship between exposure to EDCs and their long-term effects [7, 81].

The most common direct or indirect causes of female infertility are endocrine problems. EDCs alter endocrine function through various mechanisms. One of these mechanisms is that these substances directly bind to estrogen receptors and increase aromatase activity, thereby increasing estrogen sensitivity. Another mechanism is that EDCs indirectly lead to an increase in endogenous estrogen production and exert their effects through both receptor-dependent and receptor-independent mechanisms through their effects on gonadotropin-releasing hormone. Both mechanisms result in altered ovarian function by altering endocrine signaling with several processes in ovary and the other reproductive organs [3, 33, 82].

EDCs act on female reproductive hormones and receptors through estrogenic, anti-estrogenic, androgenic, and anti-androgenic mechanisms [23, 25]. Estradiol (E2) plays a very important role in female fertility. The functions of estrogens are mediated primarily by two estrogen receptors: ESR1 (ERalfa) and ESR2 (ERbeta), both of which are widely expressed in cells throughout the female reproductive system [83]. Most EDCs interfere with female reproductive function by activating or inhibiting ESRs. EDCs have different binding affinities to ESRs and therefore exert different effects in ovary. In ovary, the main function of ESR1 is to regulate steroidogenesis in theca cells. On the other hand, the function of ESR2 is granulosa cell differentiation toward FSH, follicle maturation, and ovulation. Many EDCs interfere with female reproductive function by activating or inhibiting ESRs. Different EDCs exert different effects in the ovary depending on their binding affinity to different ESRs [82, 83].

The sensitivity of the developing female reproductive system to estrogens raises the question of whether exposure to EDCs with estrogenic activity (such as heavy metals, pesticides, and cosmetics) can affect the female fertility [81].

3.1 Heavy metal (LEAD-Pb)

Lead is known to be one of potential female reproductive toxins. However, there are few studies on whether low Pb exposure causes female infertility compared with male infertility. Lead is a potent disruptor of adrenal and ovarian steroidogenesis and inhibits progesterone synthesis and activity in dose-dependent manner. The effects of lead on 17-β-estradiol, testosterone, and cortisol may cause stimulant effects after low-level exposure, while inhibiting effects after high-level exposure. Exposure to Pb causes impaired fertility in women, two key proteins in the function of the pituitary-ovarian axis. Both P-450 aromatase and ER-β-activity in granulosa cells of ovarian follicles have been shown to be strongly inhibited in women exposed to Pb [84–86].

It is known that Pb can concentrate, impair cellular processes, and cause harmful results in terms of reproductive health. Lee et al. [85] found that low blood lead level was positively associated with infertile women. It has been suggested that even low blood lead levels may be detrimental to female fertility. Silberstein et al. [87] compared lead levels in blood and follicular fluid from nine patients undergoing IVF treatment. Lead levels in follicular fluid were found to be significantly higher in non-pregnant patients compared with pregnant patients. The results of this study show that high concentrations of lead negatively affect female fertility [87]. Another researcher investigated the association between blood concentrations of Pb and risk factors for infertile or pregnant women in Taiwan. The concentration of Pb was significantly higher in the blood of infertile women than in that of pregnant women. Particularly, frequent use of Chinese herbal medicine by infertile women has been associated with elevated blood Pb levels. It is suggested that the risk-benefit of Chinese herbal medicine intake should be evaluated by women of childbearing age [88].

With the increase in the female workforce of more women in Pb production in developing countries, more women are exposed to potential reproductive hazards. In a study by Tang and Zhu [89], it was shown that Pb causes reproductive toxicity and female infertility as a result of occupational exposure (lead battery plants). In this study, it was observed that the menstrual cycle, that is, the hormonal balance of female workers exposed to lead was disturbed [89]. On the other hand, Gerhard et al. [90] investigated whether the urinary heavy metal excretion is associated with different factors of infertility. They found that accumulation of heavy metals in the ovary disturbs the production of estradiol and progesterone. The study by Srivastava et al. [91] also supports that pubertal women exposed to low levels of lead maternally have suppressed levels of both luteinizing hormone (LH) and estradiol (E2). Maternal Pb exposure changes only LH, not FSH secretion.

Endometriosis affects 10% of women of childbearing age and causes infertility in about half of these women. Recently, it has been reported that exposure to EDCs is associated with endometriosis [7]. Tanrıkut et al. [92] determined the role of endometrial concentrations of heavy metals including Pb in the unexplained infertility. Lead levels were detected in 15 and 3% of 33 infertile and 32 fertile women, respectively. Further population-based studies are needed to determine the reproductive toxicity of low-level Pb exposure [85].

3.2 Pyrethroids

Although *in vitro* and experimental animal studies show that pyrethroids may affect ovarian function, epidemiological studies in this direction are scarce. Since pyretroids are rapidly metabolized in mammals, their toxicity is reported to be very limited [93, 94]. Marettova et al. [93] reviewed the effect of pyrethroids on female reproductive system. *In vitro* and experimental animal studies have shown that pyrethroids can inhibit female endocrine functions. It has been determined that pyrethroids such as fenvalarate, deltamethrin, and cypermethrin cause morphometric and structural changes in female genital organs. It has been determined that the negative effect of toxic substances on the ovary may be caused by decreased gonadotropin secretion, impaired follicular growth, or enzymatic interaction, which may lead to decreased sex steroid hormone synthesis. As a result, it has been reported that pyrethroids/metabolities may impair the structure and function of female reproductive organs [93].

Women are normally exposed to estrogen, but the effects of ECDs on women are more difficult to monitor due to the large differences in the estrogen cycle and circulating hormone concentrations during different phases of the cycle. The presence of estrogen-mimicking compounds in adult women can interfere with natural hormone cycles, impairing reproductive capacity, potentially making women unable to conceive, or maintaining a pregnancy [5]. If fertilization does not occur or pregnancy does not occur, the corpus luteum undergoes a process of cell death known as luteolysis or corpus luteum regression. Disruption of the process of folliculogenesis and corpus luteum formation leads to adverse reproductive outcomes such as anovulation, infertility, decreased fertility, estrogen deficiency, and premature ovarian failure (POF). The POF is one of the mechanisms leading to female infertility [82, 95]. Anti-Mullerian hormone (AMH) is a marker of ovarian reserve. Whitworth et al. [96] investigated the relationship between residential spraying pyrethroid exposure and

AMH levels in African women. The authors reported that pyrethroids reduce the level of AMH, one of the predictors of female fertility. In another non-occupational exposure study in Chinese women, a positive correlation was found between increased urinary 3-PBA concentration and FSH and LH levels, and a negative correlation between AMH and 3-PBA [97]. Hu et al. [98] researched the effects of preconception exposure pyrethroids on gestational duration and infertility in the general population of couples planning to conceive in China. They found that the urinary 3-PBA concentrations in the highest quartile were correlated with longer time to pregnancy and infertility in women.

These limited study data highlight that this may be of concern due to the increasing use of pyrethroids causing non-occupational exposure among the general population and the lack of epidemiological studies.

3.3 Cosmetics (UV filters)

Residues of UV filters were also studies biological samples such as urine, breast milk, placenta, plasma, fetal cord blood, semen, and tissues [99–102]. Considering the chronic toxic effects of UV filters in terms of both their residual values and their hormone-disrupting effects, there are serious warnings in the literature. In particular, there are studies showing that organic UV filters, called "environmental estrogens-endocrine disruptors," have estrogenic and antiandrogenic activity as much as other industrial chemicals [69, 103]. Recent studies dealing with organic UV filters are mostly focused on their effect on endocrine damage. Wang et al. [68] reviewed the potential endocrine disruptors of typical UV filters including benzophenones (BPs), camphor derivatives, and cinnamate derivatives.

It has been shown that there is statistically significant relationship between exposure to endocrine-disrupting UV filters and estrogen-mediated diseases. Kunisue et al. [104] assessed the relationship between exposure to BPs and endometriozis. The association of urine concentrations of BPs with an increased probability of being diagnosed with endometriozis was studied in 600 women. Significant regional variations were found for 2OH-4MeO-BP and 2,4OH-BP urine concentrations, and monthly variations (higher concentrations in July and August) were determined based on female use. When these results are evaluated, it is reported that there may be a relationship between exposure to high 2,4OH-BP levels and endometriozsis, considering that 2,4OH-BP has a higher estrogenic activity than 2OH-4MeO-BP [104]. The most used group of UV filters is benzophenone (BP) and it has about 29 compounds. Considering the wide use of BPs in sunscreen and personal care products, as well as their estrogenic and antiandrogenic activities, BPs are reported to be a public health concern. Given the widespread use of UV filters, concerns have arisen about their potential impact on human health, including infertility [71]. Thus, further studies are needed to clarify associations between exposures to these chemicals.

Faass et al. [105] examined the pre- and postnatal effects of 4-MBC and 3-benzylidene camphor (3-BC) that are sunscreens with endocrine-disrupting properties, in rat and dog. It was observed that these UV filters disrupted female sex behaviors, estrus cycle, and gene expression of sex hormones in brain. Screening the data from this point of view, in rat exposed to endocrine-disrupturing UV filters in low doses, it was observed that these chemicals have an influence on the sexual behaviors and gene expression of sex hormones. In this study, it was additionally found that the difference is not so high when residual values of organic UV filters are compared with those in humans. It is obviously underlined that this could be a potential risk namely for women [105].

However, human data evaluating the effects of hormone disruptors of these substances are very limited and studies have been carried out recently. BP-3, which is a UV filter used in sunscreens and cosmetic products, has been detected in almost all individuals and not only during the summer season. Louis et al. [71] investigated the effects of 5 UV filters, which are most commonly used in sunscreen products and personal care products, and whose residues were detected in human urine samples, on the duration of conception. Urine samples were collected from 501 couples who stopped using contraceptives to become pregnant until they achieved pregnancy. The effect of five UV filters BP3 (its metabolites BP1, BP8), BP2, and 4-OH-BP on the duration of conception was evaulated. The results show that male exposure to selected UV filters (BP2 and 4-hydoxybenzophenone) can reduce couple's fertility, resulting in a longer time to pregnancy [71].

4. Conclusions

In general, it is being observed that the most important harmful effects of exposure to endocrine-disrupting environmental pollutants such as heavy metals, pesticides, and cosmetics are on the reproductive system in humans. Infertility is both clinical and social problems that affect the couple's life, health services, and social environment. With the awareness of these important issues, factors that increase the risk of infertility can be prevented. Further toxicological studies are needed to further understand the risk and mechanisms of action of these substances on male and especially female reproductive function, and to identify and characterize new EDCs.

Conflict of interest

The authors declare no conflict of interest.

Author details

Selma Yazar
Faculty of Pharmacy, Department of Pharmaceutical Toxicology, Istanbul Yeni Yuzyil University, Istanbul, Turkey

*Address all correspondence to: selma.yazar@yeniyuzyil.edu.tr

References

[1] Kelishadi R. Environmental pollution: Health effects and operational implications for pollutants removal. Journal of Environmental and Public Health. 2012;**2012**:1-2. DOI: 10.1155/2012/341637

[2] Kabir ER, Rahman MS, Rahman I. A review on endocrine disruptors and their possible impacts on human health. Environmental Toxicology and Pharmacology. 2015;**40**:241-258. DOI: 10.1016/j.etap.2015.06.009

[3] Canipari R, Santis L, Cecconi S. Female fertility and environmental pollution. International Journal of Environmental Research and Public Health. 2020;**17**:8802. DOI: 10.3390/ijerph17238802

[4] Leisegang K, Dutta S. Do lifestyle practices impede male fertility? Andrologia. 2020;**00**:e13595. DOI: 10.1111/and.13595

[5] Keith LH. Environmental endocrine disruptors. Pure and Applied Chemistry. 1998;**70**(12):2319-2326

[6] Di Nisio A, Foresta C. Water and soil pollution as determinant of water and food quality/contamination and its impact on male fertility. Reproductive Biology and Endocrinology. 2019;**17**(1):4. DOI: 10.1186/s12958-018-0449-4

[7] Marques-Pinto A, Carvalho D. Human infertility: Are endocrine disruptors to blame? Endocrine Connections. 2013;**2**:R15-R29. DOI: 10.1530/EC-13-0036

[8] Giudice L. Environmental toxicants: Hidden players on the reproductive stage. Fertility and Sterility. 2016;**106**(4):791-794. DOI: 10.1016/j.fertnstert.2016.08.019

[9] Balabanič D, Klemenčič AK. Endocrine-disrupting chemicals and male reproductive health: A review. Zdravstveni Vestnik. 2018;**87**(1-2):69-80. DOI: 10.6016/ZdravVestn.2456

[10] Lagos-Cabre R, Moreno RD. Contribution of environmental pollutant to male infertility: A working model of germ cell apoptosis induced by plasticizer. Biological Research. 2012;**45**:5-14. DOI: 10.4067/S0716-97602012000100001

[11] Cooke PS, Nanjappa MK, Ko C, Prins GS, Hess RA. Estrogens in male physiology. Physiological Reviews. 2017;**97**:995-1043. DOI: 10.1152/physrev.00018.2016

[12] Hess RA, Cooke PS. Estrogen in the male: A historical perspective. Biology of Reproduction. 2018;**99**(1):27-44. DOI: 10.1093/biolre/ioy043

[13] Daston GP, Gooch JW, Breslin WJ, Shuey DL, Nikiforov AI, Fıco TA, et al. Environmental estrogens and reproductive health: A discussion of the human and environmental data. Reproductive Toxicology. 1997;**11**(4):465-481. DOI: 10.1016/s0890-6238(97)00014-2

[14] Fucic A, Galea KS, Duca RC, Yamani ME, Frery N, Godderis L, et al. Potential health risk of endocrine disruptors in construction sector and plastics industry: A new paradigm in occupational health. International Journal of Environmental Research and Public Health. 2018;**15**:1229. DOI: 10.3390/ijerph15061229

[15] Kumar N, Sing AK. Trends of male factor infertility, an important cause of infertility: A review of literature. Journal of Human Reproductive Sciences. 2015;**8**(4):191-196. DOI: 10.4103/0974-1208.170370

[16] Marić T, Fučić A, Aghayanian A. Environmental and occupational exposures associated with male infertility. Arhiv za higijenu rada i toksikologiju. 2012;**72**:101-113. DOI: 10.2478/aiht-2021-72-3510

[17] Krzastek SC, Farhi J, Gray M, Smith RP. Impact of environmental toxin exposure on male fertility potential. Translational Andrology and Urology. 2020;**9**(6):2797-2813. DOI: 10.21037/tau-20-685

[18] Petersen KU, Balkiss AM, Hærvig KK, Bonde JPE, Hogaard KS, Toft G, et al. Use of personal care product and semen quality: A cross-sectional study in young Danish men. Toxics. 2020;**8**(62):1-13. DOI: 10.3390/toxics8030062

[19] Rocca CL, Tait S, Guerrati C, Busani L, Ciardo F, Bergamasco B, et al. Exposure to endocrine disruptors and nuclear receptors gene ezpression in infertile and fertile men from Italian areas with different environmental features. International Journal of Environmental Research and Public Health. 2015;**12**:12426-12445. DOI: 10.3390/ijerph121012426

[20] Arena AC, Fernandez CD, Porto EM, Bissacot DZ, Pereira OCM, Kempinas WG. Fenvalarate, a pyrethroid insecticide, adversely affects sperm production and storage in male rats. Journal of Toxicology and Environmental Health, Part A: Current Issues. 2008;**71**:1550-1158. DOI: 10.1080/15287390802392024

[21] Fisch H, Braun SR. Trends in global semen parameter values. Asian Journal of Andrology. 2013;**15**:169-173. DOI: 10.1038/aja.2012.143

[22] Carlsen E, Giwecman A, Keiding N, Skakkebaek NE. Evidence for decreasing quality of semen during past 50 years. BMJ. 1992;**305**:609-613. DOI: 10.1136/bmj.305.6854.609

[23] Kumar M, Sarma DK, Shubham S, Kumawat M, Verma V, Prakash A, et al. Environmental endocrine-disrupting chemical exposure: Upcoming global health burden. Frontiers in Public Health. 2020;**8**:549. DOI: 10.3389/fpubh.2020.553850

[24] Dobrakowski M, Kaletka Z, Machoń-Grecka A, Kasperczyk S, Horak S, Birkner E, et al. The role of oxidative stress, selected metals, and parameters of the ımmune system in male fertility. Oxidative Medicine and Cellular Longevity. 2018;**2018**:6249536. DOI: 10.1155/2018/6249536

[25] Bhatt RV. Environmental influence on reproductive health. International Journal of Gynecology & Obstetrics. 2000;**70**:69-75

[26] Roeleveld N, Bretveld R. The impact of pesticides on male fertility. Current Opinion in Obstetrics & Gynecology. 2008;**20**:229-233. DOI: 10.1097/GCO.0b013e3282fcc334

[27] Amir S, Shah STA, Mamoulakis C, Docea AO, Kalantzi O-I, Zachatiou A, et al. Endocrine disruptors acting on estrogen and androgen pathways cause reproductive disorders through multiple mechanism: A review. International Journal of Environmental Research and Public Health. 2021;**18**:1464. DOI: 10.3390/ijerph18041464

[28] Lifeng T, Shoulin W, Junmin J, Xuezhao S, Yannan L, Qianli W, et al.

Effects of fenvalarate exposure on semen quality among occupational workers. Contraception. 2006;**73**:92-96. DOI: 10.1016/j.contraception.2005.06.067

[29] Toshima H, Suziki Y, Imai K, Yoshinaga J, Shiraishi H, Mizumoto Y, et al. Endocrine disrupting chemicals in urine of Japanese male partners of subfertie couples: A pilot study on exposure and semen quality. International Journal of Hygiene and Environmental Health. 2012;**215**:502-506. DOI: 10.1016/j.ijheh.2011.09.005

[30] Sinclair S. Male infertility: Nutritional and environmental considerations. Alternative Medicine Review. 2000;**5**(1):28-38

[31] Chowdhury AR. Recent advances in heavy metals induced effect on male reproductive function-a retrospective. Al Ameen Journal of Medical Sciences. 2009;**2**(2):37-42

[32] Wu HM, Lin-Tan DT, Wang ML, Huang HY, Lee CL, Wang HS, et al. Lead level in seminal plasma may affect semen quality for men without occupational exposure to lead. Reproductive Biology and Endocrinology. 2012;**10**:91. DOI: 10.1186/1477-7827-10-91

[33] Ma Y, He X, Qi K, Wang T, Qi Y, Cui L, et al. Effects of environmental contaminants on fertility and reproductive health. Journal of Environmental Sciences. 2018;**77**:210-217. DOI: 10.1016/j.jes.2018.07.015

[34] Jamalan M, Ghaffari MA, Zeinali M. Human sperm quality and metal toxicants: Protective effects of some flavonoids on male reproductive function. International Journal of Fertility and Sterility. 2016;**10**(2):215-223. DOI: 10.22074/ijfs.2016.4912

[35] Kiziler AR, Aydemir B, Onaran I, Alici B, Ozkara H, Gulyasar T, et al. High levels of cadmium and lead in seminal fluid and blood of smoking men are associated with high oxidative stress and damage in infertile subjects. Biological Trace Element Research. 2007;**120**:82-91. DOI: 10.1007/s12011-007-8020-8

[36] He Y, Zou L, Luo W, Yi Z, Yang P, Yu S, et al. Heavy metal exposure, oxidative stress and semen quality: Exploring associations and mediation effects in reproductive-aged men. Chemosphere. 2020;**244**:125498. DOI: 10.1016/j.chemosphere.2019.125498

[37] Kahraman S, Hass H, Karatas A, Ilgın H. The effect of blood and seminal plasma heavy metal and trace element levels on sperm quality. Journal of Medical Sciences. 2012;**32**(6):1560-1568. DOI: 10.5336/medsci.2011-26578

[38] Kasperczky A, Dobrakowski M, Czuba ZP, Horak S, Kasperczyk S. Environmental exposure to lead induces oxidative stress and modulates the function of the antioxidant defense system and the immune system in the semen of males with normal semen profile. Toxicology and Applied Pharmacology. 2015;**284**(3):339-344. DOI: 10.1016/j.taap.2015.03.001

[39] Shabani K, Hosseini S, Khani AGM, Moghbelinejad S. The effects of semen parameters and age on semen motility of Iranian men. Global Journal of Fertility and Research. 2017;**2**(1):024-029. DOI: 10.17352/gjfr.000008

[40] Li C, Cao M, Ma L, Ye X, Song Y, Pan W, et al. Pyrethroid pesticide exposure and risk of primary ovarian insufficiency in Chinese women. Environmental Science & Technology. 2018;**52**(5):3240-3248. DOI: 10.1021/acs.est.7b06689

[41] Li P, Zhong Y, Jiang X, Wang C, Zuo Z, Sha A. Seminal plasma metals concentration with respect to semen quality. Biological Trace Element Research. 2012;**148**(1):1-6. DOI: 10.1007/s12011-012-9335-7

[42] Famurewa AC, Ugwuja EI. Association of blood and seminal plasma cadmium and lead levels with semen quality in non-occupational exposed infertile men in Abakaliki, south East Nigeria. Journal of Family & Reproductive Health. 2017;**11**(2):97-103

[43] Vigeh M, Smith DR, Hsu PC, PC. How does lead induce male infertility? Iran. The Journal of Reproductive Medicine. 2011;**9**(1):1-8

[44] Ji G, Xia Y, Gu A, Shi X, Long Y, Song L, et al. Effects of non-occupational environmental exposure to pyrethroids on semen quality and sperm DNA integrity in Chinese men. Reproductive Toxicology. 2011;**31**:171-176. DOI: 10.1016/j.reprotox.2010.10.005

[45] Sengupta P, Banerjee R. Environmental toxins: Alarming impacts of pesticides on male fertility. Human & Experimental Toxicology. 2014;**33**(10):1017-1039. DOI: 10.1177/0960327113515504

[46] Xia Y, Han Y, Wu B, Wang S, Gu A, Lu N, et al. The relation between urinary metabolite of pyrethroid insecticides and semen quality in humans. Fertility and Sterility. 2008;**89**:1743-1750. DOI: 10.1016/j.fertnstert.2007.05.049

[47] Song L, Wang YB, Sun H, Yuan C, Hong X, Qu JH, et al. Effects of fenvalarate and cypermethrin on rat sperm motility patterns in vitro as measured by computer-assisted sperm amalysis. Journal of Toxicology & Environmental Health Part A: Current Issues. 2008;**5**:325-332. DOI: 10.1080/15287390701738517

[48] Mehrpour O, Karrari P, Zamani N, Tsatsakis AM, Abdollahi M. Occupational exposure to pesticides and consequences on male semen and fertility: A review. Toxicology Letters. 2014;**230**:146-156. DOI: 10.1016/j.toxlet.2014.01.029

[49] Martenies SE, Perry MJ. Environmental and occupational pesticide exposure and human sperm parameters: A systematic review. Toxicology. 2013;**307**:66-73. DOI: 10.1016/j.tox.2013.02.005

[50] Pan C, Liu YP, Li YF, Hu JH, Zhang JP, Wang HM, et al. Effects of cypermethrin on the ligand-independent interaction between androgen receptor and steroid receptor coactivator-1. Toxicology. 2012;**299**:160-164. DOI: 10.1016/j.tox.2012.05.022

[51] Pan C, Wang Q, Liu YP, Xu LF, Li YF, Hu JX, et al. Anti-androgen effects of the pyrethroid pesticide cypermethrin on interactions of androgen receptor with corepressors. Toxicology. 2013;**311**:178-183. DOI: 10.1016/j.tox.2013.06.011

[52] O'Hara L, Smith LB. Androgen receptor roles in spermatogenesis and infertility. Best Practice & Research. Clinical Endocrinology & Metabolism. 2015;**29**:595-605. DOI: 10.1016/j.beem.2015.04.006

[53] Zhang J, Zhu W, Zheng Y, Yang J, Zhu X. The antiandrogenic activity of pyrethroid pesticides cyfluthrin and ß-cyfluthrin. Reproductive Toxicology. 2008;**25**:491-496. DOI: 10.1016/j.reprotox.2008.05.054

[54] Du G, Shen O, Sun H, Fei J, Lu C, Song L, et al. Assessing hormone receptor activities of pyrethroid insecticides and their metabolites in reporter gene assays. Toxicological Sciences. 2010;**116**(1):58-66. DOI: 10.1093/toxsci/kfq120

[55] Xu LC, Sun H, Chen JF, Bian Q, Song L, Wang XR. Androgen receptor activities of p,p-DDE, fenvalerate and phoxim detected by androgen receptor reporter gene assay. Toxicology Letters. 2006;**160**(2):151-157. DOI: 10.1016/j.toxlet.2005.06.016

[56] Tang W, Wang D, Wang J, Wu Z, Li L, Huang M, et al. Pyrethroid pesticide residues in the global environment: An overview. Chemosphere. 2018;**191**:990-1007. DOI: 10.1016/j.chemosphere.2017.10.115

[57] Kim KB, Barlett MG, Anand SS, Bruckner JV, Kim HJ. Rapid determination of the synthetic pyrethroid insecticide deltamethrin, in rat plasma and tissues by HPLC. Journal of Chromatography B. 2006;**834**:141-148. DOI: 10.1016/j.jchromb.2006.02.039

[58] Wu HM, Tan DTL, Wang ML, Huang HY, Wang HS, Soong YK, et al. Cadmium level in seminal plasma may affect the pregnancy rate for patients undergoing infertility evaluation and treatment. Reproductive Toxicology. 2008;**25**:481-484. DOI: 10.1016/j.reprotox.2008.04.005

[59] Xu LC, Liu L, Ren XM, Zhang MR, Cong N, Xu AQ, et al. Evaulation of androgen receptor transcriptional activities of some pesticides in vitro. Toxicology. 2008;**243**:59-65. DOI: 10.1016/j.tox.2007.09.028

[60] Han Y, Xia Y, Han J, Zhou J, Wang S, Zhu P, et al. The relationship of 3-PBA pyrethroids metabolite and male reproductive hormones among non-occupational exposure males. Chemosphere. 2008;**72**:785-790. DOI: 10.1016/j.chemosphere.2008.03.058

[61] Wang Q, Shen JY, Zhang R, Hong JW, Li Z, Ding Z, et al. Effects and mechanisms of pyrethroids on male reproductive system. Toxicology. 2020;**438**:152460. DOI: 10.1016/j.tox.2020.152460

[62] Meeker JD, Barr DB, Hauser R. Pyrethroid insecticide metabolites are associated with serum hormone levels in adult men. Reproductive Toxicology. 2009;**27**:155-160. DOI: 10.1016/j.reprotox.2008.12.012

[63] Meeker JD, Rossano MG, Protas B, Diamond MP, Puscheck E, Daly D, et al. Cadmium, lead, and other metals in relation to semen quality: Human evidence for molybdenum as a male reproductive toxicant. Environmental Health Perspectives. 2008;**116**(11):1473-1479. DOI: 10.1289/ehp.11490

[64] Sikka SC, Wang R. Endocrine disruptors and estrogenic effects on male reproductive axis. Asian Journal of Andrology. 2008;**10**(1):134-145. DOI: 10.1111/j.1745-7262.2008.00370.x

[65] Oehninger S, Kruger TF. Sperm morphology and its disorders in the context of infertility. F&S Reviews. 2021;**2**(1):75-92. DOI: 10.1016/j.xfnr.2020.09.002

[66] Merzenich H, Zeeb H, Blettner M. Decreasing sperm quality: A global problems? BMC Public Health. 2010;**10**:24. DOI: 10.1186/1471-2458-10-24

[67] Alam MF, Akhter M, Mazumder B, Ferdous A, Hossain MD, Dafader NC, et al. Assessment of some heavy metals in selected cosmetics commonly used in Bangladesh and human health risk. Journal of Analytical Science and Technology. 2019;**10**:1-8. DOI: 10.1186/s40543-018-0162-0

[68] Wang J, Pan L, Wu S, Lu L, Xu Y, Zhu Y, et al. Recent advances on endocrine disrupting effects of

UV filters. International Journal of Environmental Research and Public Health. 2016;**13**:782. DOI: 10.3390/ijerph13080782

[69] Witorsch RJ, Thomas JA. Personal care products and endocrine disruption: A critical review of the literature. Critical Reviews in Toxicology. 2010;**40**(S3):1-30. DOI: 10.3109/10408444.2010.515563

[70] Giokas DL, Salvador A, Chisvert A. UV filters: From sunscreens to human body and the environment. Trends in Analytical Chemistry. 2007;**26**:360-374. DOI: 10.1016/j.trac.2007.02.012

[71] Louis GMB, Kannan K, Sapra KJ, Maisong J, Sundaram R. Urinary concentrations of benzophenone-type ultraviolet radiation filters and couples fecundity. American Journal of Epidemiology. 2014;**180**(12):1168-1175. DOI: 10.1093/aje/kwu285

[72] Frederiksen H, Krause M, Jørgensen N, Rehfeld A, Skakkebaek N, Andersson AM. UV filters in matched seminal fluid-, urine-, and serum samples from young men. Journal of Exposure Science & Environmental Epidemiology. 2020;**31**:345-355. DOI: 10.1038/s41370-020-0209-3

[73] Nicolopoulou-Stamati P, Hens L, Sasco AJ. Cosmetics as endocrine disruptors: Are they a health risk? Reviews in Endocrine & Metabolic Disorders. 2015;**16**:373-383. DOI: 10.1007/s11154-016-9329-4

[74] Schiffer C, Müller A, Egeberg DL, Alvarez L, Brenker C, Rehfeld A, et al. Direct action of endocrine disrupting chemicals on human sperm. EMBO Reports. 2014;**15**(7):758-765. DOI: 10.15252/embr.201438869

[75] Ren D, Navarro B, Perez G, Jackson AC, Hsu S, Shi Q, et al. A sperm ion channel required for sperm motility and male fertility. Nature. 2001;**413**:603-609. DOI: 10.1038/35098027

[76] Rehfeld A, Dissing S, Skakkebaek NE. Chemical UV filters mimic the effect of progesterone on Ca2+ signaling in human sperm cells. Endocrinology. 2016;**157**(11):4297-4308. DOI: 10.1210/en.2016-1473

[77] Rehfeld A, Egeberg DL, Almstrup K, Petersen JH, Dissing S, Skakkebaek NE. EDC impact: Chemical UV filters can affect human sperm function in progesterone-like manner. Endocrine Connections. 2018;**7**:16-25. DOI: 10.1530/EC-17-0156

[78] Adoamnei E, Mendiola J, Moñino-García M, Vela-Soria F, Iribarne-Durán LM, Fernández MF, et al. Urinary concentrations of benzophenone-type ultra violet lights filters and reproductive paramaters in young men. International Journal of Hygiene and Environmental Health. 2018;**221**(3):531-540. DOI: 10.1016/j.ijheh.2018.02.002

[79] Louis GMB, Chen Z, Kim S, Sapra KJ, Phil M, Bae J, et al. Urinary concentrations of benzophenone–type ultraviolet light filters and semen quality. Fertility and Sterility. 2015;**104**(4):989-996. DOI: 10.1093/aje/kwu285

[80] Chen M, Tang R, Fu G, Xu B, Zhu P, Qiao S, et al. Association of exposure to phenols and idiopathic male infertility. Journal of Hazardous Materials. 2013;**250-251**:115-121. DOI: 10.1016/j.jhazmat.2013.01.061

[81] Joffe M. Infertility and environmental pollutants. British Medical Bulletin. 2003;**68**:47-70. DOI: 10.1093/bmb/ldg025

[82] Craig ZR, Wang W, Flaws JA. Endocrine-disrupting chemicals

in ovarian function: Effects on steroidogenesis, metabolism and nuclear receptor signaling. Reproduction. 2011;**142**(5):633-646. DOI: 10.1530/REP-11-0136

[83] Gibson DA, Saunders PTK. Endocrine disruption of oestrogen action and female reproductive tract cancers. Endocrine-Related Cancer. 2014;**21**(2):T13-T31. DOI: 10.1530/ERC-13-0342

[84] Chang SH, Cheng BH, Lee SL, Chuang HY, Yang CY, Sung FC, et al. Low blood lead concentration in association with infertility in women. Environmental Research. 2006;**101**:380-386. DOI: 10.1016/j.envres.2005.10.004

[85] Lee S, Min JY, Min KB. Female infertility associated with blood lead and cadmium levels. International Journal of Environmental Research and Public Health. 2020;**17**:1794. DOI: 10.3390/ijerph17051794

[86] Georgescu B, Georgescu C, Dărăban S, Bouaru A, Passcalău S. Heavy metals acting as endocrine disruptors. Journal of Animal Science and Biotechnology. 2011;**44**(2):89-93

[87] Silberstein T, Saphier O, Paz-Tal O, Trimarch JR, Gonzalez L, Keefe DL. Lead concentrates in ovarian follicle compromises pregnancy. Journal of Trace Elements in Medicine and Biology. 2006;**20**:205-207. DOI: 10.1016/j.jtemb.2006.05.001

[88] Lei HL, Wei HJ, Ho HY, Liao KW, Chien LC. Relationship between risk factors for infertility in women and lead, cadmium, and arsenic blood levels: A cross-sectional study from Taiwan. BMC Public Health. 2015;**15**:1220. DOI: 10.1186/s12889-015-2564-x

[89] Tang N, Zhu ZQ. Adverse reproductive effects in female workers of lead battery plants. International Journal of Occupational Medicine and Environmental Health. 2003;**16**(4):359-361

[90] Gerhard I, Monga B, Waldbrenner A, Runnebaum B. Heavy metals and fertility. Journal of Toxicology & Environmental Health Part A: Current Issues. 1998;**54**(8):593-611. DOI: 10.1080/009841098158638

[91] Srivastava V, Dearth RK, Hiney JK, Ramirez LM, Bratton GR, Dees WL. The effects of low-level Pb on steroidogenic acute regulatory protein (StAR) in the prepubertal rat ovary. Toxicological Sciences. 2004;77:35-40. DOI: 10.1093/toxsci/kfg249

[92] Tanrıkut E, Karaer A, Celik O, Celik E, Otlu B, Yilmaz E, et al. Role of endometrial concentrations of heavy metals (cadmium, lead, mercury and arsenic) in the aetiology of unexplained infertility. European Journal of Obstetrics, Gynecology, and Reproductive Biology. 2014;**179**:187-190. DOI: 10.1016/j.ejogrb.2014.05.039

[93] Marettova E, Maretta M, Legath J. Effect of pyrethroids on female genital system. Review. Animal Reproduction Science. 2017;**184**:132-138. DOI: 10.1016/j.anireprosci.2017.07.007

[94] Jurewicz J, Radwan P, Wielgomas B, Radwan M, Karwacka A, Kaluzny P, et al. Exposure to pyrethroid pesticides and ovarian reserve. Environment International. 2020;**144**:106028. DOI: 10.1016/j.envint.2020.106028

[95] Monteiro C d S, Xavier EB d S, Caetano JPJ, Marinho RM. A critical analysis of the impact of endocrine disruptors as a posisible etiology of primary ovarian insufficiency. JBRA Assisted Reproduction. 2020;**24**(3):324-331. DOI: 10.5935/1518-0557.20200005

[96] Whitworth KW, Baird DD, Steiner AZ, Bornman RMS, Travlos GS, Wilson RE, et al. Anti-Müllerian hormone and lifestyle, reproductive, and environmental factors among women in rural South Africa. Epidemiology. 2015;**26**:429-435. DOI: 10.1097/eDe.0000000000000265

[97] Li C, Cao M, Ma L, Ye X, Song Y, Pan W, et al. Pyrethroid pesticide exposure and risk of primary ovarian insufficiency in Chinese women. Environmental Science & Technology. 2018;**52**(5):3240-3248. DOI: 10.1021/acs.est.7b06689

[98] Hu Y, Ji L, Zhang Y, Shi R, Han W, Tse LA, et al. Organophosphate and pyrethroid pesticide exposure measured before conception and associations with time to pregnancy in Chinese couples enrolled in the Shanghai birth cohort. Environmental Health Perspectives. 2018;**126**(7):1-9. DOI: 10.1289/EHP2987

[99] Schlumpf M, Kypke K, Wittassek M, Angerer J, Mascher H, Mascher D, et al. Exposure patterns of UV filters, fragrances, parabens, phthalates, organochlor pesticides, PBDEs, and PCBs in human milk: Correlation of UV filters with use of cosmetics. Chemosphere. 2010;**81**:1171-1183. DOI: 10.1016/j.chemosphere.2010.09.079

[100] Jimenez-Diaz I, Molina-Molina JM, Zafra-Gomez A, Ballesteros O, Navalon A, Real M, et al. Simultaneous determination of the UV- filters benzyl salicylate, phenyl salicylate, octyl salicylate, homosalate, 3-(4-methylbenzylidene) camphor and 3- benzylidene camphor in human placental tissue by LC-MS/MS. assessment of their invitro endocrine activity. Journal of Chromatography. B, Analytical Technologies in the Biomedical and Life Sciences. 2013;**936**:80-87. DOI: 10.1016/j.jchromb.2013.08.006

[101] Zhang T, Sun H, Qin X, Wu Q, Zhang Y, Ma J, et al. Benzophenone-type UV filters in urine and blood from children, adults, and pregnant women in China: Maternal and fetal cord blood. Science of the Total Environment. 2013;**1**(461-462):49-55. DOI: 10.1016/j.scitotenv.2013.04.074

[102] Janjua NR, Mogensen B, Andersson AM, Petersen JH, Henriksen M, Skakkebaek NE, et al. The Journal of Investigative Dermatology. 2004;**123**:57-61. DOI: 10.1111/j.0022-202X.2004.22725.x

[103] Waring RH, Harris RM. Endocrine disruptors: A human risk? Molecular and Cellular Endocrinology. 2005;**244**:2-9. DOI: 10.1016/j.mce.2005.02.007

[104] Kunisue T, Chen Z, Louis GMB, Sundaram R, Hediger ML, Sun L, et al. Urinary concentrations of benzophenone-type UV filters in U.S. women and their association with endometriosis. Environmental Science & Technology. 2012;**46**(8):4624-4632. DOI: 10.1021/es204415a

[105] Faass O, Schlumpf M, Reolon S, Henseler M, Maerkel K, Durrer S, et al. Female sexual behavior, estrous cycle and gene expression şn sexually dimorphic brain regions after pre-and postnatal exposure to endocrine active UV filters. Neurotoxicology. 2009;**30**:249-260. DOI: 10.1016/j.neuro.2008.12.008

Section 5

Radioisotopes

Chapter 11

Radionuclide Contamination as a Risk Factor in Terrestrial Ecosystems: Occurrence, Biological Risk, and Strategies for Remediation and Detoxification

Peter Ostoich, Michaela Beltcheva, Jose Antonio Heredia Rojas and Roumiana Metcheva

Abstract

Radionuclide contamination poses serious hazards for terrestrial ecosystems. Beyond the readily apparent damage to the biota at high doses, low doses of ionizing radiation produce stochastic effects: mutation, carcinogenesis, and genomic instability. The proposed chapter is a review of the biological and ecological effects of radionuclides. The authors discuss, beyond the Chernobyl accident, other contamination events. The review includes the biological and ecological effects of the three principal technogenic contaminants in terrestrial ecosystems: Cs-137, Sr-90, and I-131. Ecological risks to terrestrial small mammals are assessed in detail. In addition, the chapter provides some of the lesser-known methods of remediation and detoxification, including the use of modified natural zeolites as environmental remedies and bio-sorbents. Presented herein is little-known information on environmental protection against radioactive contamination.

Keywords: radionuclides, radioecology, contamination, remediation, detoxification, zeolites

1. Introduction: the essence of radionuclides—emission types and biological effects

Radionuclides are unstable isotopes of different chemical elements. Usually, this instability is due to excess energy in the atomic nucleus, leading to the release of particles with different energies in a process called **radioactive decay**. Natural radionuclides emit three types of radiation: alpha (α), beta (β-), and gamma (γ). Of these types, α-particles have the strongest biological effects, causing 20 times more biological damage than an equivalent dose of β- or γ radiation [1, 2]. While α- and β-particles tend not to penetrate into matter, γ-radiation, especially at the higher end of the energy spectrum, penetrates deep into living and non-living matter. This means that, when considering the biological and ecological effects of radionuclide contamination, α- and β-emitters are only relevant if incorporated into living organisms. In contrast, γ-emitters are relevant as both internal and external components of the total absorbed dose. In the context of anthropogenic contamination, it needs to be taken into account that some of the man-made radionuclides emit other types of radiation. For example, radioisotopes used in medical PET scans such as ^{18}F, ^{11}C, ^{13}N, ^{15}O are positron (β^+) emitters. Other, more exotic man-made radionuclides such as Californium-252 (^{252}Cf) are capable of spontaneously emitting neutrons. Both positron and neutron emitters require specific equipment for handling and detection of the radiation sources [1]. Some radionuclides emit multiple types of particles. The anthropogenic radionuclide ^{137}Cs emits β^- particles at two energies: 511 and 1173 kiloelectronvolts (keV), and γ-rays at 32 and 661.6 keV [3, 4].

The biological effects of radionuclides are mainly due to the emitted ionizing radiation (IR). IR interacts with biomolecules directly by damaging them or indirectly—by producing reactive oxygen species (ROS), which in turn damages biomolecules. According to the paradigms of classical radiobiology, the principal target of IR on a cellular level is genomic DNA—it can be damaged directly or indirectly, leading to cell cycle arrest and an activation of DNA repair systems, followed by recovery, cell death, or mutagenesis [5, 6]. Sparsely ionizing radiations such as β- particles and γ-rays cause around 70% of DNA damage indirectly through ROS, while densely ionizing radiations, such as α-particles and high-energy cosmic particles, cause only about 30% of the biologically significant damage indirectly [7]. Researchers have elucidated the biological effects of high and medium doses of radiation. Nevertheless, biological effects at low doses remain insufficiently understood and a subject of much debate [1, 8]. Currently, radiation risk is extrapolated linearly to the low doses by using the **Linear Non-Threshold (LNT)** mathematical model [1, 9]. However, other hypotheses include **radiation hormesis**, which is the idea that small doses of radiation are beneficial [10], and **low-dose hypersensitivity**, which is the assumption that low doses of radiation are more mutagenic because they do not activate DNA repair systems [11]. While radiation hormesis has been well researched recently [10], it has still not been taken into account in radiation protection calculations, where every minimal dose of radiation is assumed to carry a small but non-negligible risk [12]. On the other hand, the low-dose hypersensitivity hypothesis is supported by recent studies, raising questions about the validity of current assumptions in radioprotection [13]. Living organisms tend to display different radiation sensitivity. Mammalian species are very sensitive to radiation, while insects tend to be comparatively radioresistant. The champion of radiation resistance is the bacterium *Deinococcus radiodurans*, which can withstand an acute dose of 5000 Gray with almost no loss of viability. Similarly, tardigrades can withstand 5000 Gray with 50% loss in viability (LD_{50} = 5000 Gy). For comparison, the LD_{50} for humans is around 6 Gray, for mice around 6.4 Gray, and for goats only around 2.4 Gray [14].

A significant concern in radionuclide-contaminated areas arises from the process of **bioaccumulation**. Similar to other chemical elements from their respective groups, radioisotopes are incorporated preferentially into different target organs and tissues. Thus, ^{137}Cs, a chemical analogue of potassium, is preferentially accumulated into nerve and muscle tissue. ^{90}Sr, an analogue of calcium, has a very strong affinity for bone and hematopoietic tissue. Some of the properties of the three most environmentally significant anthropogenic radionuclides are presented below (**Table 1**).

As evident from the table, the most significant environmental contaminants of the above are ^{137}Cs and ^{90}Sr due to their long half-lives and persistence in nature. ^{131}I was

Radionuclide	Symbol	Half-life (λ)	Emitted radiation	Target tissues and organs	Biological effects
Cesium-137	^{137}Cs	30.17 years	β-(511, 1173 keV), γ (32, 661.6 keV)	Nerve, muscle	Different cancers
Strontium-90	^{90}Sr	28.8 years	pure β-(546 keV)	Bone	Bone cancer, leukemia
Iodine-131	^{131}I	8.02 days	β-(333.8, 606.3 keV), γ (364.5, 636.9 keV)	Thyroid gland	Thyroid cancer

Table 1.
The most significant anthropogenic radionuclides and their biological effects (data adapted from [3, 4]).

only a very significant contaminant in the first year following the Chernobyl accident, causing ~4000 excess thyroid cancers in the most significantly affected populations of Russia, Belarus, and Ukraine [15].

2. Radionuclide occurrence in nature: natural and anthropogenic sources

Natural radioactivity, including external terrestrial γ radiation, internal α-, β-, and γ-radiation from naturally occurring radionuclides, cosmic radiation, and exposure to radon (^{222}Rn) and thoron (^{220}Rn) and their radioactive progeny molecules, accounts for ~95% of the annual radiation dose for the terrestrial biota [1]. The global annual dose for an average person is 3.6 millisieverts/year (mSv/a), of which 82% is due to natural radiation exposure, around 15% is due to medical exposure, and only about 0.8% is due to anthropogenic contamination of the environment. Natural radioactivity has been a subject of concern for decades. Globally, there are areas with increased natural radiation, often due to thorium (^{232}Th) deposits in the form of monazite rocks. Two such areas are Guarapari, Brazil, and the state of Kerala in southern India. The area of Ramsar, Iran, has enormously increased natural radioactivity due to radioactive hot springs containing ^{222}Rn and its progeny. Although annual doses in these areas reach an average of 35–40 mSv/a, compared to 3.6 mSv/a average in Europe and 2.5 mSv/a in Bulgaria, modern biomedical studies report no excess cancer risk, leading researchers to believe that a 10-fold increase in natural radioactivity is harmless [16].

In contrast, environmental contamination by anthropogenic radionuclides without doubt creates serious risks. The Chernobyl accident is the most prominent example of environmental damage due to technogenic sources, although it is not the only one; Chernobyl caused significant chronic morbidity and mortality in people and enormous damage to the environment and economies in Europe. This is mostly due to ^{131}I, ^{137}Cs, and ^{90}Sr, and their tendencies for **bioaccumulation** and **biomagnification** in terrestrial ecosystems [17]. Although the Chernobyl accident is the best-known example, there are many other significant contamination events in the period 1945–2011 (**Table 2**).

One aspect evident from the table is that, according to atmospheric radioactivity released, the Chernobyl accident exceeds all other INES scale 5–7 accidents combined. At the same time, during this accident, only about 30% of the core radioactivity was released, suggesting that a full-blown reactor explosion can cause even greater damage to the environment. Another noteworthy peculiarity is that most reactor accidents

Accident site, year	Country	INES scale	Date	Accident type	Radioactivity released to the atmosphere, PBq	Iodine-131 released, PBq	Cesium-137 released, PBq
Chernobyl, 1986	USSR	7	26.04.1986	Reactor meltdown	12,000	1760	85
Fukushima, 2011	Japan	7	11.03.2011	Reactor meltdown	630	<380	<37
Mayak (Chelyabinsk-40), 1957	USSR	6	29.09.1957	Nuclear waste explosion	1850	Not known	Not known
Chalk River, 1952	Canada	5	12.12.1952	Reactor meltdown	0.3	Not known	Not known
Windscale, 1957	UK	5	10.10.1957	Reactor fire	1.6	0.7	0.02
Simi Valley, 1959	USA	5	26.07.1959	Partial reactor meltdown	>200	Not known	Not known
Beloyarsk, 1977	USSR	5	1977	Partial reactor meltdown	not known	Not known	Not known
Three Mile Island, 1979	USA	5	28.03.1979	Partial reactor meltdown	1.6	<0.007	Not known

Table 2.
The most significant radioactive release accidents, their IAEA INES severity scale, and radioactivities released to the environment (data from [18]).

so far occurred either with new or experimental power plants (Chernobyl, Chalk River, Simi Valley, Beloyarsk) or military reactors (windscale). Nevertheless, the Fukushima accident in 2011 presents a new precedent—the reactors in the plant were old, nearing the end of their design life. Since this is true for many of the currently operating reactors, this presents a new, threatening perspective. Aging, crumbling nuclear infrastructure may present a new, unmitigated radiation hazard in the future.

3. Radionuclides and nature: significant risks and unknowns

Some of the risks to ecosystems posed by radionuclide contamination are well understood. They include, at high doses >1 Gray acute dose, teratogenesis in developing embryos, stunted plant growth, and visible damage to the flora and fauna. These are **deterministic effects**, and they occur definitely after exposure to strong doses of ionizing radiation and are dose dependent (**Figure 1**).

As shown in **Figure 1**, pine trees are very radiosensitive; they can serve as a bio-indicator of severe radioactive contamination at doses exceeding 3 Sv acute exposure [19]. The other depicted deterministic effect is teratogenesis in pregnant mammalian species. At doses exceeding 1 Sv acute *in utero* exposure, the number of resorbed fetuses decreases, and so does the number of offspring born with malformations [1].

Perhaps more worrying are the **stochastic effects**, which occur with a small probability even at low radiation doses. These include **radiation mutagenesis** and, as a consequence of it, **radiation carcinogenesis** [1, 12]. Based on data from experiments with specially bred laboratory mice and results from the radiobiological monitoring of humans, exposed to γ-rays and neutrons during the bombings of Hiroshima and Nagasaki, it is estimated that the doubling dose of radiation-induced mutagenesis is 1 Gy. This means that an acute exposure to 1 Gy of γ-rays doubles the spontaneously occurring rate of mutation [20, 21]. Nevertheless, this perspective is being challenged. For example, Belarussian researchers observed transmission of chromosomal damage in the progeny of wild rodents from the vicinity of Chernobyl, indicating **genomic instability** [22]. An international team observed a higher mini- and microsatellite mutation rate in the children of Chernobyl liquidators [23]. Both of these findings support the theory that even low doses of radiation can be harmful to the biota, as well as current and future generations of humans. Another, more recent venue of

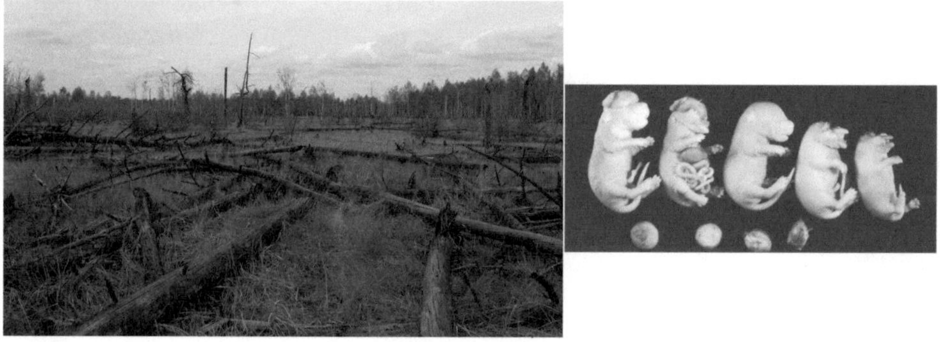

Figure 1.
Deterministic effects of ionizing radiation: Dead pine trees near Chernobyl, Ukraine in 1990 (left, taken from [19]), and experimental radiation teratogenesis in mouse embryos (right, photograph by Dr. Roberts Rugh, taken from [1]).

research with significant progress is the radiation-induced bystander effect (RIBE) phenomenon, in which non-irradiated cells show similar cytotoxicity and genetic damage to their irradiated neighbors [24, 25]. The results from bystander effect studies generally support the theory of low-dose hypersensitivity and highlight possible molecular mechanisms for increased radiation risks in the low-dose range [24, 25]. Radiation risk is still to be taken very seriously, and every effort should be made to keep radioactive contamination of ecosystems to a minimum.

4. Estimation and appraisal of radioactive contamination and its effects on the components of terrestrial ecosystems

Radioecology is a sub-discipline of ecology concerning the presence and effects of radioactivity on Earth's ecosystems. Some of the risks of ionizing radiation were known in the early twentieth century. Nevertheless, the discipline *de facto* started developing in the period following World War II and the bombings of Hiroshima and Nagasaki [26]. The advent of the Atomic Age not only gave the impetus to study radiation effects on ecosystems, but also gave them powerful tools in the form of radioactive isotopes, which could be used as tracers [26, 27]. Initially, studies were carried out by the US Atomic Energy Commission (AEC) at several sites crucial to the Manhattan Project, principally Oak Ridge, Tennessee, and Hanford, Washington; many of these studies dealt with the cycling with biogenic carbon, phosphorus and oxygen through ecosystems and were conducted with radioactive tracers (^{14}C, ^{32}P, and others) [27]. In parallel, studies were conducted in the former USSR in the closed town of Ozyorsk (Chelyabinsk-40). Some studies were conducted in secret; most of them dealt with dispersal and deposition of bomb radionuclides and with the bioaccumulation of radioactivity in crop plants and farm animals [28–30].

Without a doubt, the most significant contamination event in the context of terrestrial ecosystems is Chernobyl. It is estimated that, at the time of the accident, around 10% of the total core radioactivity was released, including 100% of all noble gases and around 30% of volatile atoms including 30% of the core radiocesium (^{134}Cs and ^{137}Cs), 55% of the core ^{131}I, and ~ 45% of the core ^{132}Te. Less volatile radionuclide species such as radiostrontium (^{89}Sr and ^{90}Sr) were also released in smaller amounts (~5% of core inventory), as well as <3.5% of the core transuranic nuclides (neptunium, plutonium, curium) [31, 32]. The core inventories and releases are summarized in **Table 3**.

The most significant release of radioactivity from the damaged reactor was in the form of noble gasses (^{85}Kr and ^{133}Xe). Nevertheless, fast atmospheric dispersal and the lack of chemical reactivity of noble gasses mean that radioactive krypton and xenon resulted only in trace global contamination. In contrast, the volatile iodine-131, released in significant quantities during the reactor fire, was the predominant problem in contaminated areas during 1986. It is estimated that up to 4000 additional thyroid cancers among people can be attributed to this nuclide [4]. In the long term, the most significant contribution of radiation dose to the biota is attributed to radiocesium (^{134}Cs, ^{137}Cs), particularly ^{137}Cs, due to its long half-life (30.17 years), its propensity to accumulate in plant and fungal matter and animal nerve and muscle tissue. The contribution of ^{90}Sr to the background dose is also significant, but much lower and often indistinguishable from pre-Chernobyl global fallout from atmospheric nuclear testing [34].

Radioecological research after 1986 in Europe involved multinational teams working in the Chernobyl exclusion zone (ChEZ) and the most contaminated areas of Belarus and Russia (Gomel and Bryansk regions), as well as many studies on a

Chernobyl core inventories at the time of accident				**Radioactive release**	
Radionuclide	**Symbol**	**Half-life (λ)**	**Core activity, PBq**	**% core activity**	**Released, PBq**
Krypton-85*	^{85}Kr	10.76 years	35	100	35
Xenon-133*	^{133}Xe	5.3 days	6500	100	6500
Iodine-131	^{131}I	8.02 days	3200	55	1760
Cesium-134	^{134}Cs	2.0 years	180	30	54
Cesium-137	^{137}Cs	30.17 years	280	30	85
Tellurium-132	^{132}Te	78 hours	2700	45	1150
Strontium-89	^{89}Sr	52.0 days	2300	5	115
Strontium-90	^{90}Sr	28.8 years	200	5	10
Barium-140	^{140}Ba	12.75 days	4800	5	240
Zirconium-95	^{95}Zr	1.4 hours	5600	3.5	196
Molybdenum-99	^{99}Mo	65.9 hours	4800	3.5	168
Ruthenium-103	^{103}Ru	39.26 days	4800	3.5	168
Ruthenium-106	^{106}Ru	1.0 year	2100	3.5	73
Cerium-141	^{141}Ce	32.5 days	5600	3.5	196
Cerium-144	^{144}Ce	284.9 days	3300	3.5	116
Neptunium-239†	^{239}Np	2.4 days	2700	3.5	95
Plutonium-238†	^{238}Pu	86.0 years	1	3.5	0.035
Plutonium-239†	^{239}Pu	24,110 years	0.85	3.5	0.03
Plutonium-240†	^{240}Pu	6580 years	1.2	3.5	0.042
Plutonium-241†	^{241}Pu	13.2 years	170	3.5	6
Curium-242†	^{242}Cm	163 days	26	3.5	0.9

**noble gases*
†transuranic nuclides

Table 3.
Core inventories and releases of the most important contaminants originating from the Chernobyl accident. Data obtained from [31–33].

national level focusing on areas with known contamination. Among the projects conducted in the ChEZ, several exemplary studies of the bioaccumulation of different radionuclides in wildlife stand out [17, 19, 34, 35]. Researchers have demonstrated that the appropriate sentinel species for radioecological studies comprise small rodents including representatives of family Cricetidae like *Myodes glareolus* Schreber, 1870, *Microtus arvalis* Pallas, 1778, *Microtus oeconomus* Pallas, 1776 as well as European murid species: the yellow-necked wood mouse *Apodemus flavicollis* Melchior, 1834 and the wood mouse *Apodemus sylvaticus* Linnaeus, 1758.

During the 200 s, researchers reported very high internal doses in Cricetidae, particularly the bank vole (*M. glareolus*) due to high dietary intake of ^{137}Cs [17, 34]. This has been confirmed by subsequent monitoring studies in the ChEZ [19, 35, 36], as well as in Alpine ecosystems in Bulgaria [37, 38]. Recent monitoring data suggest that *M. glareolus* is potentially the best rodent zoo monitor for residual contamination in Europe. A selection of results from two groups of monitoring programs, mentioned above is presented in **Table 4**.

Study	Location	Result
Chesser et al., 2001 [17]	Six different biotopes within the Chernobyl Exclusion Zone	Very high internal doses from ^{137}Cs in dry muscle of *M. glareolus* from areas with high and medium contamination; average ^{137}Cs body burden in *M. glareolus* 2902–24,720 Bq/g. High body burden of ^{137}Cs in *Sorex araneus*—2592–5901 Bq/g).
Beresford et al., 2008 [36]	Three different biotopes within the Chernobyl Exclusion Zone	High total-body internal doses from ^{137}Cs in *M. glareolus* 2260 ± 1290 Bq/g; much lower doses from ^{90}Sr in different species of small rodents (for *M. glareolus* 81.3 ± 22.1 Bq/g, for *Microtus* sp. 107 ± 35.0 Bq/g, for *Apodemus* sp. 66.6 ± 28.3 Bq/g).
Beresford et al., 2020a [19]	Reference (low-contamination) biotopes within the Chernobyl Exclusion Zone	Comparatively high doses from ^{137}Cs in *M. glareolus* from low-contamination "reference areas" in the ChEZ, total body burden of ^{137}Cs in *M. glareolus* = 649 Bq/g; comparatively high total body burden of ^{137}Cs in *Microtus* sp. (952 Bq/g); Much lower doses from ^{137}Cs in Soricidae (161 Bq/g for *S. araneus*, 121 Bq/g for *S. minutus*).
Iovtchev et al., 1996 [37]	Two localities (Musala peak and Skakavtsite), Rila Mountain, Bulgaria	Comparatively high whole-body total β-activities in wild rodents from both localities (2.5–3.0 Bq/g for *Apodemus* species, 3.25 Bq/g for *Chionomys nivalis* from Musala Peak, 2.75 Bq/g for *M. glareolus* from Skakavtsite).
Beltcheva et al., 2019 [38]	Two localities (Musala peak and Skakavtsite), Rila Mountain, Bulgaria	Overall 10-fold reduction in whole-body total β-activities in wild rodents from both localities. Highest residual activities observed in *M. glareolus* (0.52 Bq/g). β-activities in other rodents show more significant reduction (0.23–0.37 Bq/g for *Apodemus* sp., 0.38 Bq/g for *Ch. nivalis*).

Table 4.
A summary of the findings of five radioecological studies using small mammals as zoo monitors.

The summarized works show evidence for the high value of *M. glareolus* as a monitoring species for residual radioactivity from the Chernobyl accident due to its propensity to accumulate radiocesium. While accounting for the differences in values obtained by the various research groups, and the different time frames, another aspect of Chernobyl contamination becomes apparent: There are significantly higher depositions and animal body burdens of radiostrontium (^{90}Sr) within the Chernobyl exclusion zone, as opposed to very low amounts of ^{90}Sr present at greater distances from the accident site; this can be explained by the much lower volatility of strontium compared to cesium. This is one of the main reasons why ^{90}Sr is still a significant contaminant within the ChEZ, but in most of Europe the largest part of the Chernobyl-associated dose burden to the biota comes from ^{137}Cs.

During recent monitoring studies, conducted in Bulgaria in the period 1996–2020, small mammals such as rodents and insectivores were selected mainly due to their positions in the food chain like primary consumers, rapid maturity, large population number, and rapid biological reaction to the environmental changes [38]. The possible biological response of the organism was studied at different levels of organization of living matter, and evaluated the population number and structure, food spectrum, total beta-activity in target tissues, and organs of the investigated animals, standard hematological methods—to determine hemoglobin contents, hematocrit, and morphological characterization of erythrocytes, as well as cytogenetic methods. The food spectrum was analyzed as a basis for further investigations on the transfer of beta-emitters through the rodent populations and the whole ecosystem.

Moussala Peak 2925 m a.s.l.		β-activity /mean ± SD/, Bq/kg	Beli Iskar (Skakavtsite area), 1400–1500 m a. s. l.		β-activity /mean ± SD/, Bq/kg
Ap. flavicollis	**n = 12**	**230.3 ± 7.2**	*Ap. flavicollis*	**n = 13**	**366.3 ± 8.1**
Ch. nivalis	n = 12	382.0 ± 8.3	*M. glareolus*	n = 22	424.2 ± 5.3

Table 5.
Whole-body total β-beta activities at two localities (Rila Mountain, Bulgaria), 2019–2020 [38].

The total body burden of β-emitters of a species depends on the trophic chain position, food, life mode, physicochemical composition of the atmospheric precipitation, total suspended dust content in atmospheric air, and other factors. The total β-activities in Bq/kg of some small mammal species were investigated at two different altitudes in Rila Mountain, Bulgaria. The results, obtained in 2019–2020, are presented on **Table 5**.

All values were below 480 Bq/kg and were considered as referent.

Significant differences between mice and voles were obtained only due to the difference in their food specialization. Mice are omnivorous, while voles are mainly herbivorous species. Green vegetable parts accumulate radiocesium more actively than seeds and the quantity of the consumed low-caloric green food by animals is higher.

The comparison of the results obtained with the data 20 years ago makes it obvious that the values of total β-activity decreased by about 10 times in the period 1995–2019. Data obtained in the bodies of different monitor species of small mammals from Rila Mountain during 1995 varied from about 3500 Bq/kg in the yellow-necked wood mouse to 5000 Bq/kg in the snow vole. The total level of beta-activity in bank vole and yellow-necked wood mouse from Beli Iskar region during 1995 was between 2000 and 3000 Bq/kg [37].

High doses of radiation can influence the normal function of the blood and disturb the hematopoiesis. These were possible basophilic granulations that appear in enhanced, but also disturbed erythropoiesis, basophilic DNA fragments observed in a blood smear, frequently as a result of decreased spleen function, anemia, and overloaded bone marrow. However, the given results do not suggest such changes, and they have not been established.

A correlation between total beta-activity loading and chromosome aberration frequency in bone marrow cells was established. The percentage of chromosome aberrations in mice was about 1.6% and breaks were 0.2% and in herbivorous voles respectively 7.0 and 2.5%. The percentage of aberrant bone marrow cells of mice from the investigated regions is visibly lower than in vole species. This fact correlates with the recorded total body burden of β-emitters in herbivorous species in comparison with the omnivorous murids.

5. Principal remediation strategies for radioactive contamination

The issue of remediating radioactively contaminated terrestrial ecosystems dates back to the early years of the Atomic Age (1945–1965) when protection measures were a secondary consideration to weapons production. Tests were conducted in contaminated areas such as near Hanford, Washington, and Ozyorsk (Chelyabinsk-40) [27, 29].

After 1986, to protect the environmental health and resolve the liabilities due to eventual radioactive contamination, severely contaminated countries and the responsible institutions have undertaken certain remediation and protection measures:

1. mechanical/physical methods—creation of barriers, burial/demobilization of radioactive sources; deep tilling of agricultural fields for facilitating downward migration of radioisotopes;

2. forestry management—clearing and burial of severely contaminated coniferous forests presenting a fire hazard, natural succession/ecosystem restoration, and manual afforestation of contaminated agricultural areas with deciduous trees;

3. selective use of soil additives—addition of lime to increase soil pH and limit the uptake of ^{90}Sr by plants, use of fertilizers containing phosphorus, and potassium in order to reduce ^{137}Cs bioaccumulation in plant matter, the addition of complexing agents such as powdered zeolites, and other aluminosilicate minerals in order to demobilize ^{137}Cs; addition of hydroxyapatite (HAP) to prevent ^{90}Sr cycling in ecosystems;

4. crop selection in agricultural areas—production of non-food/feed crops such as cotton, flax, timber, and biofuels; use of land with low levels of contamination for sugar and oil production, whereby most residual radioactivity is removed during the refining processes;

5. careful livestock farming—feeding farm animals clean fodder, administration of powdered zeolites as bio-sorbents, the addition of salt licks containing Prussian Blue to reduce ^{137}Cs uptake by grazing animals.

Most of these strategies are discussed in detail elsewhere [39–44]. All of the methods were applied to some degree within the ChEZ and the highly contaminated areas of the former USSR [42]. By far, the most widespread method used was the deep tilling of agricultural fields. Nevertheless, one of the strategies for remediation, the use of zeolites for demobilization and biodetoxification of ^{137}Cs has only been tested on a small scale in the ChEZ, while, at the same time, being the most promising approach for countering the toxicity of radiocesium [39, 45].

6. Zeolites as bio-detoxifiers of radionuclides

Natural zeolites are one of the most interesting groups among minerals, some of which (clinoptilolite, mordenite, chabazite) have enormous potential in science and technology due to their high sorption capacity and the presence of deposits with huge reserves in many countries, including Bulgaria. In the early years of zeolite research, Ames (1960) found that clinoptilolite from the Hector deposit, California, is highly selective for Sr^{2+} and Cs^+ [46]. Other heavy metals, especially monovalent ones, were also well adsorbed—respectively ion-exchanged by this natural zeolite. The author introduced an order of selectivity of clinoptilolite, which is:

$$Cs^+ > Rb^+ > K+ > NH_4^+ > Ba^+ > Sr^{2+} > Na^+ > Ca^{2+} > Fe^{2+} > Al^{3+} > Mg^{2+} > Li^+$$

The ion exchange properties of clinoptilolite and its selective sorption are especially valuable in the control of radioactive waste from nuclear energy production. The mineral has been successfully used as a sorbent of radionuclides from water and contaminated soils, as well as a food additive to limit ^{137}Cs absorption in livestock [39, 41, 45].

Very significant research on zeolites has been conducted in Bulgaria for the past five decades, with two deposits of clinoptilolite in the Eastern Rhodope Mountains—Beli Plast and Beliya Bair-Zhelezni Vrata—being particularly suitable for bio-sorbents of heavy metals and radionuclides in the form of additives to food and livestock feed [47]. Recently, it was demonstrated that modified natural clinoptilolite from the Golobradovo deposit in the Eastern Rhodopes was practically non-toxic to laboratory mice and facilitated significantly the excretion of Pb^{2+}ions from the gastro-intestinal tract of the experimental animals, thus protecting them against lead toxicity [48, 49]. In parallel, other Bulgarian researchers validated the use of zeolites from the Eastern Rhodopes in decontamination procedures and as soil fertilizer and even developed a clinoptilolite-based artificial soil ("Balkanin") that was used for growing vegetables in space onboard the Mir station [50]. In the early 1990s, researchers from the Bulgarian Academy of Sciences developed a specially modified natural clinoptilolite (CLS-5) as a bio-sorbent for radiocesium (^{134}Cs and ^{137}Cs) and radiostrontium (^{89}Sr and ^{90}Sr) [51]. In a modified form and labeled KS-3, CLS-5 was used in the production of over 55,000 personal radiation protection emergency kits, most of which were distributed among the personnel of the Kozloduy Nuclear Power Plant and the people from the surrounding areas (**Figure 2**).

Two plastic vials containing CLS-5 with a quantity of 7 grams each have been integrated in the radiation emergency kit. The other components of the radiation protection kit are a painkiller syrette, a syrette with an antiemetic, a broad-spectrum antibiotic, potassium iodide (KI) tablets, and CBT (a radioprotector for abating acute exposure to radiation), bandages, and ethanol for disinfection [51].

As evident from the material presented, research into zeolites as bio-sorbents of radionuclides and heavy metals is fairly advanced in Bulgaria. The past achievements in developing modified clinoptilolite derivatives as ^{90}Sr and ^{137}Cs sorbents, and current and ongoing basic research in clinoptilolites as a countermeasure to Pb^{2+} and Cd^{2+} intoxication in mammalian species promise to yield the interesting results.

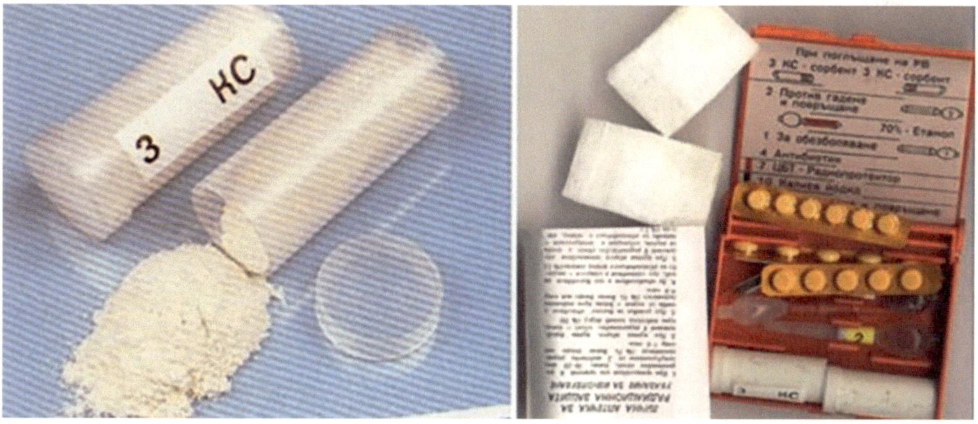

Figure 2.
Modified natural zeolites as part of a radiation protection emergency kit: Plastic vials containing CLS-5 (left), and the entire emergency kit (right) [51].

7. Conclusion

Ionizing radiation is one of the best understood cytotoxic and genotoxic agents. Nevertheless, much remains to be understood about the behavior of radionuclides in nature and the biological responses they induce. The radiobiology of low-dose, protracted irradiation is still an open area of research.

At the same time, bioaccumulation of certain radioisotopes along food chains poses serious ecosystem risks, or as the doyen of modern ecology Eugene Odum stated: "we could give nature an apparently innocuous amount of radioactivity and have her give it back to us in a lethal package!" [26].

The mitigation of environmental risks from radionuclides involves responsible management of the nuclear fuel cycle, as well as careful monitoring and safeguarding of nuclear installations. Among the strategies discussed in the chapter, all have been applied to a varying degree in severely contaminated agroecosystems and forest ecosystems. Perhaps the most promising venue of detoxication research is the application of zeolites as immobilizers and bio-detoxifiers for radiocesium and radiostrontium. Nevertheless, no method can fully remediate a contaminated ecosystem, meaning that prevention of radioactive contamination remains the first and best defense against anthropogenic radioactive pollution.

Acknowledgements

This work is supported by the National Science Fund of the Republic of Bulgaria, Project KP-06-PN44/3, 12.12.2020: "Crystal-chemical and structural characteristics of modified natural clinoptilolite and correlation between its sorption properties, ion exchange capacity for heavy metals and biological response in vivo and in vitro".

Author details

Peter Ostoich[1*], Michaela Beltcheva[1], Jose Antonio Heredia Rojas[2] and Roumiana Metcheva[1]

1 Institute of Biodiversity and Ecosystem Research, Bulgarian Academy of Sciences, Sofia, Bulgaria

2 Faculty of Biological Sciences, Autonomous University of Nuevo León, San Nicolás de los Garza, Nuevo León, Mexico

*Address all correspondence to: p.ostoich@gmail.com

References

[1] Hall E, Giaccia A. Radiobiology for the Radiologist. New York, London: Lippincott Williams and Wilkins; 2006. p. 576

[2] UNSCEAR. Sources, Effects and Risks of Ionizing Radiation, Annex B. New York: United Nations; 2020. p. 240

[3] Besson B, Pourcelot L, Lucot E, Badot PM. Variations in the transfer of radiocesium (^{137}Cs) and radiostrontium (^{90}Sr) from milk to cheese. Journal of Dairy Science. 2009;**92**(11):5363-5370

[4] Holm LE. Thyroid cancer after exposure to radioactive ^{131}I. Acta Oncologica. 2006;**45**(8):1037-1040

[5] Puck TT, Marcus PI. Action of X-rays on mammalian cells. The Journal of Experimental Medicine. 1956;**103**(5):653-666

[6] Blakely E, Chang P, Lommel L, Bjornstad K, Dixon M, Tobias C, et al. Cell-cycle radiation response: Role of intracellular factors. Advances in Space Research. 1989;**9**(10):177-186

[7] Pettersen EO, Wang H. Radiation-modifying effect of oxygen in synchronized cells pre-treated with acute or prolonged hypoxia. International Journal of Radiation Biology. 1996 Sep;**70**(3):319-326

[8] National Academies of Sciences, Engineering, and Medicine; Division on Earth and Life Studies; Nuclear and Radiation Studies Board. In: Kosti O, editor. The Future of Low Dose Radiation Research in the United States: Proceedings of a Symposium. Washington (DC): National Academies Press (US); 2019

[9] Trott KR, Rosemann M. Molecular mechanisms of radiation carcinogenesis and the linear, non-threshold dose response model of radiation risk estimation. Radiation and Environmental Biophysics. 2000 Jun;**39**(2):79-87

[10] Schirrmacher V. Less can be more: The hormesis theory of stress adaptation in the global biosphere and its implications. Biomedicine. 2021;**9**(3):293

[11] Joiner MC, Marples B, Lambin P, Short SC, Turesson I. Low-dose hypersensitivity: Current status and possible mechanisms. International Journal of Radiation Oncology, Biology, Physics. 2001;**49**(2):379-389

[12] Hawk C, Hyland J, Rupert M, Colonvega M, Hall S. The 2007 recommendations of the International Commission on Radiological Protection. ICRP publication 103. Annals of the ICRP. 2007;**37**(2-4):1-332

[13] Heuskin AC, Michiels C, Lucas S. Low dose hypersensitivity following *in vitro* cell irradiation with charged particles: Is the mechanism the same as with X-ray radiation? International Journal of Radiation Biology. 2014 Jan;**90**(1):81-89

[14] Bond VP, Robertson JS. Comparison of the Mortality Response of Different Mammalian Species to X-Rays and Fast Neutrons. *Technical Report BNL-7603*. NY, United States: Brookhaven National Laboratory; 1963

[15] Williams ED. Chernobyl and thyroid cancer. Journal of Surgical Oncology. 2006;**94**(8):670-677

[16] Dobrzyński L, Fornalski KW, Feinendegen LE. Cancer mortality among people living in areas with various levels of natural background

radiation. Dose Response. 2015;**13**(3):1559325815592391

[17] Chesser RK, Rodgers BE, Wickliffe JK, Gaschak S, Chizhevsky I, Phillips CJ, et al. Accumulation of ^{137}Cesium and ^{90}Strontium from abiotic and biotic sources in rodents at Chornobyl, Ukraine. Environmental Toxicology and Chemistry. 2001;**20**(9):1927-1935

[18] Lelieveld J, Kunkel D, Lawrence MG. Global risk of radioactive fallout after major nuclear reactor accidents. Atmospheric Chemistry and Physics. 2012;**12**:4245-4258

[19] Beresford NA, Barnett CL, Gashchak S, Maksimenko A, Guliaichenko E, Wood MD, et al. Radionuclide transfer to wildlife at a 'Reference site' in the Chernobyl Exclusion Zone and resultant radiation exposures. Journal of Environmental Radioactivity. 2020a;**211**:105661

[20] Russell WL, Russell LB, Kelly EM. Radiation dose rate and mutation frequency. Science. 1958;**128**(3338): 1546-1550

[21] Sankaranarayanan K. Estimation of the hereditary risks of exposure to ionizing radiation: History, current status, and emerging perspectives. Health Physics. 2001;**80**(4):363-369

[22] Goncharova RI, Riabokon' NI. Biological effects in natural populations of small rodents in radiation-polluted territories. Dynamics of chromosome aberration frequency in a number of generations of European bank vole (*Clethrionomys glareolus* Schreber). Radiatsionnai Biologiia Radioecologiia. 1998;**38**(5):746-753

[23] Dubrova YE, Nesterov VN, Krouchinsky NG, Ostapenko VA, Neumann R, Neil DL, et al. Human minisatellite mutation rate after the Chernobyl accident. Nature. 1996;**380**(6576):683-686

[24] Osterreicher J, Prise KM, Michael BD, Vogt J, Butz T, Tanner JM. Radiation-induced bystander effects. Mechanisms, biological implications, and current investigations at the Leipzig LIPSION facility. Strahlentherapie und Onkologie. 2003;**179**(2):69-77

[25] Wang R, Zhou T, Liu W, Zuo L. Molecular mechanism of bystander effects and related abscopal/cohort effects in cancer therapy. Oncotarget. 2018;**9**(26):18637-18647

[26] Odum E. Fundamentals of Ecology. Philadelphia: W. B. Saunders Company; 1959. p. 546

[27] Creager A. Life Atomic: A History of Radioisotopes in Science and Medicine. Chicago: University of Chicago Press; 2013. p. 512

[28] Bradley DJ, Schneider KJ. Radioactive Waste Management in the USSR: A Review of Unclassified Sources, 1963-1990: Technical Report. Richland, WA, United States: Pacific Northwest National Lab (PNNL); 1990. p. 235

[29] Ilyin L. Chernobyl: Myth and Reality. Moscow: Megapolis Publishing; 1995. p. 358

[30] Akleyev AV, Kostyuchenko VA, Peremyslova LM, Baturin VA, Popova IY. Radioecological impacts of the Techa River contamination. Health Physics. 2000;**79**(1):36-47

[31] Kirchner G, Noack CC. Core history and nuclide inventory of the Chernobyl core at the time of accident (TPR-NS--29-No1). Nuclear Safety. 1988;**29**(1):1-5

[32] Güntay S, Powers D, Devell L. The Chernobyl reactor accident source term:

Development of a consensus view. IAEA: INIS. 1995;**41**(8):183-193

[33] Kai M, Homma T, Lochard J, Schneider T, Lecomte JF, Nisbet A, et al. ICRP Publication 146: Radiological protection of people and the environment in the event of a large nuclear accident: Update of ICRP PUBLICATIONS 109 AND 111. Annals of the ICRP. 2020;**49**(4):11-135

[34] Chesser R, Sugg D, Lomakin M, Van den Bussche R, DeWoody A, Jagoe C, et al. Concentrations and dose rate estimates of 134,137-cesium and 90-Strontium in small mammals at Chornobyl, Ukraine. Environmental Toxicology and Chemistry. 2000;**19**(2):305-312

[35] Beresford NA, Scott EM, Copplestone D. Field effects studies in the Chernobyl Exclusion Zone: Lessons to be learnt. Journal of Environmental Radioactivity. 2020;**211**:105893

[36] Beresford NA, Gaschak S, Barnett CL, Howard BJ, Chizhevsky I, Strømman G, et al. Estimating the exposure of small mammals at three sites within the Chernobyl exclusion zone-a test application of the ERICA Tool. Journal of Environmental Radioactivity. 2008;**99**(9):1496-1502

[37] Iovtchev M, Metcheva R, Atanasov N, Apostolova M, Bogoeva L, Zivkov M, et al. Investigation on total β-activity of indicator vertebrate species from Rila National Park. OM2. 1996;**4**:38-42

[38] Beltcheva M, Metcheva R, Geleva E, Aleksieva I, Ostoich P, Ravnachka I, et al. Total β - activity in monitor species small rodents from two different altitudes in Rila Mountain (Bulgaria). AIP Conference Proceedings. 2019;**2075**:130004

[39] Phillippo M, Gvozdanovic S, Gvozdanovic D, Chesters JK, Paterson E, Mills CF. Reduction of radiocaesium absorption by sheep consuming feed contaminated with fallout from Chernobyl. The Veterinary Record. 1988;**122**(23):560-563

[40] IAEA. Technologies for Remediation of Radioactively Contaminated Sites. Vol. **1086**. Vienna: IAEA publications; 1999. pp. 1-110

[41] Jacob P, Fesenko S, Firsakova SK, Likhtarev IA, Schotola C, Alexakhin RM, et al. Remediation strategies for rural territories contaminated by the Chernobyl accident. Journal of Environmental Radioactivity. 2001;**56**(1-2):51-76

[42] Vidal M, Camps M, Grebenshikova N, Sanzharova N, Ivanov Y, Vandecasteele C, et al. Soil- and plant-based countermeasures to reduce ^{137}Cs and ^{90}Sr uptake by grasses in natural meadows: The REDUP project. Journal of Environmental Radioactivity. 2001;**56**(1-2):139-156

[43] Smiciklas I, Dimovic S, Plecaš I. Removal of $Cs1^{+}$, Sr^{2+} and Co^{2+} from aqueous solutions by adsorption on natural clinoptilolite. Applied Clay Science. 2007;**35**:139-144

[44] Handley-Sidhu S, Mullan TK, Grail Q, Albadarneh M, Ohnuki T, Macaskie LE. Influence of pH, competing ions, and salinity on the sorption of strontium and cobalt onto biogenic hydroxyapatite. Scientific Reports. 2016;**18**(**6**):23361

[45] Pöschl M, Balás J. Reduction of radiocaesium transfer to broiler chicken meat by a clinoptilolite modified with hexacyanoferrate. Radiation and Environmental Biophysics. 1999;**38**(2):117-124

[46] Ames L. The cation sieve properties of clinoptilolite. American Mineralogist. 1960;**45**(5-6):689-700

[47] Djourova E, Aleksiev B. Zeolitic rocks related to the second acid Paleogene volcanism to the east of the town of Kardzhali. In: Konstantinos S, editor. Geologica Rhodopica 2. Thessaloniki: Aristotel University; 1990. pp. 489-499

[48] Beltcheva M, Metcheva R, Popov N, Teodorova SE, Heredia-Rojas JA, Rodríguez-de la Fuente AO, et al. Modified natural clinoptilolite detoxifies small mammal's organism loaded with lead I. Lead disposition and kinetic model for lead bioaccumulation. Biological Trace Element Research. 2012;**147**(1-3):180-188

[49] Beltcheva M, Metcheva R, Topashka-Ancheva M, Popov N, Teodorova S, Heredia-Rojas J, et al. Zeolites versus lead toxicity. Journal of Bioequivalence & Bioavailability. 2015;7(1):12-29

[50] Ivanova T, Stoyanov I, Stoilov G, Kostov P, Sapunova S. Zeolite gardens in space. In: Kirov G, Filizova L, Petrov O, editors. Natural Zeolites. Proceedings of the Sofia Zeolite Meeting' 95, PENSOFT, Sofia. 1997: 3-10

[51] Popov N, Jilov G, Popova T. Study of the use of natural clinoptilolites and their modifications as effective sorbents of Sr and Cs and heavy metals from water solutions and drinking waters. In: Proceedings of the 5th International Conference of Natural Zeolites "Zeolite-97", September 21-29, 1997. Ischia (Naples), Italy; 1997

Section 6

Tools for Evaluating Environmental Contaminations

Chapter 12

Marine Free-Living Nematodes as Tools for Environmental Pollution Assessment: A Special Focus on Emerging Contaminants Impact in the Tunisian Lagoon Ecosystems

Ahmed Nasri, Amel Hannachi, Mohamed Allouche, Abdelwaheb Aydi, Patricia Aïssa, Hamouda Beyrem and Ezzeddine Mahmoudi

Abstract

Coastal ecosystems are exposed to pollution by various contaminants due to several anthropogenic activities. Numerous pollutants, such as pesticides, drugs, metals, Polycyclic Aromatic Hydrocarbons (PAHs), Brominated flame retardants (BFRs), and Microplastics (MPs), transported in the water column tend to persist in the sediments. Among the Tunisian coastal areas, the Bizerte and Ghar El Melh lagoons are exposed to several pollutants resulting from different activities, such as agriculture, urbanization, and industrialization. Consequently, sediments are intensely dirtied by a wide range of pollutants. Due to their relatively short life cycles and high turnover rates, free-living nematodes reacted quickly to environmental changes. This most dominant meiobenthic taxon, has been mainly exploited as indicator of disturbance because of its ubiquity, high abundance, and taxonomic diversity. In this current chapter, we cited the different environmental pollutants effects and show the importance of nematodes as bio-indicator species in environmental monitoring.

Keywords: Tunisian Lagoon ecosystems, free-living nematodes, emerging contaminants (ECs), risk assessment, experimental approach

1. Introduction

Emerging contaminants (ECs), including drugs, polycyclic aromatic hydrocarbons (PAHs), metals, pesticides, brominated flame retardants (BFRs), and microplastics (MPs), resulting from the rise of industrial production and anthropogenic activities around lagoon ecosystems are transported toward the water column and adsorbed on sediments particles [1]. Coastal lagoons are considered to be distinct systems rather than adjoining ones [2]. As interfaces between land and sea, they exhibit high primary and secondary productions that promote the development of extensive fisheries and aquaculture [3]. As semi-enclosed systems, coastal lagoons are strongly influenced by freshwater input [4] and are usually impacted by agricultural, industrial, and tourism activities [5]. These unique features allow lagoon waters to acquire significantly different characteristics compared to the nearby seawater, which leads to greater diversity in the biological communities in these ecosystems. In Tunisia, the Bizerte and Ghar El Melh lagoons are exposed to several contaminants resulting from different activities, such as agriculture, urbanization, and industrialization [6].

Free-living marine nematodes sheltering the marine sediment matrices can accumulate these chemicals and then transfer them to higher trophic levels through the food chain causing widespread contamination of the trophic chain [7]. These species constitute the dominant meiobenthic group in marine areas. They are characterized by their high abundance (up to 20 million individuals per m^2) [8] and species richness (approx. 8000 species) [9], their ubiquity and holobenthic lifestyle [10], and their small size (1–5 mm in average length), which make them easily manipulated in laboratory studies [11]. Nematodes have also high fecundity and metabolic rates and their short generation time, less than a year [12], which allow fast experimental outcomes (e.g., a month) laboratory assays based on the rapid responses to pollutants [13–17].

The objective of this chapter is to describe previous studies and to show the ecological risks of emerging contaminants in two different Tunisian lagoon ecosystems " Bizerte and Ghar El Melh lagoons" by focusing on the responses of benthic meiofauna more particularly marine nematodes to experimental various environmental pollutants exposure.

2. Materials and methods

2.1 Bizerte and Ghar el Meleh lagoons

In Tunisia, lagoon milieus cover a total space of 1100 km^2 and are distributed over the entire Mediterranean coastline [18]. These lagoons are of high ecological and economic importance but are experiencing rising anthropogenic pressure, being exposed to various types of environmental degradation resulting from agricultural, manufacturing, and touristic activities [19]. Among its many lagoons, two are the best known and are located in northern Tunisia (**Figure 1**):

The Ghar El Melh is a shallow coastal lagoon, which is isolated by a narrow-vegetated sand strip from the Mediterranean Sea. It is located in the southern Mediterranean Sea on the northeastern coast of Tunisia (37°06–37°10 N and 10°08′–10°15 E) and is influenced by regional water circulation patterns [20]. It covers a surface area of about 3000 ha, including two small sub-lagoons, El Ouafi Lagoon to which it is permanently connected, and Sidi Ali El Meki Lagoon from which it is separated by embankments. The Ghar El Melh is linked to the Mediterranean Sea via a permanent channel. The lagoon displays different levels of salinity with the highest registered in the lagoon still areas. Freshwater inflows are cyclical, restricted in summer, and tall in winter, occasionally with the existence of exceptional floods generating a link between the lagoon and the Mejerda River. The benthic vegetation is dominated by *R. cirrhosa* that extensively covers (80–100%) the lagoon bottom in summer [21]. The benthic fauna has important biodiversity, such as the presence of molluscs, crustaceans, and fishes (26 species) [22].

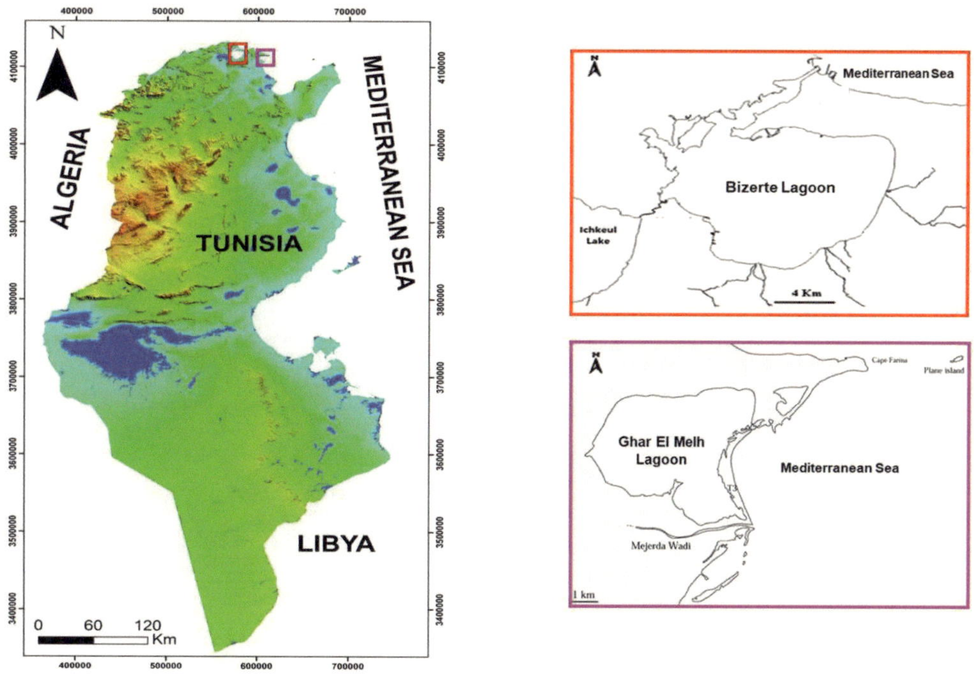

Figure 1.
Location of the Bizerte and Ghar ElMelh lagoons (Northern Tunisia).

The Bizerte lagoon is situated in the north of Tunisia in the latitudinal and longitudinal extensions of 37°8′–37°16′N and 9°46′ and 9°56′E. It has a 150 km^2 complete surface, an 8 m mean depth, and a 380 km^2 catchment area. It is connected with the Mediterranean Sea through a channel 12 m deep and communicates in the south with the Lake of Ichkeul (140 km^2) by the Tinja river. This ecosystem has great biodiversity (30 teleosts and eight elasmobranch fish species have been described) and its socio-commercial revenues in the animals' sale (mussel and oyster farming) [23]. Unfortunately, it receives freshwater inputs via eight rivers [24], urban (bounded by six cities) and industrial activity discharges as well as the products of agricultural activity. In addition, this lagoon is exposed to high biotic and abiotic variations [25].

2.2 Experimental nematodes study

Free-living marine nematodes are known to be well suited as bioindicators for monitoring studies in marine environments and bioassays (**Figure 2**) [26]. These worms are ubiquitous and occupy an important link in the food chain, feeding on microalgae and bacteria and, in turn, being preyed upon by macrobenthic predators, such as polychaetes, crabs, and fishes [27]. They are expected to be highly susceptible to sediment-associated pollutants because they live and feed on the sediment [8].

Technically, sediments containing meiofauna were collected from a coastal site in the Tunisian lagoon. Before being enriched with ECs, the sediment was arranged using the method of Austen et al. [28]. Then, large substrate particles (>63 mm) were removed by wet sieving, and appropriate concentrations of ECs were supplemented with sediment (100 g dry weight; dw). The microcosms used in this experiment were based on the original design of Austen et al. [28] and consisted of 570 mL glass bottles.

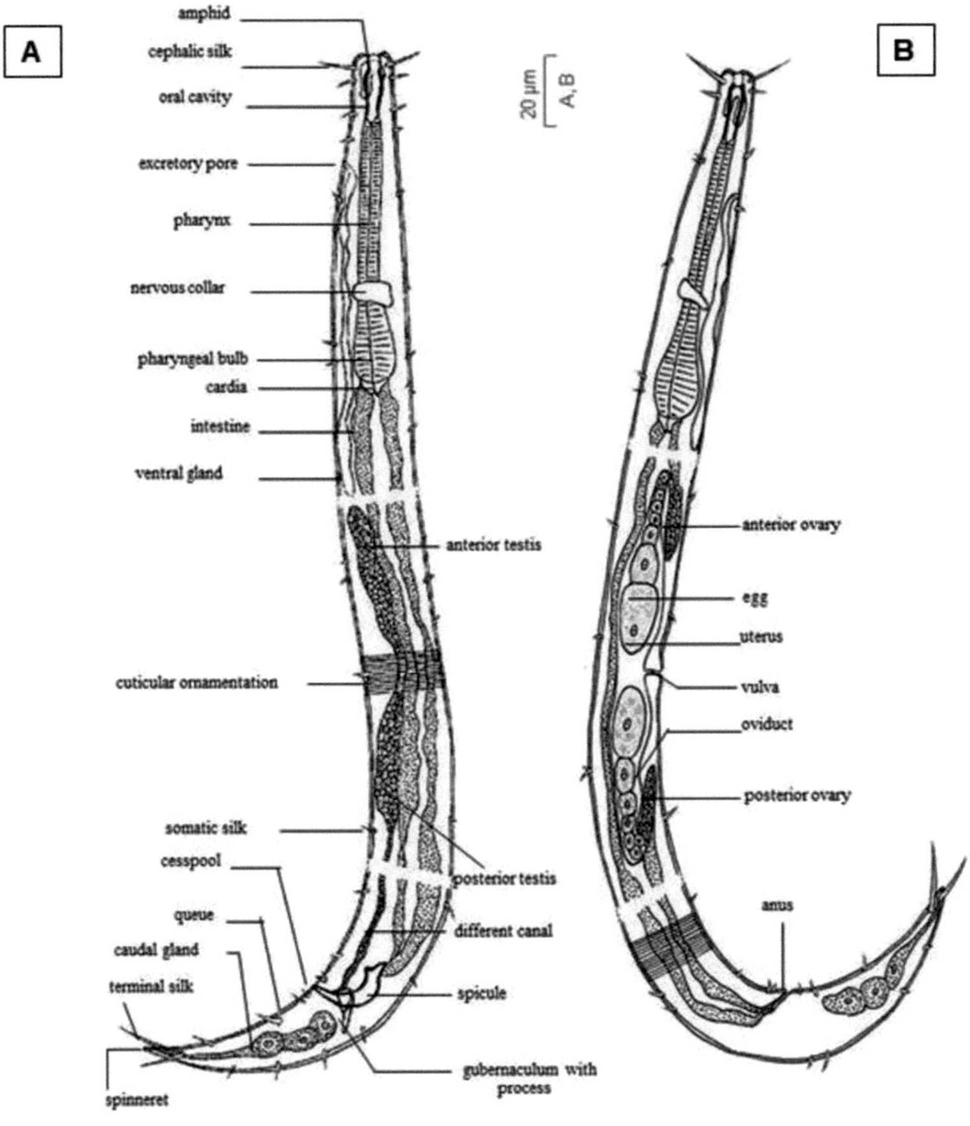

Figure 2.
General organization of nematodes species"Odontophora villoti" *(Axonolaimidae); A: male; B: gravid female.*

Treated microcosms were occupied by 300 g of homogenized sediments (200 g of natural sediment + 100 g of contaminated sediment) topped up with filtered natural water (0.1 mm). The control microcosm consisted of not treated and azoic sediments. Treatments were set up, each with minimum of three replications (control [(C)] and "treated by ECs" microcosm [29]. During the 30 days of the experiment, each microcosm was constantly aerated with an oxygen pump (**Figure 3**) [13].

At the end of the experiment, the sediment samples were fixed in a 4% buffered formalin solution. Nematodes were extracted by centrifuging with Ludox-TM three times and stained with Rose Bengal (0.2 g l^{-1}) for one day [30]. The nematofauna taxa were counted on a stereomicroscope (50×, Wild Heerbrugg M5A Model), and a

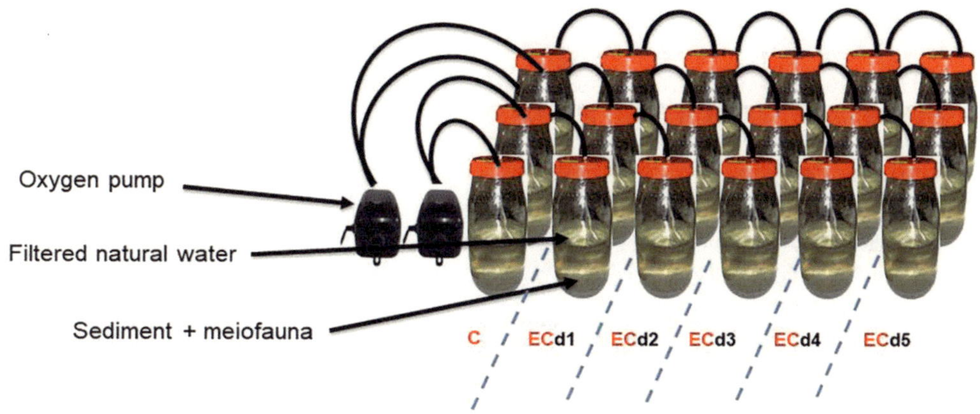

Figure 3.
*The experimental design. [C]: control; [***ECd1, ECd2, ECd3, ECd4, ECd5***]: increasing doses of emerging contaminant.*

maximum of 100 individuals/replicates were randomly taken. Animals were slowly evaporated in anhydrous glycerol, mounted on slides under an oil immersion objective (100×). The Platt and [31–33] pictorial guides and NeMys database [34] were used to species identify, respectively.

2.3 Biological parameters analysis

Nematodes are the most diverse and numerically dominant metazoans in aquatic ecosystems, and, because of their rare ability to survive in extremely polluted conditions, they are usually the only persistent taxon in heavily polluted/disturbed habitats [35]. To assess the effect of chemical pollutants on the benthic fauna, the research work has focused on studying ecological indices of nematodes, such as the spatial or temporal diversity of a taxonomic group (Shannon–Wiener diversity (H')), the distribution of the relative species abundances (Pielou's evenness (J')), the species number present (Margalef's species richness (d)), Maturity Index [36] (MI; based on the ecological characteristics and reproductive strategies of nematodes), and Index of Trophic Diversity [37] (ITD; expressed in an index calculated on the basis of the percentage of each feeding type) were studied.

In addition, the functional and morphological attributes of each species (i.e., trophic diet, tail shape, amphid shape, and life history) were considered. Trophic diet was categorized based on the characteristics of the buccal cavity [38], as epigrowth feeders (2A), selective deposit feeders (1A), non-selective deposit feeders (1B), and omnivores/predators (2B). The tail shape was illustrated into four types: conical (co), clavate/conico-cylindrical (cla), short/round (s/r), and elongated/filiform (e/f) [39]. The Amphid shape was distinguished into eight categories based on the shape of the amphidial fovea, of which four categories were used in our study—circular (Cr), spiral (Sp), pocket (Pk), and indistinct (Id) [8]. The life strategy (c–p scale) was estimated on a scale of c–p=1 (good colonizers: short life cycle, great reproduction rates, resistant to various types of stress) to c–p=5 (good persisters: lengthy life cycles, limited offspring, sensitive to stress), analogous to K/r-strategists, following [36, 40, 41]. The adult length was assigned to four groups (<1 mm, 1–2 mm, 2–4 mm, and >4 mm) [10].

Supplementary studies were conducted for the analysis of bacterial abundance. Density (per gram) was calculated for each sediment sample. Aliquots of 100 μL were successively diluted in PBS and then displaced on duplicate bacterial agar plates (Difco), which were later incubated at 37°C (overnight). Using the plaque method, 30 to 300 colonies were counted and the amounts were expressed as colony-forming units per gram of sediment (CFU g^{-1}) [14].

2.4 Statistical data analysis

Statistical analyses were executed using the Plymouth Routines in Multivariate Ecological Research (Primer v5.0) software package [42, 43]. For each microcosm treatment, all univariate indices were considered—abundance, species number (S), Shannon-Wiener diversity index (H'), Margalef's species richness (d), and Pielou's evenness (J'). Data were first tested to fulfill parametric requirements, Gaussian normality, and homogeneity of variances. Two tests were necessary: The Kolmogorov–Smirnov test to evaluate the first condition and the Bartlett to check the second condition. Once our data approximated normality, one-way ANOVA (1-ANOVA) was useful to determine the total significant difference between conditions. For multiple comparisons, the test of Tukey's HSD was applied (Statistica version 5.1).

For multivariate analyses: a non-metric Multi-Dimensional Scaling ordination (nMDS) by the Bray-Curtis matrix of similarity (square-root transformed abundance) were performed to detect a possible trend in the distribution of treatment, depending on the responses of nematode taxa or those of biological traits after ECs exposure. Hierarchical cluster analyses (CLUSTER) were used to confirm the results provided by the nMDS. The analysis of Similarity (ANOSIM) was considered to test the dissimilarities significance eventually noted between the nematode assemblages or each biological trait. Finally, The SIMPER analysis was useful in determining the contribution (cumulative contribution of 70%) of each species or functional group to the mean dissimilarity between treatments.

To detect the different relationships between nematode taxa and functional groups, PAST v3.26 software was used to perform correspondence analysis (CA) using two-dimensional plots. Also, the principal component analysis (PCA) (performed after transforming the data into log (x + 1)) is associated with the Pearson correlation (adopted via XLSTAT. 2019) to determine the targeted relationships.

3. Results and discussion

Emerging pollutants (ECs) from industrial production or agricultural runoff enter coastal waters and cause negative impacts on benthic organisms. Meiobenthic organisms, particularly free-living marine nematodes, because of their short life cycles and rapid metabolic rates, are considered ideal for laboratory experiments [13–17]. Many studies have investigated the impact of various ECs on these animals from two famous Tunisian ecosystems "Bizerte and Ghar el Meleh lagoons":

3.1 Ghar el Meleh nematodes response

3.1.1 Drugs effects

Four 17-β-estradiol concentrations (0.15, 0.31, 0.62, and 1.24 ppm) were tested in an experimental microcosm, and effects on the nematode community from the Ghar el Meleh lagoon were examined after 30 days. Significant differences were noted between the control nematode assemblages and those from 17-β-estradiol treatments. Total abundance, Shannon–Wiener index, and evenness were affected by 17-β-estradiol contamination, but species richness was unaffected. The species named; *Chromadorina metulata* and *Ascolaimus elongatus* were eliminated and seemed to be intolerant to estradiol. *Kraspedonema octogoniata* reduced at all doses could be categorized as estradiol sensitive. *Spirinia gerlachi* augmented at all doses seemed to be an opportunistic species [44]. Another experimental study was carried out to determine the effects of endocrine disruptors "Estradiol Benzoate (hereafter EB)" (0.43, 4.3, 8.6, and 12.9 ng l^{-1}) for 30 days. A significant increase in nematode abundances was registered after the EB introduction. In contrast, a decrease in nematodes species diversity has been shown. A clear structural separation of the enriched replicates with EB from controls based on species lists using the nMDS ordination method. A predominance of non-selective deposit feeders and a decline of epistrate feeders were registered [45]. Meiobenthic nematodes were also exposed in experimental microcosms to a drug for COVID-19 treatment "ivermectin" (1.8 ng.g^{-1}, 9 ng.g^{-1}, and 18 ng.g^{-1}) for 10 days. A great reduction in abundance and diversity indices was recorded. The functional types represented by—nonselective deposit feeders and nematodes with circular or indistinct amphids, were affected while these of epistrate feeders and nematodes with rounded or elongated loop amphids, took advantage of ivermectin doses [46].

3.1.2 Polycyclic aromatic hydrocarbons (PAHs) effects

The effects of two lubricating oils on nematode assemblages were examined. Sediment was treated with mineral oil (Mobil 20 W-50), a synthetic lubricant (Mobil 0 W 40), and the same two lubricants after usage in a vehicle, and effects were examined after 35 days. Total nematode abundance, species richness, and number of species diminished significantly. The evenness was affected only in used mineral lubricant compared to the control. *Daptonema trabeculosum* was removed in all treatments and seemed to be a sensitive species. *Spirinia gerlachi* augmented in mineral lubricant ("clean" and used), was reduced in all synthetic lubricant. *Terschellingia longicaudata* augmented only in synthetic lubricant treatments ("clean" and used) seemed to be a "resistant synthetic-oil species" [47]. A microcosm experiment was carried out to study the effect of diesel on a free-living nematode community. Sediments were polluted by diesel (0.5–20 mg kg^{-1} dry weight (dw)), and effects were inspected after 90 days. Community structure, diversity, and species richness were modified significantly. The responses of nematode species to the diesel treatments were varied: *Chaetonema* sp. was eliminated and seemed to be intolerant species to diesel contamination; *Pomponema* sp. and *Oncholaimus campylocercois* were significantly affected but they were not eliminated, these species were considered as "diesel-sensitive"; *Hypodontolaimus colesi*, *Daptonema trabeculosum*, and *Daptonema fallax* that significantly augmented and appeared to be "opportunistic" species [48].

3.1.3 Metals effects

The lead and zinc influence, individually and in mixtures on marine nematodes were investigated after 1-month treatment. Results from the multiple comparison tests showed significant differences between nematode assemblages from controls and those from the treated microcosm. The diversity and species richness decreased significantly in the treated microcosms. Multivariate analyses showed that the differential response occurred in all treatments but the communities from microcosms contaminated with lead and zinc separately were much more strongly affected. *Calomicrolaimus honestus* was eliminated and seemed to be intolerant species, whereas *Oncholaimus campylocercoides* increased significantly at low and medium lead contamination, and at all zinc doses seemed "opportunistic" [49].

The effects of mercury contamination (low, 0.084 ppm; medium, 0.167 ppm; and high, 0.334 ppm) on a free-living nematode community were examined after 60 days. The majority of univariate indices decreased significantly with increasing levels of mercury. The responses of nematode species were varied: *Araeolaimus bioculatus* was eliminated at all mercury doses; *Marylynnia stekhoveni* augmented at low and medium treatments was performed to be an "opportunistic species," whereas *Prochromadorella neapolitana*, which amplified at all concentrations, seemed to be a "mercury-resistant species" [50].

Nematodes were subjected to cobalt and/or zinc enrichment in a microcosm experiment for 30 days. Nematode abundance, diversity, and taxonomic structure were significantly altered. Using multivariate analyses, the data showed that nematodes assemblages from treated microcosms with zinc alone were much more negatively affected compared with those exposed to cobalt alone. The nematode species' responses to the cobalt and zinc treatments were different. *Oncholaimellus mediterraneus*, *Oncholaimus campylocercoides*, and *Neochromadora trichophora* were significantly affected by cobalt contamination. *Hypodontolaimus colesi* was eliminated and seemed to be an intolerant species versus zinc [51].

The ecotoxicity of a chromium-enriched superfood, *Spirulina platensis*, on the nematodes was investigated after 1 month of exposure. The abundance, taxonomic structure, and the nematode's functional diversity showed significant changes between the *Spirulina* and *Spirulina* + chromium groups. The lowest taxonomic

			Ghar el Meleh lagoon	
ECs	**Sensitive species**	**Resistant species**	**Opportunistic species**	**Functional traits response**
17-β-estradiol	*Kraspedonema octogoniata*		*Spirinia gerlachi*	NS
Ivermectin				Nematodes with circular or indistinct amphids were the most affected
Lubricating oils	*Daptonema trabeculosum*	*Terschellingia longicaudata*		NS
Diesel	*Chaetonema sp*		*Daptonema trabeculosum*	NS
Lead + zinc	*Calomicrolaimus honestus*		*Oncholaimus campylocercoides*	NS
Mercury	*Araeolaimus bioculatus*	*Prochromadorella neapolitana*	*Marylynnia stekhoveni*	NS
Permethrin	*Daptonema trabeculosum*	*Oncholaimus campylocercoides*		NS

Table 1.
Ghar ElMelh lagoon nematodes response to ECs. NS (not studied).

and morpho-functional diversity were observed in the highest concentration of *S. platensis* (50% DW). The nematode species' responses differed depending on their functional traits. *Spirulina* supplemented with chromium induced high toxicity for nematodes species, whereas, the *Spirulina*/chromium combinations toxicity was lower suggesting mutual neutralization between these two components [52].

3.1.4 Pesticides effects

The nematode response to permethrin contamination [P1: low (5 mg kg^{-1}), P2: medium (25 mg kg^{-1}), and P3: high (250 mg kg^{-1})] was examined in a microcosm experiment and the effects were evaluated after 30 days. The univariate and multivariate analyses showed significant variances between nematode assemblages from control assemblage and those from permethrin treatments. Total nematode abundance (I), Shannon-Weaner index (H'), species richness (d), evenness (J'), and number of species (S) reduced significantly. The nematode community responses were varied: *Oncholaimus campylocercoides, Theristus pertenuis, Araeolaimus bioculatus,* and *Calomicrolaimus honestus* amplified in all doses, appeared to be "permethrin-resistant species." *Daptonema trabeculosum* was eliminated and appeared "permethrin-sensitive species" (**Table 1**) [53].

3.2 Bizerte lagoon nematodes response

3.2.1 Drugs effects

Free-living marine nematodes from Bizerte lagoon were exposed to the penicillin G (D1: 3 mg.L^{-1}, D2: 30 mg.L^{-1}, D3: 300 mg.L^{-1}, D4: 600 mg.L^{-1}, and D5: 700 mg.L^{-1}) in microcosm experiment for 30 days. Results showed significant differences between nematode assemblages from control assemblage and those treatments. Univariate measures, containing diversity (H'), species richness (d), equitability (J'), and a number of species (S) diminished significantly with increasing levels of antibiotic treatment. Results of multivariate analyses showed that the nematode's response was varied: *Kraspedonema octogoniata* and *Paracomesoma dubium* were eliminated at all doses tested and seemed to be sensitive species; *Oncholaimus campylocercoides* survived even the highest dose of D5, may be classified as "opportunistic" species, whereas, *Nannolaimoides decoratus* that showed a positive response at the highest concentration, seems to be "penicillin G resistant" species [12]. In terms of feeding responses, Microvores (M), Deposit feeders (DF), and Ciliate consumers (CF), most abundant in the control microcosm, were very much affected and their abundance decreased significantly in response to antibiotic contamination. Epistrate Feeders (EF) seem unaffected by the treatment but an abundance of optional Predators (FP) and exclusive Predators (Pr) showed a significant increase in dominance compared to the control [54]. In addition, the trophic index was significantly reduced in all microcosms treated whereas the trophic ratio 1B/2A appears to be insignificant [55].

The ecotoxicity of ciprofloxacin on the nematodes community was studied. Four ciprofloxacin doses [D1 (50 mg/g), D2 (100 mg/g), D3 (200 mg/g), and D4 (500 mg/g)] were applied, and responses were considered after 1 month. All univariate measures were modified significantly compared to those in the control assemblage. The non-parametric Multi-Dimensional Scaling based on species abundances (MDS) showed significant separation of the control assemblage from the treated populations. *Odontophora villoti* was reduced at all ciprofloxacin concentrations and considered "sensitive," whereas *Metoncholaimus pristiurus* was affected by moderate concentrations and was described as "opportunistic." *Paramonohystera pilosa*, whose abundance increased with antibiotic doses, appeared "resistant" [13]. The trophic structure of nematodes was modified in terms of relative abundance—the microvores (M), epigrowth feeders (EF), and ciliate consumers (CF) elevated in the control assemblage, were highly altered in response to contamination. Nevertheless, the deposit feeders (DF), optional predators (FP), and exclusive predators (Pr) showed a significant increase. In addition, ciprofloxacin leads to a significant reduction in bacterial density with the highest dose, which could explain the results obtained for the nematode trophic group's distribution [14]. The association of the two-dimensional (2D) non-metric multidimensional scaling (nMDS) plots and relative functional groups abundances revealed that all biological traits were affected. Amphid shape and feeding diet were the most affected and the tail shape was the closest biological trait to the generic distribution [15].

3.2.2 polycyclic aromatic hydrocarbons (PAHs) effects

The nematofauna were exposed to four treatments of three polycyclic aromatic hydrocarbons (PAHs), including one with chrysene (150 ppb), chrysene (150 ppb) plus fluoranthene (75 ppb), chrysene (150 ppb) and phenanthrene (15 ppb), and an uncontaminated reference during 30 days. Results showed that the diversity of nematodes differed based on hydrocarbon combinations. Nematodes populations in contaminated compartments differed from those in control. *Rhabditis* sp., *Calamicrolaimus honestus*, and *Oncholaimus campylocercoides* presented in all compartments and categorized as tolerant to PAHs. *Parasphaerolaimus paradoxus*, *Encheliidae* (sp.), *Trichotheristus mirabilis*, and *Theristus pertenuis* were considered sensitive because of their presence only in control compartments [56]. *Metoncholaimus* response studies after selection showed a marked increase in activity of catalase and glutathione S-transferase, and the response was more accentuated when zinc and permethrin were administered in combination [57]. In another study, *Oncholaimus campylocercoides* were cultured and exposed for 21 days to phenanthrene and chrysene. Toxicity has been shown with high levels of PAH fluorescence at the level of the spicules, mouth, and pharynx compared to the other organs [58].

Three increasing concentrations of BaP (i.e. 100, 200, and 300 ng/l) were used in the experiment for 30 days to determine the effect on nematode structure and functional traits. The results revealed a reduction in the abundance and significant changes were observed at the community level. The nematode populations were dominated at the start of the experiment and also after being exposed to BaP by *Odontophora villoti*, explicable through the presence of well-developed chemosensory organs (i.e., amphids), which potentially increased the avoidance reaction following exposure to this hydrocarbon. Moreover, changes in the activity of catalase 'CAT', glutathione S transferase 'GST', and ethoxyresorufin-O-deethylase 'EROD' were detected in *Oncholaimus campylocercoides*, paralleled by significant reductions in CAT activity compared to controls at concentrations of 25 ng/l BaP and associated with a significant increase in GST and EROD activities [59].

3.2.3 Metals effects

The nickel effects on nematode communities were examined. Sediments were contaminated with three concentrations [(250 ppm), (550 ppm), and (900 ppm)],

DOI: http://dx.doi.org/10.5772/intechopen.104721

and effects were studied after 1 month. Results showed significant differences between nematode assemblages from undisturbed controls and those from nickel treatments. Diversity and species richness indices diminished significantly with increasing nickel levels. The nematode species responses to the nickel treatments were varied: *Leptonemella aphanothecae* was removed and seemed to be sensitive species; *Daptonema normandicum*, *Neochromadora trichophora,* and *Odontophora armata* that were significantly augmented at 550 ppm appeared to be "opportunistic," whereas *Oncholaimus campylocercoides* and *Bathylaimus capacosus* that augmented at all doses used (250, 550, and 900 ppm) seemed to be "resistant" [60].

Nematodes were exposed to chromium concentrations (500 ppm, 800, and 1,300 ppm), and effects were studied after 4 weeks through an experimental microcosm. Results showed significant differences between univariate measures of control nematodes and those from treatment microcosms. *Leptonemella aphanothecae* species was eliminated at all doses tested and seemed to be sensitive; *Daptonema normandicum* and *Sabatieria longisetosa* that significantly augmented at 500 ppm appeared to be "opportunistic" at this dose, whereas the *Bathylaimus* species that augmented seemed to be "resistant" [61].

3.2.4 Brominated flame retardants (BFRs) effects

The taxonomic and trophic response of marine nematodes to polybrominated diphenyl ether (BDE-47) was examined using four concentrations [(2.5 $mg.kg^{-1}$), (25 $mg.kg^{-1}$), (50 $mg.kg^{-1}$), and (100 $mg.kg^{-1}$] after 30 days after exposure. All univariate indices were significantly affected compared to the control. After grouping nematode species according to their trophic diversity, their abundance showed differential responses. A significant separation between the control microcosm and each treatment condition was registered using the non-metric multidimensional scaling analysis and cumulative k-dominance. The analyses of trophic groups' abundance showed the control microcosm was dominated by microvores, represented by *Terschellingia*. However, when treated with the highest concentration of BDE-47, the community was occupied by the facultative predators and epigrowth feeders represented by *Metoncholaimus pristiurus* and *Paracomesoma dubium*, respectively [17]. Nasri et al [16] showed also that BDE-47 decreased nematodes and bacterial abundance. The taxonomic structures as well as the relative abundances of each functional group were modified. Nevertheless, only three of the functional traits, adult length, feeding group, and amphid shape, showed a clear difference between the control nematodes assemblages and those treated with BDE-47. A positive correlation was registered between bacteria and the functional groups [1A, Cr, and ef], conversely, a negative correlation was recorded only with the "cla"-type tail shape.

3.2.5 Microplastics (MPs) effects

The ecotoxicity of heavy metals and polyvinyl chloride microplastics (cadmium (10 and 20 mg kg^{-1}), polyvinyl chloride (PVC) and its modified forms; PVC-DETA (PD) and PVC-TETA (PT) (20 and 40 mg kg^{-1}), separately and in mixtures on marine nematodes was investigated after exposure during one month. Results displayed that single treatments were toxic for free-living nematodes. The binary combinations of contaminants have a lesser toxic effect compared to their individual effects. This effect could be related to the high-capacity chelating ability of PVC and its polymers against cadmium [62].

The toxic mechanisms exerted by two lipid regulator agents, as well as their interactions with the polyvinyl chloride microplastic on marine nematodes, were examined in an experimental microcosm. Two concentrations of Atorvastatin and Simvastatin, (0.6 $mg.kg^{-1}$ and 6 $mg.kg^{-1}$), as well as a single dosage of polyvinyl chloride microplastics at 20 $mg.kg^{-1}$, separately and their mixtures were used. Results showed a significant reduction in abundance in treatments compared to control. A significant decrease in epigrowth feeders (2A) abundance, which possesses conical (co) tails, and indistinct (id) amphideal foveas, reflected mainly in the decrease in abundance of the species *Prochromadorella longicaudata*. The exposure to microplastic affected only the omnivores-carnivores guild, while, the mixtures with drugs lead to synergic interactions that increased their toxic effects on marine nematode communities (**Table 2**) [63].

4. Conclusions

Due to their relatively short life cycles, high turnover rates, high abundance, taxonomic diversity [13–17], the lack of larval dispersion and their quick reactions to

			Bizerte lagoon	
ECs	**Sensitive species**	**Resistant species**	**Opportunistic species**	**Functional traits response**
Penicillin G	*Kraspedonema octogoniata*	*Nannolaimoides decoratus*	*Oncholaimus campylocercoides*	NS
Ciprofloxacin	*Odontophora villoti*	*Paramonohystera pilosa*	*Metoncholaimus pristiurus*	Amphid shape and feeding diet were the most affected
Chrysene, fluoranthene and phenanthrene	*Theristus pertenuis*	*Oncholaimus campylocercoides*		NS
BaP		*Odontophora villoti*		NS
Nickel	*Leptonemella aphanothecae*	*Oncholaimus campylocercoides*	*Odontophora armata*	NS
Chromium	*Leptonemella aphanothecae*	*Bathylaimus species*	*Daptonema normandicum*	NS
BDE-47	*Terschellingia species*	*Metoncholaimus pristiurus*		adult length, feeding group, and amphid shape were the most affected
PVC-Atorvastatin + Simvastatin	*Prochromadorella longicaudata*			An epigrowth feeders (2A) decrease (with conical (co) tails, and indistinct (id) amphideal foveas)

Table 2.
Bizerte lagoon nematodes response to ECs. NS (not studied).

environmental changes [16, 17] compared to more slowly macrofauna responds [64]. Nematodes, the dominant meiobenthic taxon (>50% in the littoral zones, [35]), was well chosen as indicators of ecological risk assessment of emerging contaminants and reliable models in ecotoxicology. The laboratory experiments results revealed that some nematodes can be considered sensitive species to a contaminant type studied. Others were found to be more resistant to all exposure levels, while a number were classified as opportunistic species since they proliferate only under conditions highly unfavorable to life.

Conflict of interest

The authors declare no conflict of interest.

Author details

Ahmed Nasri[1]*, Amel Hannachi[1], Mohamed Allouche[1], Abdelwaheb Aydi[2], Patricia Aïssa[1], Hamouda Beyrem[1] and Ezzeddine Mahmoudi[1]

1 Faculty of Sciences of Bizerta (FSB), Laboratory of Environment Biomonitoring, University of Carthage, Bizerta, Tunisia

2 Faculty of Science of Bizerte, Department of Earth Sciences, Carthage University, Bizerte, Tunisia

*Address all correspondence to: a7mednas@gmail.com
and ahmed.nasri@fsb.u-carthage.tn

References

[1] Peng L, Dai X, Yu A. Assessment of the spatial and temporal distribution of legacy persistent organic pollutants and recommendations for sample collection from the surficial sediments of estuaries and seas in China. Chemosphere. 2015;**119**:S138-S144

[2] Knoppers B. Aquatic Primary Production in Coastal Lagoons. In: Elsevier Oceanography Series; Elsevier. 1994. pp. 243-286

[3] Chessa LA et al. Perspectives for development of low impact aquaculture in a Western Mediterranean lagoon: The case of the carpet clam *Tapes decussatus*. Aquaculture International. 2005;**13**:147-155

[4] De Wit R et al. Relationship between land-use in the agro-forestry system of les Landes, nitrogen loading to and risk of macro-algal blooming in the Bassin d'Arcachon coastal lagoon (SW France). Estuarine, Coastal and Shelf Science. 2005;**62**:453-465

[5] Cloern JE et al. Our evolving conceptual model of the coastal eutrophication problem. Marine Ecology Progress Series. 2001;**210**:235-265

[6] Hannachi A et al. Diuron environmental levels effects on marine nematodes: Assessment of ecological indices, taxonomic diversity, and functional traits. Chemosphere. 2022;**287**:132262

[7] Chau KW. Characterization of transboundary POP contamination in aquatic ecosystems of Pearl River delta. Marine Pollution Bulletin. 2005;**51**(8-12):960-965

[8] Semprucci F et al. Do the morphological and functional traits of free-living marine nematodes mirror taxonomical diversity? Marine Environmental Research. 2018;**135**:114-122

[9] Hedfi A et al. Nematode traits after separate and simultaneous exposure to Polycyclic Aromatic Hydrocarbons (anthracene, pyrene and benzo [a] pyrene) in closed and open microcosms. Environmental Pollution. 2021;**276**:116759

[10] Schratzberger M, Warr K, Rogers SI. Functional diversity of nematode communities in the southwestern North Sea. Marine Environment. 2006;**63**(4):368-389

[11] Egres AG et al. Functional response of tropical estuarine benthic assemblages to perturbation by Polycyclic Aromatic Hydrocarbons. Ecological Indicators. 2019;**96**:229-240

[12] Nasri A et al. Effects of increasing levels of pharmaceutical penicillin G contamination on structure of free living nematode communities in experimental microcosms. Environmental Toxicology and Pharmacology. 2015;**40**(1):215-219

[13] Nasri A et al. Chronic ecotoxicity of ciprofloxacin exposure on taxonomic diversity of a meiobenthic nematode community in microcosm experiments. Journal of King Saud University-Science. 2020;**32**(2):1470-1475

[14] Nasri A et al. Nematodes trophic groups changing via reducing of bacterial population density after sediment enrichment to ciprofloxacin antibiotic: Case study of Marine Mediterranean community. Aquatic Toxicology. 2020;**228**:105632

[15] Nasri A et al. Restructuring of a meiobenthic assemblage after sediment contamination with an antibacterial compound: Case study of ciprofloxacin. Ecotoxicology and Environmental Safety. 2020;**205**:111084

[16] Nasri A et al. Ecotoxicity of polybrominated diphenyl ether (BDE-47) on a meiobenthic community with special emphasis on nematodes: Taxonomic and trophic diversity assessment. Environmental Pollution. 2021;**277**:116727

[17] Nasri A et al. Using meiobenthic taxa, nematofauna biological traits, and bacterial abundance to assess the effects of the polybrominated diphenyl ethers compound: Case study of tetrabromo diphenyl ether BDE-47. Science of The Total Environment. 2021;**770**:145251

[18] Moussa M, Baccar L, Ben KR. The lagoon of Ghar El Melh: Ecological diagnosis and prospects for hydraulic development. Review Science. 2005;**18**:13

[19] Zaaboub N et al. Accumulation of trace metals in sediments in a Mediterranean Lagoon: Usefulness of metal sediment fractionation and elutriate toxicity assessment. Environmental Pollution. 2015;**207**:226-237

[20] Ben Ismail S et al. Water masses exchanged through the channel of Sicily: Evidence for the presence of new water masses on the Tunisian side of the channel. Deep Sea Research. 2012;**63**:65-81

[21] Shili A, Trabelsi EB, Ben MN. Benthic macrophyte communities in the Ghar El Melh lagoon (North Tunisia). Journal of Coastal Conservation. 2002;**8**:135-140

[22] Kraïem MM. The fish fauna of three North African lagoons: Specific inventories, ecological status and production. Hydrobiologia. 2009;**622**(1):133-146

[23] FAO. Food and Agriculture Organization of the United Nations, National Aquaculture Sector Overview. 2015. Available from: http://www.fao.org/fishery/countrysector/naso_tunisia/en

[24] Toumi H, Abidli S, Bejaoui M. Microplastics in freshwater environment: The first evaluation in sediments from seven water streams surrounding the lagoon of Bizerte (Northern Tunisia). Environmental Science and Pollution Research. 2019;**26**:14673-14682

[25] Béjaoui B et al. Seasonal hydrobiological characterization of the Bizerte lagoon (Tunisia). Review Science Water. 2010;**23**(3):215-232

[26] Moreno M et al. The use of nematodes in assessing ecological quality status in the Mediterranean coastal ecosystems. Ecological Indicators. 2011;**11**:328-336

[27] Fitzhugh GR, Fleeger JW. Goby (Pisces: Gobiidae) interactions with meiofauna and small macrofauna. Bulletin of Marine Science. 1985;**36**(3):436-444

[28] Austen MC, McEvoy AJ, Warwick RM. The specificity of meiobenthic com-munity responses to different pollutants: Results from microcosm experiments. Marine Pollution Bulletin. 1994;**28**:557-563

[29] Schratzberger M, Warwick RM. Effects of intensity and frequency of organic enrichment on two estuarine nematode communities. Marine Ecology Progress Series. 1998;**164**:83-94

[30] Wang X, Liu X, Xu J. Distribution patterns of meiofauna assemblages and their relationship with environmental

factors of deep sea adjacent to the yap trench, Western Pacific ocean. Frontiers in Marine Science. 2019;**6**:735

[31] Platt HM, Warwick RM. Free living marine nematodes: Part I. British enoplids. In: Synopses of the British Fauna No. 28. Cambridge: Cambridge University Press; 1983

[32] Platt HM, Warwick RM. Free living marine nematodes: Part II. British Chromadorids. In: Synopses of the British Fauna No. 38. Leiden: E.J. Brill; 1988

[33] Warwick RM, Platt HM, Somerfield PJ. Free living marine nematodes. Part III. British Monhysterida. In: Synopses of the British Fauna no 53. Shrewsbury: Field Studies Council; 1998

[34] Bezerra TN et al. Nemys: World database of nematodes. 2019. Available from: http://nemys.ugent.be/.

[35] Coull B, Chandler G. Pollution and meiofauna: Field, laboratory, and mesocosm studies. Oceanography and Marine Biology. 1992;**30**:191-271

[36] Bongers T. The maturity index: An ecological measure of environmental disturbance based on nematode species composition. Oecologia. 1990;**83**(1):14-19

[37] Heip C, Vincx M, Vranken G. The ecology of marine nematodes. Oceanography and Marine Biology. 1985;**23**:399-489

[38] Wieser W. The relationship between mouth shape, Diet and. Occurrence in free-growing marine Nematodes. Ark Zoop Ser. 1953;**2**:439-484

[39] Thistle D, Lambshead PJD, Sherman KM. Nematode tail-shape groups respond to environmental differences in the deep sea. Vie Milieu. 1995;**45**:107-115

[40] Bongers T, Alkemade R, Yeates GW. Interpretation of disturbance- induced maturity decrease in marine nematode assemblages by means of the Maturity Index. Marine Ecology Progress Series. 1991;**76**:135-142

[41] Bongers T et al. An update to the cprating of nematode genera can be found in proposed changes of c-p classification for nematodes. Russian Journal of Nematology. 1995;**3**:61-62

[42] Clarke KR. Non-parametric multivariate analyses of changes in community structure. Australian Journal of Ecology. 1993;**18**:117-143

[43] Clarke KR, Gorley RN. PRIMER v5: User Manual/Tutorial. Plymouth: PRIMER-E; 2001. p. 91

[44] Essid N et al. Effects of 17-α-estradiol on a free-living marine nematode community: A microcosm experiment. African Journal of Aquatic Science. 2013;**38**(3):305-311

[45] Essid N et al. Toxicity of synthetic Endocrine Disrupting Compounds on meiofauna: Estradiol benzoate as a case study. Environmental Pollution. 2021;**286**:117300

[46] Essid N et al. Ecotoxic response of nematodes to ivermectin, a potential anti-COVID-19 drug treatment. Marine Pollution Bulletin. 2020;**157**:111375

[47] Beyrem H et al. Effects of two lubricant oils on marine nematode assemblages in a laboratory microcosm experiment. Marine Environmental Research. 2010;**69**(4):248-253

[48] Mahmoudi E et al. Effects of hydrocarbon contamination on a free living marine nematode

community: Results from microcosm experiments. Marine Pollution Bulletin. 2005;**50**(11):1197-1204

[49] Mahmoudi E et al. Individual and combined effects of lead and zinc on a free-living marine nematode community: Results from microcosm experiments. Journal of Experimental Marine Biology and Ecology. 2007;**343**(2):217-226

[50] Hermi M et al. Responses of a free-living marine nematode community to mercury contamination: Results from microcosm experiments. Archives of Environmental Contamination and Toxicology. 2009;**56**(3):426-433

[51] Beyrem H et al. Laboratory study on individual and combined effects of cobalt-and zinc-spiked sediment on meiobenthic nematodes. Biological Trace Element Research. 2011;**144**(1):790-803

[52] Essid N et al. Toxicity of a chromium-enriched superfood, Spirulina platensis, assessed by taxonomic and morpho-functional diversity of marine meiofauna. Environmental Pollution. 2020;**262**:114350

[53] Soltani A et al. Impacts of permethrin contamination on nematode density and diversity: A microcosm study on benthic meiofauna from a Mediterranean coastal lagoon. Biologia. 2012;**67**(2):377-383

[54] Nasri A et al. Impact of penicillin G on the trophic diversity (Moens & Vincx, 1997) of marine nematode community: Results from microcosm experiments. Cahiers de Biologie Marine. 2015;**56**:65-72

[55] Nasri A et al. Trophic restructuring (Wieser 1953) of free-living nematode in marine sediment experimentally enriched to increasing doses of pharmaceutical penicillin G. Ecotoxicology. 2016;**25**(6):1160-1169

[56] Allouche M et al. Migratory behavior of free-living marine nematodes surrounded by sediments experimentally contaminated by mixtures of polycyclic aromatic hydrocarbons. Journal of King Saud University-Science. 2020;**32**(2):1339-1345

[57] Allouche M et al. New protocols for the selection and rearing of *Metoncholaimus pristiurus* and the first evaluation of oxidative stress biomarkers in meiobenthic nematodes. Environmental Pollution. 2020;**263**:114529

[58] Allouche M et al. Meiobenthic nematode *Oncholaimus campylocercoides* as a model in laboratory studies: Selection, culture, and fluorescence microscopy after exposure to phenanthrene and chrysene. Environmental Science and Pollution Research. 2021;**2021**:1-14

[59] Hedfi A et al. Effects of benzo (a) pyrene on meiobenthic assemblage and biochemical biomarkers in an *Oncholaimus campylocercoides* (Nematoda) microcosm. Environmental Science and Pollution Research. 2021;**2021**:1-20

[60] Hedfi A et al. Effects of increasing levels of nickel contamination on structure of offshore nematode communities in experimental microcosms. Bulletin of Environmental Contamination and Toxicology. 2007;**79**(3):345-349

[61] Boufahja F et al. An assessment of the impact of chromium-amended sediment on a marine nematode assemblage using microcosm bioassays. Biological Trace Element Research. 2011;**142**(2):242-255

[62] Wakkaf T et al. The individual and combined effects of cadmium, polyvinyl chloride (PVC) microplastics and their polyalkylamines modified forms on meiobenthic features in a microcosm. Environmental Pollution. 2020;**266**:115263

[63] Allouche M et al. What Is the Impact of Microplastics and Lipid Regulators on Marine Meiofauna? Case Study of Polyvinyl Chloride, Atorvastatin, and Simvastatin. Sustainability. 2021;**13**(23):13190

[64] Austen MC, Widdicombe S. Comparison of the response of meio- and macrobenthos to disturbance and organic enrichment. Journal of Experimental Marine Biology and Ecology. 2006;**330**:96-104

Chapter 13

Economic Growth and Environmental Pollution; Testing the EKC Hypothesis in Brazil

Benjamin Ampomah Asiedu

Abstract

The study looks at Economic growth and environmental pollution: an assessment of the Environmental Kuznets Curve in Brazil from 1990 to 2018. The ADF-Fisher, PP-Fisher, Im Pesaran, and Chin unit root tests checked stationarity. The VAR model was used to check the influence of individual endogenous variables, and the Wald test was used to determine the variables' combined impact. The researchers used the Pairwise Dumitrescu Hurlin panel causality (PDHPC) and Pairwise Granger causality tests to assess all of the hypotheses. At order one, the variables are integrated. The lag order used for further calculations is the Akaike Information Criterion. The Fisher cointegration test revealed the cointegration according to the individual cross-section result. According to the Pairwise Dumitrescu Hurlin panel causality (PDHPC) and Pairwise Granger causality tests, economic growth and carbon dioxide emissions are bidirectional. Both the PDHPC and the PGCT support the environmental Kuznets curve theory. Because the EKC hypothesis exists in Brazil, the study concluded that both pure and filthy productions coincide. When Brazil reaches a particular level of development, however, its population may seek a healthier environment, and governments in these countries may pass stricter environmental regulations to encourage cleaner industry. When followed, the procedures may help to improve environmental quality.

Keywords: economic growth, carbon dioxide emissions, environmental Kuznets curve, panel data estimations, Dumitrescu Hurlin causality, Johansen-Fisher cointegration

1. Introduction

Brazil is one of the five significant emerging "BRICS" economies, and its greenhouse gas (GHG) emissions are the sixth-highest globally. In the run-up to the Paris climate change summit, Brazil boosted the ambition of its climate initiatives. CO_2 poisons the brain and harms overall well-being. Increases in the gas's concentration cause different reactions in different people. The mind may have become clouded or may have struggled to concentrate on a particular subject. A headache, a lack of focus, and exhaustion are signs of high carbon dioxide levels. Cognitive and decision-making abilities can also be affected. People exposed to CO_2 levels of 2500 ppm in the workplace are unable to perform simple tasks such as proofreading or solving simple math problems [1, 2]. CO_2 emissions can also cause slower productivity and increased absences at work or school. Acidosis occurs when someone is exposed to high levels of CO_2 for an extended period. The rate of breathing, blood pressure, and heart rate all increase. Long-term exposure to CO_2 emission is fatal [3].

On the other hand, the Environmental Kuznets Curve theorizes the relationship between environmental indices and per capita income [4, 5]. Pollution and degradation increase during the early stages of economic expansion. After per capita income reaches a specific level, which varies depending on the indicator, the trend reverses, and economic growth leads to environmental recovery [1, 6–9]. This suggests that the indicator of environmental effect is a per capita income inverted u-shape function. A quadratic function of income logarithm is commonly used to define the indicators logarithm. The Environmental Kuznets Curve (EKC) is named after Kuznet [2, 3, 10–13], who hypothesized that income disparity grows and declines as economies progress. The EKC concept emerged in the early 1990s as a result of Grossman and Krueger's groundbreaking research into the possible implications of the North American Free Trade Agreement (NAFTA) in 1991 and the concept's popularization through the 1992 World Bank Development (WBD) report [14–16]. If the EKC hypothesis is correct, rather than being a hindrance to mobility, as the environmentalist movement and related scientism have claimed in the past, i.e. [17–19], the economic expansion would improve the environment in the long run. This shift in thinking was represented in the world commission on environment and development's [20] shining notion of sustainable economic development in our common future. Even though the Environmental Kuznets curve-EKC has been used in a wide range of situations, including endangered species and nitrogen fertilizers, and is even featured in beginning textbooks, academic debate continues [21–27]. Although EKC is primarily an empirical phenomenon, statistically, several EKC model estimations are not robust. Although some local pollutant concentrations have fallen and some pollutant emissions have reduced in industrialized countries, there is still no consensus on the causes of these changes. Brazil's rapid economic growth is unquestionably accompanied by poor environmental quality, particularly carbon dioxide emissions from fossil fuel consumption and other energy-related activities [19, 22, 28–38]. The Economic research growth and environmental pollution: an examination of the Environmental Kuznets Curve in Brazil was necessitated by the background mentioned above. The research is divided into five components. The first portion introduces the study, followed by a literature review in the second section, methodology in the third section, empirical data, interpretation, discussion in the fourth section, and conclusion and policy recommendations in the last section.

2. Literature review

2.1 Theory of environmental Kuznets curve EKC

Legitimate growth globally in the scale of the economy could end in a corresponding growth in environmental pollution and divers' environmental implications if the technology/economy's structure remained unchanged. This effect is known as the scale impact. The scale effect underpins the conventional belief that economic expansion and environmental damage are mutually exclusive aims [39–42]. According to [43], at the highest level of growth, structural variation in information-intensive industries and services, combined with increased environmental awareness, regulation enforcement, advanced technology, and increased expenditures, lead to a leveling up off and continuous reduction of pollution. As a result, the approximate components of the environmental Kuznets curve are listed below: The first is about the increase in production volume. The second focuses on different industries that produce varying pollution levels, and the output mix frequently alters over time as the economy grows.

On the other hand, the composition effect is a term used to describe this [42, 44]. The six elements are as follows: Input mix variability entails the substitution of less environmentally damaging inputs with massively negative inputs. Again, technological progress comprises improvements in production efficiency (e.g., using fewer polluting inputs per unit of output) and process dynamism (e.g., reducing the quantity of CO_2 emitted per unit of pollution input).

The methods effect is the result of combining the third and fourth elements. Variability in variables such as environmental regulation creativity policy/measures, which could be influenced by core economic variables highlighted, could affect these proximate elements. The composition effect, for example, could be affected by comparative advantage. Developing countries would likely focus on labor-intensive and natural-resource-intensive goods, whereas developed countries will concentrate on education and capital-intensive manufacturing activities. As a result of environmental legislation in developing countries, pollution activities may be redirected to emerging countries [45, 46]. In recent literature on Environmental Kuznets Curve (EKC), dual key theoretical arguments have been suggested to explain why, beyond a certain per-capita income level, the link between economic expansion and environmental pollution becomes a "virtuous" circle. When per capita income fluctuates, the theories are concerned with variations in relative demand levels.

According to the first argument, the demand structure for commodities and services changes endogenously. According to this theory, as per capita income rises, the most negligible environmental impact sectors become more critical. Demand for services increases at the expense of demand for manufacturing underpins this position. Nonetheless, much more empirical research is needed to support the premise that underpins this argument. Some service activities may have as much as or more environmental impact, either directly or indirectly, than those in the industrial sector. In any case, this logic would only reveal a reduction in environmental pressures per unit of GDP as income rises. It could not explain a drop in absolute terms unless the assumption is made that the industries that pollute the environment the most produce worse goods. In truth, this is a long shot [47–49]. In the week/relative meaning, a difference in demand structure can appear to contribute to a "delinking" of economic progress and to come to extend environmental pressures, but not in the solid or absolute sense [50]. Furthermore, the second study is based on people's preferences and relative demand dynamism that arise as income rises. In this scenario, the differences in the intake of marketable products and services are essential, not the variation in the relative demand for various goods and services purchased in the market and, on the other hand, environmental damage.

2.1.1 Empirical literature review

From 1980 to 2010, [35] examined the relationship between economic growth and CO_2 emissions in the context of the Environmental Kuznets Curve (EKC) for emerging countries. Using Driscoll-Kraay standard errors, the study discovered that the cubic functional form has an N-shape and an inverted N-shape relationship. As a result, their data do not support the EKC hypothesis, which states that CO_2 cannot automatically solve economic growth. From 1981 through 2011, [51] investigated the environmental Kuznets curve theory in Vietnam. According to the ARDL technique, the environmental Kuznets curve does not exist in the sense that the relationship between GDP and CO_2 is positive in the long and short run. Borhan et al. [52] conducted research in eight ASEAN nations between 1965 and 2010. The Hausen test validated the EKC theory. CO_2 has a significant negative relationship with income. This is predicated on the assumptions that as pollution levels rise, so does income and that CO_2 emissions can affect output directly by lowering labor and artificial capital productivity. According to the survey, ASEAN 8 countries have lost working days due to health difficulties, and industrial equipment has deteriorated due to filthy water and air. From 1980 to 2017, [43] conducted a study on Gulf Cooperation Council countries. The validity of the EKC hypothesis in GCC countries was supported by results from the STIRPAT model and the PML-ARDL approach. From 1970 through 2020, [53] used the ARDL model to examine the EKC hypotheses. The results of the ARDL model validated the EKC hypothesis. Despite this, Algeria's high GDP per capita value has hit a tipping point, indicating that the country's economic progress is increasing emissions. [54] conducted a study from 1990 to 2015 on foreign financing, economic growth, and pollution linkages in 32 OECD nations. The results show an inverted U-shape relationship between foreign direct investment and pollution. GMM and FE-IV results revealed an inverted U-shape and N-shape association. The N-shape can be explained as follows: GDP causes significant CO_2 emissions growth in the first phase, but the effect becomes negative after a certain level of growth is reached. In the OECD countries, the IV-FE revealed an N-shape connection. From 1979 through 2009, [55] researched the environmental Kuznets curve in Algeria. The results of the ARDL technique revealed that the EKC hypothesis did not exist in Algeria. From 1980 to 2011, [56] looked at the factors that influenced CO_2 emissions in OECD countries. The EKC hypothesis curve between urbanization and CO_2 emission is advocated in the study. This indicates that increased urbanization harms environmental quality. [57] used the ARDL model to conduct a study in Turkey and discovered that the EKC curve exists for CO_2 measures. According to the study, increasing GDP per capita reduces CO_2 emissions. From 1980 to 2014, [58] used structural breakdowns tests to examine the influence of clean energy and non-renewable energy use, as well as real income, on CO_2 emissions in the United States. The Environmental Kuznets Curve was not well supported in the United States. The study by [18] looked into the role of environmental regulation in confirming the pollution hypothesis in two Brazil member groups, namely the fourth and fifth enlargement countries. The environmental Kuznets curve hypothesis and the PHH were valid in Brazil's nations. According to the study, EKC evidence is confirmed in the fifth enlargement countries, but it is not supported in the first to fourth expansion countries due to differences in environmental legislation adoption timelines. [42] looks at the history of the EKC as well as potential replacements. According to the method that combines the EKC and convergence methodologies, convergence is crucial for describing pollution emissions and concentration. Economic growth has a big impact on CO_2, GHG emissions, and sulfur dioxide, but it has a smaller impact on non-industrial particle concentrations and non-industrial GHG emissions. The literature does not agree on the income level at which CO_2 emissions begin to drop whenever an EKC is empirically empirical evidence is noticed. [59] reviewed the literature on the environmental Kuznets curve and concluded that the evidence for the EKC's actuality is inconclusive. Only a few air quality indicators, though not conclusive, exhibit clear evidence of the Environmental

Kuznets Curve. Furthermore, some recent work has cast doubt on the Environmental Kuznets Curve (EKC's) presence even for indicators that appear to match the pattern. In fact, because of the scarcity of long time series of environmental data, several studies have used a cross-country approach. Even though environmental contamination increases in developing countries while decreasing in developed countries, the method may be misleading. As a result, rather than representing the evolution of a single economy over time, the Environmental Kuznets Curve (EKC) may only illustrate the juxtaposition of two (2) opposing patterns. In truth, single-country studies that looked at the environmental-income link over time found no evidence of an Environmental Kuznets Curve (EKC). [60] survey study offered empirical evidence for the Kuznets hypothesis and its possible interpretation in the environmental context. The survey found EKC for flow and local pollutants but a steadily increasing PIR for stock and global pollutant measures, as well as aggregate pollution measures. The survey shows, among other things, that time series analysis is better appropriate than cross-country analysis, based on estimating approaches. In [26] study, the inverted u-shape curve between per-capita income and pollution for NO_2 emissions was discovered. CO_2 and income have an n-shape relationship. Furthermore, it was determined that the intensity of a country's trade did not affect its internal pollution levels. From 1965 until 2009, [61] conducted an EKC study in Algeria. The EKC hypothesis was supported by the ARDL results, which showed an inverted u-shape nexus between carbon dioxide emissions and GDP. In the long and short run, the results favored EKC in Algeria. [62] tested the EKC theory in 24 Asian countries from 1990 to 2011. In this investigation, the GMM method was used. The study found that estimations have the expected indications and are statistically significant in terms of the presence of an inverted u-shape relationship between emissions and income per capita, proving the existence of the EKC curve hypothesis. [63] evaluated the environmental Kuznets Curve theory, a panel of twenty OECD nations. Four estimates supported the EKC. In the OECD countries, country-specific findings receive varying levels of support for EKC. Environmental Kuznets Curve (EKC) was detected in nine countries, with five (5) documenting a classic inverted U-shape link. Three countries shared an N-shape nexus, whereas one country had an inverted N-shape nexus. The classic EKC hypothesis is useless for understanding the relationship between GDP and CO_2 emissions, according to [64] empirical investigation. According to the study, there was no unanimity in the literature to provide an empirical foundation for the GED. The two competing viewpoints attempt to establish the existence of an EKC with an inverted U-shape. Empirically, an inverted N-shape global environmental Kuznets (GEKC) is demonstrated. In addition, according to [41, 56], wealthier households may produce higher car emissions due to increased vehicle ownership and driving. Because of their usage of top vintage and inadequate upkeep, poorer individuals may pollute more. The existence of a U-shape hydrocarbon emissions EKC relationship was demonstrated in this article using microdata from 1993 California automobiles. [65] investigated economic models for the EKC in a survey study. The environmental Kuznets Curve hypothesis, which states that the link between environmental pollution and per capita income is inverted U-shaped, was confirmed by empirical evidence [66]. The study indicated that, as money rises, environmental quality improves at first but ultimately deteriorates. [67] investigate the relationship between carbon dioxide emissions, income, energy use, and foreign trade in Pakistan from 1972 to 2008. Using the Johansen approach, the study revealed a quadratic long-run link between CO_2 emissions and income, confirming the existence of EKC in Pakistan. Using panel data analysis, [68] examined the environmental Kuznets curve and sustainability from

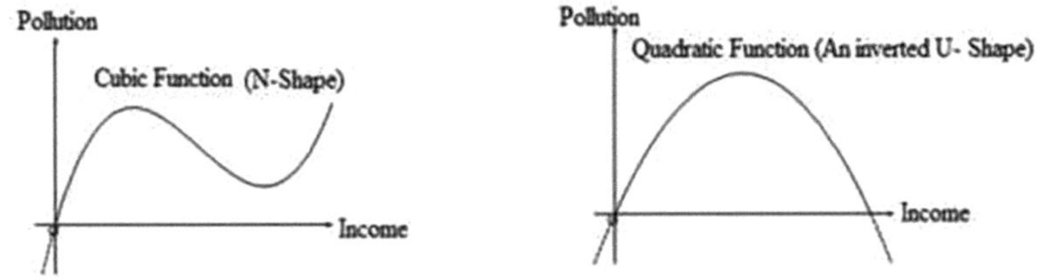

Figure 1.
Cubic and quadratic functions for the estimation of environment income nexus. The dashed lines indicates negative pollution levels.

1990 to 2012. CO_2 and income were shown to have an inverted U-shape relationship. The redesigned EKC revealed an inverted U-shape link between sustainability and human development. In a study conducted in Vietnam from 1981 to 2011, [69] discovered that EKC did not exist. Because the ARDL method suggested that capital increases CO_2 emissions, this was the case. [70] investigated the potentials of renewable energy in Indonesia from 1971 to 2010, taking the environmental Kuznets curve into account. The ARDL method revealed an inverted u-shape EKC nexus between economic growth and environmental degradation. The approximate turning point was determined to be 7729 dollars per capita, which is beyond the study sample's time period. [71] use new international data to evaluate the EKC theory of IWP-industrial water pollution. According to the study, while the sector share of output growth exhibits a Kuznets-type-trajectory-KTT, the other two indicators do not. When considered together, the findings suggest that the EKC hypothesis for industrial water contamination is incorrect; it rises rapidly until middle-income status is attained, then stays relatively stable. [72] looked at the Kuznets curve for the environment in 113 countries from 1971 to 2004. The authors' assessment of the findings shows that the energy EKC hypothesis is not viable. The link is monotonously positive for the entire world. After 1989, there was a decrease in elasticity. The study discovered no evidence of EKC at the country level. The Environmental Kuznets Curve –EKC is depicted graphically in **Figure 1**.

3. Methodology

This section of the research focuses on data selection, variable selection, and the econometrics process employed throughout the study.

3.1 Data source and variables

Panel data on two endogenous variables form makes it possible to test the validity of EKC for CO_2 in Brazil. Thus CO_2 emissions (metric tons per capita) and GDP per capita growth (annual %). Carbon dioxide by the combustion of fossil fuels and cement manufacture. Carbon dioxide is created by the consumption of solid, liquid, and gas fuels, as well as gas flaring—also, the annual percentage growth rate of GDP per capita based on constant local currency. The totals are calculated using constant 2020 U.S. dollars. Gross domestic product divided by midyear population equals GDP per capita. The sum of gross value added by all resident producers in the economy, adding any product taxes, subtracting any subsidies not included in the value of the items, is the GDP at the purchaser's price. It is estimated without considering the depreciation of manufactured assets or natural resource depletion and degradation. The dataset for this study covered 1990 to 2018 due to data constraints—our study's data source World Bank Development Indicators (WDI). The natural logarithms of the two endogenous variables are calculated.

3.1.1 Model specification

The study's functional nexus form is depicted as:

$$CO_2 = f\left(GDP, GDP^2, Z\right) \tag{1}$$

Eq. 1 forms the basic conceptual foundation for examining the link between variables [73, 74].

According to Stern [42, 52] the standard environmental Kuznets curve hypothesis model is specified as:

$$E_{it} = \alpha_i + \gamma_t + \beta_1 Y_{it} + \beta_2 Y^2_{it} + \varepsilon_{it} \tag{2}$$

Where E is the natural logarithm of carbon dioxide emissions, Y is the natural logarithm of GDP per capita, and t is the error term. I and t are nation indices and time, respectively. The use of logarithm necessitates a positive or negative prognosis for the experimental variable, which is appropriate.

The first two (2) terms on the right-hand side of the model are country and time impacts. While CO_2 per capita may vary by the county at any particular income level, the sensitivity of all pollutants to income in almost all of Brazil at that level, according to country effects. The timing implications are viewed as time-varying omitted variables and random shocks that Brazil is experiencing.

3.1.2 Lag length selection

The initial step in cointegration is to choose an appropriate lag length criteria. As a result, we conducted a joint test of lag selection, which implies that we should take the two lags of each variable (based on AIC).

3.1.3 Vector auto-regression estimates

The word Autoregressive comes from the fact that the dependents variable's lagged values show on the right-hand side, and the term vector comes from the fact that the model includes a vector of two or more variables. By treating every variable in the model as endogenous and a function of the actual values of all endogenous variables in the system, the VAR approach avoids the necessity for structural modeling. The VAR is frequently used to anticipate systems of interconnected time series and to analyze the dynamic influence of random disturbances on the system of variables. The VAR model is specified as:

$$LnCO_{2t} = a + \sum_{i=1}^{k} \beta_i lnCO_{2t-I} + \sum_{j=1}^{k} \varphi_j lnGDP_{t-j} + \sum_{m=1}^{k} \phi_m lnGDP^2_{t-m} + \mu_{1t} \tag{3}$$

$$\mathrm{LnGDPi_t} = \mathrm{b} + \sum_{i=1}^{k} \beta_i lnGDP_{t-I} + \sum_{j=1}^{k} \varphi_j \mathrm{lnCO_{2t-j}} + \sum_{m=1}^{k} \phi_m \mathrm{lnGDP^2}_{\mathrm{t-m}} + \mu_{2t} \quad (4)$$

$$\mathrm{LnGDP^2}_{\mathrm{it}} = \mathrm{c} + \sum_{i=1}^{k} \beta_i lnGDP^2_{t-I} + \sum_{j=1}^{k} \varphi_j \mathrm{lnGDP_{t-j}} + \sum_{m=1}^{k} \phi_m \mathrm{lnCO_{2t-m}} + \mu_{3t} \quad (5)$$

In the model, the dependent variable is a function of its lagged values and other variables' lagged values. Where k = the optimal lag length, a,b,c, = intercept, $\mathrm{Lngdp_t} = \beta_i, \varphi_j, \phi_m$,= short run dynamic coefficients of the model's adjustment long run equilibrium,

μ_{1t} μ_{2t}, μ_{3t} represent the impulses, innovation or shocks often called the stochastic error term.

3.1.4 Panel causality

In the classical sense, regression does not imply causal interaction. As a result, investigating the causal flow within the variables. This is correct, given the test's predictive power. This study applies the widely utilized Granger causality test technique among the elements under investigation. When one variable, for example, X, Granger causes another, the implication is that variable X and its previous expression can forecast the outcome of variable Y, rather than only the historical variable of Y alone, as is generally thought in the literature. A bivariate relationship between (X, Y) can be expressed in a Granger-causality test.:

$$\mathrm{X_t} = \mathrm{n_0} + \mathrm{n_1 X_{t-1}} + \mathrm{n_2 Y_{t-1}} + \varepsilon_t \quad (6)$$

$$\mathrm{Y_t} = \mathrm{n_0} + \mathrm{n_1 Y_{t-1}} + \mathrm{n_2 X_{t-1}} + \varepsilon_t \quad (7)$$

3.2 Data analysis techniques

The data analysis techniques adopted for the study follow the following simple steps. First, prior to examining the nature of the link between carbon dioxide emissions and economic growth, the study examined the sequences in which the two variables were integrated. The ADF unit root test by [75], PP-Fisher by [76] Im Pesaran, and Chin unit root test were used to check for stationarity. VAR model was used to check the individual endogenous variables' impact and the Wald test determined the collective impact of the variables. The model will prove to be stable through the VAR stability checks. The study made use of Pairwise Dumitrescu Hurlin panel causality (PDHPC) and Pairwise Granger causality test to test all the hypotheses. The Akaike Information Criterion is the lag order utilized for further estimations. Our study will employ the Pairwise Dumitrescu Hurlin panel causality (PDHPC) and Pairwise Granger causality test in the fourth and final phase based on the parameters stability test findings performed in the third phase.

4. Empirical result, interpretation, and discussions

The information on the unit root test is presented in **Table 1**. The variables are non-stationary in their level form, according to **Table 1**, but they become stationary after the first difference I. (1). Because all variables are integrated at order one I, we may proceed with cointegration analysis (1). In **Table 2**, the lag order selection criteria are used to decide which criterion best fits the study—the icteric (*) number with the lowest value is chosen as the criterion for selecting the delays. One SC reported −24.55327* under lag, according to the table. With icteric (*) in lag two, four criteria were identified: LR-36.39728, FPE-1.55e-05*, AIC-2.560914*, and HC - 2.507760*. Among the criteria, the AIC with the number − 2.560914 is the lowest number with icteric (*) under lag two. As a result, the Akaike Information Criterion is chosen as the lag order for future estimations.

Table 3 provides Vector Auto-regression estimates-VAR estimate$_{s.}$ Given that C (1) is the coefficient of the first lag of CO_2 and it is a log-log formation, the interpretation will be on elasticity form. The coefficient signs tell us the direction of the impact; negative signs indicate a decrease, and positive signs indicate an increase.

Variables	At level		At First Difference		Conclusion
	I	I&T	I	I&T	
ADF-Fisher Chi-square					
$LgCO_2$	0.9912(no)	0.6177(no)	0.0000***	0.0000**	I(I)
LgGDP	0.0050***	0.0107**	0.0000***	0.0000***	I(I)
$LgGDP^2$	0.0130***	0.0262***	0.2088***	0.6752***	I(I)
PP-Fisher Chi-square					
$LgCO_2$	0.9751(no)	0.2719(no)	0.0000***	0.0000**	I(I)
LgGDP	0.0050***	0.0104**	0.0001***	0.0000***	I(I)
$LgGDP^2$	0.0130***	0.0368***	0.0000***	0.0000***	I(I)
Im, Pesaran and Shin W-stat					
$LgCO_2$	1.405(no)	0.027(no)	−11.806***	−10.728***	I(I)
LgGDP	−8.855***	−6.880***	−21.002***	−17.912***	I(I)
$LgGDP^2$	−8.873***	−6.9487***	−22.0883***	−19.135***	I(I)

I- denote intercept, I&T- represent intercept and trend (*) Significant at the 10%(**)Significant at the 5%(***) Significant at the 1%(No)Not significant. Lag length based on SIC. Probability based on MacKinnon (1996) one sided p-value.

Table 1.
Unit root test.

LAG	LOGL	LR	FPE	AIC	SC	HC
0	−573.5986	NA	0.001057	1.661668	1.681304	1.669261
1	891.2532	2912.818	1.59e-05	−2.533871	−24.55327*	−2.503497
2	909.6373	36.39728*	1.55e-05*	−2.560914*	−2.423462	−2.507760*
3	3914.1947	8.98339	1.57e-05	−2.548111	−2.351751	−2.472176

** Indicates lag order selected by the criterion, LR: sequential modified LR test statistics (each test at 5% level), FPE: Final prediction error, AIC: Akaike information criterion, SC: Schwarz information criterion, HQ: Hannan-Quinn information criterion.*

Table 2.
Lag order selection criteria.

		$LGCO_2$	LGGDP	LGGDPSQ
$LGCO_2(-1)$	Coefficients	1.001878	1.526624	3.082094
	Standard errors	(0.03792)	(0.48075)	(1.11605)
	T-statistics	[26.4216***]	[3.17553]	[2.76162]
$LGCO_2(-2)$	Coefficients	−0.014756	−1.685399	−3.384602
	Standard errors	(0.03793)	(0.48092)	(1.11644)
	T-statistics	[−0.38902***]	[−3.50456*]	[3.03161*]
LGGDP(−1)	Coefficients	−0.003035	−1.685399	−3.384602
	Standard errors	(0.00517)	(0.06549)	(0.15203)
	T-statistics	[−0.58753]	[4.80273***]	[1.79354***]
LGGDP(−2)	Coefficients	0.014185	0.161283	0.468169
	Standard errors	(0.00495)	(0.06275)	(0.14567)
	T-statistics	[2.86608***]	[2.57035*]	[3.21396*]
LGGDPSQ(−1)	Coefficients	0.004306	0.061816	0.285895
	Standard errors	(0.00219)	(0.02771)	(0.06434)
	T-statistics	[1.96983*]	[2.23055*]	[0.06434***]
LGGDPSQ(−2)	Coefficients	−0.004597	−0.061609	−0.133240
	Standard errors	(0.00569)	(0.07209)	(0.06187)
	T-statistics	[−2.18715**]	[−2.31176]	[−2.15363***]
C	Coefficients	0.003280	0.301598	0.584892
	Standard errors	(0.00569)	(0.07209)	(0.16736)
	T-statistics	[0.57690***]	[4.18350**]	[3.9479***]

(*) depicts Significant at 10%, (**) denotes Significant at 5%, (***) represents Significant at 1% level.

Table 3.
Vector auto-regression estimates.

Therefore, looking at CO_2, we can see that CO_2 strongly influences itself at LGGDPSQ (−1). The past realization of CO_2 is associated with a 100% increase in CO_2 emissions on average certris paribus. LGGDPSQ(−1) recorded t-statistic value of 1.96983* and its corresponding coefficient of 0.004306. Therefore, a percent increase in GDP per capita is associated with a 0.431 percent increase in carbon dioxide emissions on average. The findings from **Table 4**- the VAR estimates indicated that economic growth increase environmental pollution cetris paribusThe Wald test is shown in **Table 4**. **Table 4** shows that the P-value is significant at the 1% level; as a result, we reject the null hypothesis; (5) = C (6), since the Wald test shows that the coefficient of log GDP data to the first and second lags of GPD have a statistical impact on the log of CO_2. We may conclude that GDP GDPSQ has a combined significant effect on CO_2 based on the results of the Walt test. It can also be observed in **Table 5** that no root lies outside the unit circle. This indicates that VAR meets the stability requirement.

The Pairwise Dumitrescu Hurlin panel causality (PDHPC) and Pairwise Granger causality tests are estimated in **Table 6**. Economic growth and carbon dioxide emissions are bidirectional, according to the PDHPC. The Zbar-stat and its probability values (2.21122, 0.0270; 3.41367, 0.0006) respectively verified this. This finding

Test statistics	**Value**	**Df**	**Probability**
Chi-square	7.470434	1	0.0063
Null hypothesis:C(5) = (6)			
Null hypothesis summary:			
Normalized Restriction(=0)		Value	Std.Err.
C(5)-C(6)		0.008927	0.003266
Restriction are linear in coefficients.			

Table 4.
Wald test.

Root	**Modulus**
0.982854	0.982854
0.502592	0.502592
0.146208	0.146208
−0.035224 - 0.107841i	0.113448
−0.035224 + 0.107841i	0.113448
−0.102302	0.102302

Table 5.
VAR stability conditions checks.

Granger causality: Pairwise Dumitrescu Hurlin Panel Causality Test and Pairwise Granger causality test			
1.Pairwise Dumitrescu Hurlin Panel Causality Test			
Null Hypothesis	**W-Stat**	**Zbar-Stat**	**Prob.**
LGGDP→$LGCO_2$	2.81152	1.30380	0.1923
$LGCO_2$→LGGDP	3.46328	2.69518	0.0070
$LGGDP^2$→$LGCO_2$	3.23502	2.21122	0.0270
$LGCO_2$→$LGGDP^2$	3.79785	3.41367	0.0006
$LGGDP^2$→LGGDP	2.67254	1.00711	0.3139
LGGD→$LGGDP^2$	4.19400	3.41367	0.0000
2.Pairwise Granger causality test			
Null Hypothesis:	**Obs**	**F-statistics**	**Prob.**
LGGDP→$LGCO_2$	723	6.23136	0.0021
$LGCO_2$→LGGDP		6.72034	0.0013
$LGGDP^2$→$LGCO_2$	723	6.01514	0.0026
$LGCO_2$→$LGGDP^2$		8.31827	0.0003
$LGGDP^2$→LGGDP	723	3.17036	0.0426
LGGD→$LGGDP^2$		10.1542	0.00004
→Depicts X does not Granger cause Y and Y does not Granger cause X.			

Table 6.
Pairwise Dumitrescu Hurlin panel causality test.

agrees with [77–80], who believe that economic expansion leads to increased pollution. The Pairwise Granger causality test (PGCT) also revealed a bidirectional association between economic growth and pollution. The findings are in line with those of [6, 14, 15, 56, 81–90], who discovered a similar link between economic growth and pollution. The findings are confirmed by PGCT F-statistics and their probability values (F-stat 6.01514, p-value 0.0026; F-stat 8.31827,P-value 0.0003). Both the PDHPC and the PGCT support the environmental Kuznets curve theory.

5. Conclusion and policy direction

The study looks at economic growth and CO_2 emissions: an assessment of the Environmental Kuznets Curve in Brazil. ADF-Fisher, PP-Fisher, Im Pesaran, and Chin unit root test checked stationarity. VAR model was used to check the individual endogenous variable's impact and the Wald test determined the collective impact of the variables. The model proved to be stable through the VAR stability checks. The study used Pairwise Dumitrescu Hurlin panel causality (PDHPC) and Pairwise Granger causality test to test all the hypotheses. The variables are integrated in order one. The Akaike Information Criterion is the lag order utilized for other estimations. Pairwise Dumitrescu Hurlin panel causality (PDHPC) and Pairwise Granger causality test indicated bidirectional causality between economic growth and carbon dioxide emissions. Both the PDHPC and PGCT validate the environmental Kuznets curve hypothesis.

The following recommendation was made based on the study's findings; the investigation supported the EKC concept. Because the EKC hypothesis exists in Brazil, both pure and filthy productions are taking place simultaneously. However, after Brazil has reached a certain level of development, its inhabitants may seek a healthier environment, and the Brazilian Government may impose stricter environmental regulations to encourage a cleaner industry. The measures listed above can help to reduce pollution in Brazil. The Brazilian Government could enhance collaboration among industry, institutions, and researchers, as well as the formation of a single alliance. Creating a safe and ecologically friendly energy usage structure will remain a goal as alternative energy sources become more widely used, could reduce the reliance on fossil fuels and other sources for economic development. As a result, it is critical to strengthen ties between tertiary research institutions and enterprises because joint tertiary and industry-based research would aid in the translation of scientific and technological advances into actual output in the Brazilian economy. The findings of this study and other existing research show that economic growth has a primarily positive impact on emissions, reaffirming an earlier dilemma that the environmental Kuznets literature would lead policymakers to overlook ecological policies in favor of developing a solution. The data imply that environmental quality may suffer significantly and that the economic impact of expansion on certain pollutants is more negligible in Brazil. The most practical application of these discoveries is to notify businesses about their emission forecasts, which can then be used as benchmarks for evaluating environmental policies.

Acknowledgements

I thank the Almighty God for granting me strength and wisdom. Inputting this chapter together, I realized how true this gift of writing is for me. You have given me the power to believe in my passion and pursue my dreams. I could never have done this without the faith I have in God. I want to express my gratitude to IntetchOpen for the opportunity granted me. Heartfelt thanks go to my family and friends for their encouragement and support in diverse ways.

Authors contributions

BAA wrote the introduction section and methodology and interpreted the data with a conclusion. The author'(s) read and approved the final manuscript.

Funding

This current study did not receive any funding from anybody or an organization.

Conflict of interest

The author(s) declare that they have no competing interest.

Author details

Benjamin Ampomah Asiedu[1,2]

1 Cyprus International University, Nicosia, North Cyprus

2 Valley View University, Faculty of Accounting and Finance, Ghana, West Africa

*Address all correspondence to: asieduampomab@gmail.com

References

[1] Stern DI. The rise and fall of the environmental Kuznets curve. World Development. 2004;**32**(8): 1419-1439

[2] Sulaiman J, Azman A, Saboori B. The potential of renewable energy: Using the environmental Kuznets curve model. American Journal of Environmental Sciences. 2013;**9**(2):103

[3] Wagner M. The environmental Kuznets curve, cointegration and nonlinearity. Journal of Applied Econometrics. 2015;**30**(6):948-967

[4] Cheikh NB, Zaied YB, Chevallier J. On the nonlinear relationship between energy use and CO2 emissions within an EKC framework: Evidence from panel smooth transition regression in the MENA region. Research in International Business and Finance. 2021;**55**:101331

[5] Cuthbert MC, Jackson K, Jhonna M. Econometrics of the environmental Kuznets curve in the face of climate change and sustainability in Zambia. Environmental Challenges. 2021;**5**: 100289

[6] Dasgupta S, Laplante B, Wang H, Wheeler D. Confronting the environmental Kuznets curve. Journal of economic perspectives. 2002;**16**(1): 147-168

[7] Gray W, Shadbegian R. Economics of environmental compliance and enforcement. Oxford Research Encyclopedia of Environmental Science. 2021

[8] Stern DI, Common MS. Is there an environmental Kuznets curve for sulfur? Journal of Environmental Economics and Management. 2001;**41** (2):162-178

[9] Stern DI, Common MS, Barbier EB. Economic growth and environmental degradation: The environmental Kuznets curve and sustainable development. World Development. 1996;**24**(7): 1151-1160

[10] Ali MU, Gong Z, Ali MU, Wu X, Yao C. Fossil energy consumption, economic development, inward FDI impact on CO2 emissions in Pakistan: Testing EKC hypothesis through ARDL model. International Journal of Finance & Economics. 2021;**26**(3):3210-3221

[11] Balsalobre-Lorente D, Leitão NC, Bekun FV. Fresh validation of the low carbon development hypothesis under the EKC scheme in Portugal, Italy, Greece and Spain. Energies. 2021;**14**(1): 250

[12] Barbier EB. Introduction to the environmental Kuznets curve special issue. Environment and Development Economics. 1997;**2**(4):369-381

[13] Kuznets S. Economic growth and income inequality. The American Economic Review. 1955;**45**(1):1-28

[14] Işik C, Ahmad M, Pata UK, Ongan S, Radulescu M, Adedoyin FF, et al. An evaluation of the tourism-induced environmental Kuznets curve (T-EKC) hypothesis: Evidence from G7 countries. Sustainability. 2020;**12**(21):9150

[15] Iwata H, Okada K, Samreth S. Empirical study on the environmental Kuznets curve for CO2 in France: The role of nuclear energy. Energy Policy. 2010;**38**(8):4057-4063

[16] World Bank. World Development Report 1992: Development and the Environment. The World Bank; 1992

[17] Bengochea A, Faet O. Renewable energies and CO2 emissions in the European Union. Energy Sources, Part B: Economics, Planning, and Policy. 2012;**7** (2):121-130

[18] Mert M, Bölük G, Çağlar AE. Interrelationships among foreign direct investments, renewable energy, and CO 2 emissions for different European country groups: A panel ARDL approach. Environmental Science and Pollution Research. 2019;**26**(21):21495-21510

[19] Minlah MK, Zhang X. Testing for the existence of the environmental Kuznets curve (EKC) for CO 2 emissions in Ghana: Evidence from the bootstrap rolling window granger causality test. Environmental Science and Pollution Research. 2021;**28**(2):2119-2131

[20] Watson CL. Income, trade, and environmental quality: An environmental Kuznets curve approach

[21] Beşe E, Kalayci S. Environmental Kuznets curve (EKC): Empirical relationship between economic growth, energy consumption, and CO2 emissions: Evidence from 3 developed countries. Panoeconomicus 2021(00):4-

[22] Bilgili F, Koçak E, Bulut Ü. The dynamic impact of renewable energy consumption on CO2 emissions: A revisited environmental Kuznets curve approach. Renewable and Sustainable Energy Reviews. 2016;**54**:838-845

[23] Chow GC, Li J. Environmental Kuznets curve: Conclusive econometric evidence for CO2. Pacific Economic Review. 2014;**19**(1):1-7

[24] Dogan E, Seker F, Bulbul S. Investigating the impacts of energy consumption, real GDP, tourism and trade on CO2 emissions by accounting for cross-sectional dependence: A panel study of OECD countries. Current Issues in Tourism. 2017;**20**(16):1701-1719

[25] Kaika D, Zervas E. The environmental Kuznets curve (EKC) theory. Part B: Critical issues. Energy Policy. 2013;**62**:1403-1411

[26] Wood BJ. Editor. Mineral resources and the limits to growth. Elements: An International Magazine of Mineralogy, Geochemistry, and Petrology. 2017;**13** (5):291-292

[27] Zhang X, Davidson EA, Mauzerall DL, Searchinger TD, Dumas P, Shen Y. Managing nitrogen for sustainable development. Nature. 2015;**528**(7580): 51-59

[28] Alola AA, Donve UT. Environmental implication of coal and oil energy utilization in Turkey: Is the EKC hypothesis related to energy? Management of Environmental Quality: An International Journal. 2021

[29] Aziz N, Sharif A, Raza A, Jermsittiparsert K. The role of natural resources, globalization, and renewable energy in testing the EKC hypothesis in MINT countries: New evidence from method of moments quantile regression approach. Environmental Science and Pollution Research. 2021;**28**(11):13454-13468

[30] Baloch MA, Ozturk I, Bekun FV, Khan D. Modeling the dynamic linkage between financial development, energy innovation, and environmental quality: Does globalization matter? Business Strategy and the Environment. 2021; **30**(1):176-184

[31] Bibi F, Jamil M. Testing environment Kuznets curve (EKC) hypothesis in different regions. Environmental Science

and Pollution Research. 2021;**28**(11): 13581-13594

[32] Erdogan S, Adedoyin FF, Bekun FV, Sarkodie SA. Testing the transport-induced environmental Kuznets curve hypothesis: The role of air and railway transport. Journal of Air Transport Management. 2020;**89**:101935

[33] Panasiuk A, Wszendybył-Skulska E. Social aspects of tourism policy in the European Union. The example of Poland and Slovakia. Economies. 2021;**9**(1):16

[34] Onifade ST, Erdoğan S, Alagöz M, Bekun FV. Renewables as a pathway to environmental sustainability targets in the era of trade liberalization: Empirical evidence from Turkey and the Caspian countries. Environmental Science and Pollution Research. 2021;**30**:1-2

[35] Ozcan B, Ulucak R. An empirical investigation of nuclear energy consumption and carbon dioxide (CO2) emission in India: Bridging IPAT and EKC hypotheses. Nuclear Engineering and Technology. 2021;**53**(6):2056-2065

[36] Pata UK, Caglar AE. Investigating the EKC hypothesis with renewable energy consumption, human capital, globalization and trade openness for China: Evidence from augmented ARDL approach with a structural break. Energy. 2021;**216**:119220

[37] Sun Y, Li M, Zhang M, Khan HS, Li J, Li Z, et al. A study on China's economic growth, green energy technology, and carbon emissions based on the Kuznets curve (EKC). Environmental Science and Pollution Research. 2021;**28**(6): 7200-7211

[38] Wang K, Zhu Y, Zhang J. Decoupling economic development from municipal solid waste generation in China's cities: Assessment and prediction based on Tapio method and EKC models. Waste Management. 2021;**133**:37-48

[39] Farhani S, Mrizak S, Chaibi A, Rault C. The environmental Kuznets curve and sustainability: A panel data analysis. Energy Policy. 2014;**71**:189-198

[40] Jiang Q, Khattak SI, Rahman ZU. Measuring the simultaneous effects of electricity consumption and production on carbon dioxide emissions (CO2e) in China: New evidence from an EKC-based assessment. Energy. 2021;**229**: 120616

[41] Kahn ME. A household level environmental Kuznets curve. Economics Letters. 1998;**59**(2):269-273

[42] Stern DI. The environmental Kuznets curve after 25 years. Journal of Bioeconomics. 2017;**19**(1):7-28

[43] Özokcu S, Özdemir Ö. Economic growth, energy, and environmental Kuznets curve. Renewable and Sustainable Energy Reviews. 2017;**72**: 639-647

[44] Cole MA, Rayner AJ, Bates JM. The environmental Kuznets curve: An empirical analysis. Environment and Development Economics. 1997;**2**(4): 401-416

[45] Murshed M, Ali SR, Banerjee S. Consumption of liquefied petroleum gas and the EKC hypothesis in South Asia: Evidence from cross-sectionally dependent heterogeneous panel data with structural breaks. Energy, Ecology and Environment. 2021;**6**(4): 353-377

[46] Stern DI. Progress on the environmental Kuznets curve? Environment and Development Economics. 1998;**3**(2):173-196

[47] Roca J. Do individual preferences explain the environmental Kuznets curve? Ecological Economics. 2003; **45**(1):3-10

[48] Saint Akadırı S, Alola AA, Usman O. Energy mix outlook and the EKC hypothesis in BRICS countries: A perspective of economic freedom vs. economic growth. Environmental Science and Pollution Research. 2021;**28** (7):8922-8926

[49] Torras M, Boyce JK. Income, inequality, and pollution: A reassessment of the environmental Kuznets curve. Ecological Economics. 1998;**25**(2): 147-160

[50] De Bruyn SM, Opschoor JB. Developments in the throughput-income relationship: Theoretical and empirical observations. Ecological Economics. 1997;**20**(3):255-268

[51] Al-Mulali U, Ozturk I. The investigation of environmental Kuznets curve hypothesis in the advanced economies: The role of energy prices. Renewable and Sustainable Energy Reviews. 2016;**54**:1622-1631

[52] Borhan H, Ahmed EM, Hitam M. The impact of CO2 on economic growth in ASEAN 8. Procedia-Social and Behavioral Sciences. 2012;**35**: 389-397

[53] Bouznit M, Pablo-Romero MD. CO2 emission and economic growth in Algeria. Energy Policy. 2016;**96**:93-104

[54] Alshubiri F, Elheddad M. Foreign finance, economic growth and CO2 emissions nexus in OECD countries. International Journal of Climate Change Strategies and Management. 2019

[55] Lacheheb M, Rahim AS, Sirag A. Economic growth and CO2 emissions: Investigating the environmental Kuznets curve hypothesis in Algeria. International Journal of Energy Economics and Policy. 2015;**5**(4)

[56] Shafiei S, Salim RA. Non-renewable and renewable energy consumption and CO2 emissions in OECD countries: A comparative analysis. Energy Policy. 2014;**66**:547-556

[57] Haug AA, Ucal M. The role of trade and FDI for CO2 emissions in Turkey: Nonlinear relationships. Energy Economics. 2019;**81**:297-307

[58] Dogan E, Ozturk I. The influence of renewable and non-renewable energy consumption and real income on CO2 emissions in the USA: Evidence from structural break tests. Environmental Science and Pollution Research. 2017;**24** (11):10846-10854

[59] Borghesi S. The environmental Kuznets curve: a survey of the literature

[60] Lieb CM. The environmental Kuznets curve and satiation: A simple static model. Environment and Development Economics. 2002;**7**(3): 429-448

[61] Latifa L, Yang KJ, Xu RR. Economic growth and CO2 emissions nexus in Algeria: A cointegration analysis of the environmental kuznets curve. International Journal of Economics, Commerce Research. 2014;**4**(4):1-4

[62] Apergis N, Ozturk I. Testing environmental Kuznets curve hypothesis in Asian countries. Ecological Indicators. 2015;**52**:16-22

[63] Churchill SA, Inekwe J, Ivanovski K, Smyth R. The environmental Kuznets curve in the OECD: 1870–2014. Energy Economics. 2018;**75**:389-399

[64] Jha R, Murthy KB. An inverse global environmental Kuznets curve. Journal of Comparative Economics. 2003;**31**(2): 352-368

[65] Kijima M, Nishide K, Ohyama A. Economic models for the environmental Kuznets curve: A survey. Journal of Economic Dynamics and Control. 2010; **34**(7):1187-1201

[66] Shahbaz M, Khan S, Ali A, Bhattacharya M. The impact of globalization on CO2 emissions in China. The Singapore Economic Review. 2017; **62**(04):929-957

[67] Nasir M, Rehman FU. Environmental Kuznets curve for carbon emissions in Pakistan: An empirical investigation. Energy Policy. 2011;**39**(3): 1857-1864

[68] Farhani S, Shahbaz M. What role of renewable and non-renewable electricity consumption and output is needed to mitigate CO2 emissions in MENA region initially? Renewable and Sustainable Energy Reviews. 2014;**40**:80-90

[69] Al-Mulali U, Saboori B, Ozturk I. Investigating Vietnam's environmental Kuznets curve hypothesis. Energy Policy. 2015;**76**:123-131

[70] Sugiawan Y, Managi S. The environmental Kuznets curve in Indonesia: Exploring the potential of renewable energy. Energy Policy. 2016; **98**:187-198

[71] Hettige H, Mani M, Wheeler D. Industrial pollution in economic development: The environmental Kuznets curve revisited. Journal of Development Economics. 2000;**62**(2):445-476

[72] Luzzati T, Orsini M. Investigating the energy-environmental Kuznets curve. Energy. 2009;**34**(3):291-300

[73] Agboola MO, Bekun FV. Does agricultural value-added induce environmental degradation? Empirical evidence from an agrarian country. Environmental Science and Pollution Research. 2019;**26**(27):27660-27676

[74] Gokmenoglu KK, Taspinar N. Testing the agriculture-induced EKC hypothesis: The case of Pakistan. Environmental Science and Pollution Research. 2018;**25**(23):22829-22841

[75] Dickey DA, Fuller WA. Likelihood ratio statistics for autoregressive time series with a unit root. Econometrica: Journal of the Econometric Society. 1981; **1**:1057-1072

[76] Phillips PC, Perron P. Testing for a unit root in time series regression. Biometrika. 1988;**75**(2):335-346

[77] Asiedu BA, Hassan AA, Bein MA. Renewable energy, non-renewable energy, and economic growth: Evidence from 26 European countries. Environmental Science and Pollution Research. 2021;**28**(9):11119-11128

[78] Bekun FV, Alola AA, Gyamfi BA, Yaw SS. The relevance of EKC hypothesis in energy intensity real-output trade-off for sustainable environment in EU-27. Environmental Science and Pollution Research. 2021:1-2

[79] Gyamfi BA, Adedoyin FF, Bein MA, Bekun FV. Environmental implications of N-shaped environmental Kuznets curve for E7 countries. Environmental Science and Pollution Research. 2021:1-1

[80] Ntow-Gyamfi M, Bokpin GA, Aboagye AQ, Ackah CG. Environmental sustainability and financial development in Africa; does institutional quality play any role? Development Studies Research. 2020;7(1):93-118

[81] Adebayo TS. Testing the EKC hypothesis in Indonesia: Empirical evidence from the ARDL-based bounds and wavelet coherence approaches. Applied Economics Journal. 2021;**28**(1):78-100

[82] Bölük G, Mert M. Fossil & renewable energy consumption, GHGs (greenhouse gases) and economic growth: Evidence from a panel of E.U. (European Union) countries. Energy. 2014;**74**:439-446

[83] Bölük G, Mert M. The renewable energy, growth and environmental Kuznets curve in Turkey: An ARDL approach. Renewable and Sustainable Energy Reviews. 2015;**52**:587-595

[84] Brundtland GH. Our common future—Call for action. Environmental Conservation. 1987;**14**(4):291-294

[85] Dogan E, Seker F. The influence of real output, renewable and non-renewable energy, trade and financial development on carbon emissions in the top renewable energy countries. Renewable and Sustainable Energy Reviews. 2016;**60**:1074-1085

[86] Gao J, Xu W, Zhang L. Tourism, economic growth, and tourism-induced EKC hypothesis: Evidence from the Mediterranean region. Empirical Economics. 2021;**60**(3):1507-1529

[87] Grossman GM, Krueger AB. Environmental impacts of a North American free trade agreement.

[88] Jebli MB, Youssef SB, Ozturk I. Testing environmental Kuznets curve hypothesis: The role of renewable and non-renewable energy consumption and trade in OECD countries. Ecological Indicators. 2016;**60**:824-831

[89] Sarkodie SA, Strezov V. Empirical study of the environmental Kuznets curve and environmental sustainability curve hypothesis for Australia, China, Ghana and USA. Journal of Cleaner Production. 2018;**201**:98-110

[90] Zmami M, Ben-Salha O. An empirical analysis of the determinants of CO2 emissions in GCC countries. International Journal of Sustainable Development & World Ecology. 2020; **27**(5):469-480